Sex Trafficking

Mary de Chesnay, DSN, RN, PMHCNS-BC, FAAN, is professor of nursing at Kennesaw State University, Kennesaw, Georgia. Her experience with victims of trafficking dates to the early 1970s when she served as a pro bono family therapist to the Juvenile Court of Pima County, Arizona. For the past 40 years, she has treated several hundred traumatized survivors of child sexual abuse, including forced prostitution. She currently serves on the Human Trafficking Task Force of the American Academy of Nursing and the Commercial Sex Exploitation of Children (CSEC) Task Force in the state of Georgia. She educates nurses, other health care providers, and mental health professionals on the topic of violence against women and children and teaches an honors course in human trafficking at Kennesaw State University.

Sex Trafficking

A Clinical Guide for Nurses

Mary de Chesnay, DSN, RN, PMHCNS-BC, FAAN
Editor

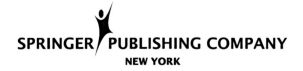

SPRINGER PUBLISHING COMPANY
NEW YORK

Springer Publishing Company, LLC
11 West 42nd Street
New York, NY 10036
www.springerpub.com

Acquisitions Editor: Margaret Zuccarini
Production Editor: Joseph Stubenrauch
Composition: Techset

ISBN: 978-0-8261-7115-3
E-book ISBN: 978-0-8261-7116-0

12 13 14 15 / 5 4 3 2 1

The author and the publisher of this Work have made every effort to use sources believed to be reliable to provide information that is accurate and compatible with the standards generally accepted at the time of publication. Because medical science is continually advancing, our knowledge base continues to expand. Therefore, as new information becomes available, changes in procedures become necessary. We recommend that the reader always consult current research and specific institutional policies before performing any clinical procedure. The author and publisher shall not be liable for any special, consequential, or exemplary damages resulting, in whole or in part, from the readers' use of, or reliance on, the information contained in this book. The publisher has no responsibility for the persistence or accuracy of URLs for external or third-party Internet websites referred to in this publication and does not guarantee that any content on such websites is, or will remain, accurate or appropriate.

Library of Congress Cataloging-in-Publication Data

Sex trafficking : a clinical guide for nurses / Mary de Chesnay, editor.
    p. ; cm.
  Includes bibliographical references and index.
  ISBN 978-0-8261-7115-3 — ISBN 978-0-8261-7116-0 (e-book)
  I. De Chesnay, Mary.
  [DNLM: 1. Emigrants and Immigrants—United States—Nurses' Instruction. 2. Sex Workers—United States—Nurses' Instruction. 3. Child Welfare—United States—Nurses' Instruction. 4. Women's Health—United States—Nurses' Instruction. WA 300 AA1]
  610.73—dc23

                                               2012035691

Printed in the United States of America by Gasch Printing.

For Aunt Lorraine, Aunt Dot, and Uncle Bob—thanks for the many years of love, support, and warm welcomes

—MdC

Contents

Biographies of Contributors   **xi**

Foreword   Senator Renee S. Unterman   ***xvii***

Foreword   Melanie S. Percy   ***xxi***

Preface   ***xxv***

Acknowledgments   ***xxvii***

I: THEORETICAL PERSPECTIVES

1. Sex Trafficking as a New Pandemic   **3**
    Mary de Chesnay

2. Human Trafficking   **23**
    Mark Hoerrner and Keisha Hoerrner

3. Community Models and Resources   **51**
    Mary de Chesnay

4. Working With Law Enforcement   **63**
    Mark Hoerrner

5. Legislation Efforts: The Foundation in the Fight Against
    Sex Trafficking   **73**
    Jennifer McMahon-Howard and Tara Tripp

6. Trials and Tribulations: The Prosecution of Sex Traffickers   **87**
    Jennifer McMahon-Howard and Tara Tripp

7. Sexual Trafficking: Designing Experiential Learning
    for Health Professional Students   **101**
    Barbara A. Anderson

8. Trafficking and Women of Color: Hidden in Plain Sight   **113**
    Vanessa Robinson-Dooley and Edwina Knox-Betty

II: CLINICAL PERSPECTIVES

9. First-Person Accounts of Illnesses and Injuries Sustained
    While Trafficked   **131**
    *Mary de Chesnay, Cheryse Chalk-Gaynor, Jennifer Emmons,
    Emily Peoples, and Chandler Williams*

10. Health Issues and Interactions With Adult Survivors   **151**
    Donna Sabella

11. A Human Trafficking Toolkit for Nursing Intervention   **167**
    Patricia Crane

12. Malnutrition   **183**
    Nicole Mareno and Mary de Chesnay

13. Pregnancy and Termination of Pregnancy   **191**
    Mary de Chesnay and Lacie Szekes

14. Drug-Abused Women and Children   **203**
    Kimberly Groot

15. Sexually Transmitted Infections   **239**
    Gloria Taylor and Barbara Blake

16. Physical Trauma   **263**
    Mary de Chesnay and Jordan Greenbaum

17. Pediculosis, Scabies, and Tuberculosis: Effects
    of Overcrowding in Trafficked Children   **281**
    Rebecca L. Shabo

18. Policy and Procedures Guide for Emergency Departments
    and Community-Based Clinics   **295**
    Mary de Chesnay and Nancy Capponi

19. Mental Health Perspectives on the Care of Human Trafficking Victims Within Our Borders   *305*
Cheryl Ann Lapp and Natalie Overmann

20. Mental Health Intervention: Clinical Cases   *321*
Mary de Chesnay

Appendices   341

   *Appendix A: Policy and Procedures for the ED on Human
            Trafficking   342*
   Appendix B: Principles and Definitions   349
   Appendix C: Patient Referrals   350
   Appendix D: Tertiary Screening and Interviewing   351
   *Appendix E: Curriculum Plan for Staff Development on Human
            Trafficking   352*
   Appendix F: Common Emergency Room Lab Values   354

Index   357

Biographies of Contributors

Barbara A. Anderson, DrPH, RN, CNM, FACNM, FAAN is Director of the Doctor of Nursing Practice (DNP) at Frontier Nursing University. Her consistent career theme has been human vulnerability. She has guided students from the U.S. and from multiple other nations in on-site community health experiences in over 20 countries exploring these issues, including gender issues, sexual trafficking, trafficking of children, and the health consequences of sexual violence. She has led graduate level curriculum development in all of these areas and she has published on community-based educational approaches to enhancing learning about human vulnerability.

Barbara Blake, RN, PhD, ACRN is a Professor of Nursing at Kennesaw State University. Her expertise in nursing is community health. Dr. Blake's research focuses on HIV and related risk factors, such as sexually transmitted infections. Dr. Blake has co-authored numerous HIV related publications, presented at national and international conferences, and developed workshops for nurses and the community about HIV and sexually transmitted infections.

Nancy Capponi, MSN, RN is a clinical faculty member of nursing at Clayton State University, Morrow, GA. She teaches undergraduate pediatrics nursing students at Egleston Hospital in Atlanta, GA. Her experience with victims of trafficking is relatively new but she has worked as an emergency nurse for more than 25 years and has seen many traumatized survivors of child abuse and neglect. She has written a detailed doctoral paper on the topic of human trafficking which included a review of the literature. Additionally, she is assisting a group of health care professionals from the Stephanie V. Blank Center for Safe and Healthy Children in Atlanta, GA with guidelines for medical evaluations of child victims of commercial sexual exploitation. She is passionate about this topic and plans to assist in the dissemination of information about human trafficking throughout Georgia.

Cheryse Chalk-Gaynor is an undergraduate student nurse at Kennesaw State University. She served as the author's unofficial research assistant on the study reported in Chapter 9. She expects to graduate at the end of the year and practice nursing in the Atlanta area.

Patricia Crane, PhD, MSN, RN, WHNP-BC, DF-IAFN is Associate Professor in Nursing at the University of Texas Medical Branch–Galveston. As a forensic nurse, she pioneered the education of health care providers in assessment procedures for human trafficking, conducts research and teaches about victims of violence and trafficking to nurses and other health care professionals. She works closely with Senator Leticia Van de Putte who was instrumental in getting the legislative changes in place in Texas that have improved higher prosecution rates of traffickers and protection of victims. She maintains a practice as a women's health care nurse practitioner and takes students to Texas border clinics and Central America for clinical experiences.

Katrina Embrey, MSN, RN is a nursing instructor at Armstrong Atlantic University, Savannah, GA and a doctoral student at Kennesaw State University. Her doctoral studies include an interest in alternative therapies in health promotion and disease prevention.

Jennifer Emmons is an undergraduate nursing student at Kennesaw State University whose interest in human trafficking began during an honors course she took with Dr. de Chesnay. Her project involved helping on the research in Chapter 9.

Jordan Greenbaum, MD is a nationally recognized forensic pathologist who serves as Medical Director of the Stephanie V. Blank Child Protection Center at the Children's Hospital of Atlanta. A specialist in child abuse and past-President of the International Society for Prevention of Child Abuse and Neglect, Dr. Greenbaum conducts medical evaluations of children suspected to be victims of physical or sexual abuse or neglect. She conducts research and has given papers on such child abuse topics as head trauma and Shaken Baby Syndrome. A member of the Georgia Governor's Office Task Force on the Commercial Sex Exploitation of Children (CSEC) Dr. Greenbaum actively participates in training law enforcement, prosecutors, social service providers and medical professionals on human trafficking and she is currently preparing a book on best practices for physicians on treating victims of CSEC.

Kimberly Groot, RN, MSN is an Adjunct Professor, at University of Hartford College of Education, Nursing, and Health Professions, in West Hartford, CT.

Her expertise developed working in the State of Connecticut Department of Mental Health and Addiction Service, Capital Region Mental Health Center, in Hartford, CT. There she was responsible for a variety of intensive inpatient and outpatient clinical case management services, to adults with a history of severe mental illness and substance abuse disorders. She has provided individual, group, and family counseling, psychotherapy, community outreach, and crisis intervention. In her 36-year career, she also practiced emergency nursing care and triage services and trained and mentored RNs and paraprofessionals in emergency procedures and policies.

Keisha Hoerrner, PhD is Associate Dean in University College and a Professor of Communication at Kennesaw State University. She is also Co-Chair of KSU's American Democracy Project initiative, which promotes students' civic and political engagement. In addition to her work with students, Dr. Hoerrner is also personally dedicated to global political advocacy. She works with the ONE Campaign, a national grassroots advocacy group working to end extreme poverty and hunger. She served as the 2007 Chair of the Darfur Urgent Action Coalition of Georgia, a statewide coalition of faith-based, human rights and advocacy groups. She has held leadership roles in modern-day abolitionist organizations working to end human trafficking locally, nationally, and internationally. Dr. Hoerrner and her husband, Mark, ran E-Living, Inc., an organization that supported the economic viability of populations vulnerable to slavery as well as survivors of slavery through the sale of fair-trade and survivor-made goods. She has written and lectured on the topic of human trafficking for the past five years.

Mark Hoerrner spent two decades in the fields of human resources, communication and investigation. He's now putting those corporate experiences into the fight against human trafficking by pursuing non-governmental routes to solving key challenges in the field. Hoerrner served as the Southeast Regional Director of an anti-trafficking organization, overseeing an international slavery mapping initiative, leading investigations resulting in federal prosecution and training individuals and organizations on how to mobilize community resources. In 2009, he wrote the Georgia Human Trafficking Operations Report, or GAHTOR, as a comprehensive overview of trafficking in the state of Georgia. He has trained law enforcement officers in the Southeast U.S. on identifying victims, case-building and active patrolling. He has communicated with agencies and government officials in Israel, Ireland, Peru, and Cambodia on human trafficking issues and has traveled extensively to see the conditions that drive modern-day slavery firsthand. Hoerrner also serves as a board member and past-Chair of the Executive Board of the Georgia Rescue & Restore Coalition, a U.S. Department of Health & Human Services-promoted coalition of dozens of organizations fighting human trafficking within the state. He has advised and mentored other coalitions and has lectured across the nation on the subject of modern-day slavery. He co-founded Ethical Living, Inc, a non-profit organization that markets goods made by and benefits survivors of human trafficking.

Edwina Knox-Betty, LCSW, is a Licensed Clinical Social Worker (LCSW) with over twenty years' experience working with at-risk populations including survivors of domestic violence. Edwina's area of expertise is women's issues. She has served as the Director of Programs for domestic violence organizations in Florida and Georgia. Edwina currently works as a clinician with a public community mental health agency where she provides psychotherapy to individuals with clinically diagnosed mental health disorders. Edwina has trained DFCS staff, educators, domestic violence advocates and community members on the effects of domestic violence, the intersection of family violence and child welfare, teen dating violence, women and self-esteem, ethical communication and group dynamics. Edwina is a qualified Supervisor of LMSWs working towards state licensure. She received her MSW from University of Georgia and is a member of NASW and NABSW. In 2007, Edwina was recognized by Georgia State University School of Social Work for her commitment and contributions to the community. Edwina serves on the board of Rainbow Village a non-profit agency with a vision to break the cycle of homelessness, poverty, and domestic violence. In 2010 Edwina co-founded M&E Counseling and Consulting with her partner Zuri Murphy. Edwina is committed to social justice and social change.

Cheryl Ann Lapp, PhD, MPH, RN, is a Professor of nursing at the University of Wisconsin–Eau Claire. She teaches Family Health Nursing in both undergraduate and graduate programs, has travelled extensively and taught nursing courses internationally. She has recently established a domestic intercultural immersion experience in northern Wisconsin, for family nurse practitioner students. It was during her development of an interdisciplinary honors course in Global Health, that she developed a commitment to helping her profession address issues of human trafficking both domestically and internationally. She is currently collaborating with colleagues to advance scholarship and develop a theory of the process of human trafficking within the Sri Lankan housemaid industry. Pending successful funding, research will be conducted on-site to better understand and document the domestic labor situation in Sri Lanka. Dr. Lapp currently serves on the Board of the Children's Mental Health Alliance in Eau Claire WI, and is a clinician and interdisciplinary faculty supervisor at the Human Development Center of the University of Wisconsin–Eau Claire.

Nicole Mareno, PhD, RN is an Assistant Professor of nursing at Kennesaw State University in Kennesaw, GA. Dr. Mareno has studied wellness, childhood obesity, and family weight management since 2006. She has worked with families to improve nutrition in schools and community health settings for the past six years. Dr. Mareno's current research interests include parental perceptions of child weight, and family weight management interventions to improve healthy eating and exercise.

Jennifer McMahon-Howard, PhD, is an Assistant Professor of Sociology at Kennesaw State University. She earned her MA and PhD in Sociology, with a concentration in Crime, Law, and Deviance, from the University of Georgia. Her research focuses on violence against women and children and she teaches courses on criminology, victimology, and violence. She currently serves on the Governor's Office for Children and Families' Commercial Sex Exploitation of Children (CSEC) Task Force in the state of Georgia. She also has practical experience working with child and adult victims of sexual exploitation.

Natalie Overmann, MSN, RN is a recent graduate of the University of Wisconsin–Eau Claire. She completed her scholarly project identifying the need for health care providers to better identify and assist victims of human trafficking. She developed policies, procedures, and guidelines for health care providers after identifying that Minneapolis/St. Paul is one of the top ten U.S. cities for sex trafficking. She currently works as a Registered Nurse in the Emergency Department of Region's Hospital in St. Paul, MN.

Emily Peoples is an undergraduate nursing student at Kennesaw State University, who was inspired to learn about human trafficking by taking her honors elective with Dr. de Chesnay. Her fieldwork for the course involved collecting data for the research presented in Chapter 9.

Melanie S. Percy, PhD, RN, CPNP, FAAN is an Associate Professor at the University of Medicine & Dentistry of New Jersey. She has been a certified pediatric nurse practitioner for more than 20 years. Her practice and research have been with low income parents and their children, especially in the areas of child abuse and resilience. For 10 years she worked with Dr. T. Berry Brazelton on his Touchpoints project, applying the concepts to low-income families. She has published her work in a variety of journals and provided consultation on nursing education and research throughout the U.S., as well as, India, Uganda, and Turkey. Currently, she is the committee chair for the Global Health Care Task Force on Human Trafficking for the American Academy of Nursing.

Vanessa Robinson-Dooley, PhD, MPA, LCSW is an Assistant Professor of social work at Kennesaw State University, Kennesaw, GA. In addition to her teaching and research activities, she currently provides mental health services in a free community health clinic. Her work includes behavioral assessments, counseling, and clinical training. Her career has included working with trauma survivors in the area of domestic violence prevention/intervention. As a licensed clinical social worker and therapist, she provided assessments and treatment recommendations for children dealing with physical and sexual abuse. She has also worked with trauma survivors in her private practice.

Donna Sabella, MEd, MSN, PhD, RN is a mental health nurse and the Assistant Dean of Health Sciences in The College of Global Studies at Arcadia University, Glenside, PA. She is a founding member and former Program Director for Dawn's Place, a residential treatment program for trafficked and prostituted women in Philadelphia, PA. She is currently the Director of Project Phoenix which offers counseling to trafficked and prostituted women and trainings on human trafficking. In addition, she teaches courses at various universities on human trafficking and is the Director of Education for the National Research Consortium on Commercial Sexual Exploitation (NRC-CSE).

Rebecca L. Shabo, PhD, RN, PNP-BC is an associate professor of child health nursing at Kennesaw State University, Kennesaw, GA. A pediatric nurse practitioner, she has over 25 years of nursing experience working in primary care, acute care and public health in Georgia and Alabama.

Lacie Szekes, BSN, RN is a graduate in nursing of Kennesaw State University who has conducted research on substance abusing adolescents and has a particular interest in pregnancy. She assisted in the preparation of Chapter 13.

Gloria Taylor, DSN, RN is a Professor of Nursing at Kennesaw State University. She has a strong background in public/community health and engages in scholary activities related to infectious disease, cancer, and school health. Recently she completed a workshop on breast cancer for nurses associated with the National Cancer Institute in Cairo, Egypt. Dr. Taylor has contributed to numerous publications and has presented at varied conferences both national and international.

Tara Tripp, BA is a Master's candidate in Criminal Justice at Kennesaw State University, Kennesaw, GA. She obtained a BA in Spanish and a BA in International Affairs from the University of Georgia. She has observed and assisted in trial preparation for sex trafficking cases. Her research interests include human trafficking, transnational crime, and organized crime.

Senator Renee S. Unterman, (R-45, GA) has dedicated the past 22 years to public service and is currently the Republican Senator for District 45 in Georgia. She chairs the Health and Human Services Committee and has been honored as a Public Health Hero by the Georgia Public Health Association. Educated as both a nurse and social worker, she has dedicated her career to ending exploitation of the young and elderly vulnerable. With every legislative session she has fought to end the sexual exploitation of children and to change the legal perception of exploited children as victims and not criminals.

Chandler Williams is an undergraduate nursing student at Kennesaw State University who was inspired to work on the research chapter for her project in the honors course on human trafficking.

Foreword

While sitting at my Capitol office desk in Atlanta, Georgia about 5 years ago, my administrative assistant, Debra, came to my door and told me a preacher wanted to visit with me and he was waiting in the Capitol hall. Little did I realize at the time that preacher Reverend Scott Reimer, from North Avenue Presbyterian Church on Peachtree Street, would change not only my life but the system of care in Georgia government that takes care of Georgia's most vulnerable citizens. Citizens who have always, until that time, been overlooked and trampled upon by a system that did not even acknowledge their existence. This preacher changed the course of my legislative career and sent me on a personal journey asking how can a society that cares more about animal rights and taking care of animals in shelters, not see little children on the downtown streets of Atlanta selling sex just to have a place to reside and put food in their hungry stomachs.

Reverend Reimer explained to me his perspective and why he took the time to find a legislator who might be sympathetic and could effect a change. He started by saying, "Senator, do you know what is happening just two blocks from where you sit in your office every day?" Of course, I said, "Yes sir, I live downtown four months every year while the Georgia General Assembly is in session. I ride to work every day and see what is happening on the streets of Atlanta." And I said to myself ... I'm tired, it's been a long day, doesn't this guy understand I grew up just a few blocks from here working at Grady Memorial Hospital seeing the tragedy of what living on the street is all about. I know tragedy. I've seen hunger. I've taken care of the health of the under-served. Reverend Reimer stated, "No Senator, I don't believe you really do understand and that is why I am here today waiting to see you." He further stated, "Senator just blocks from here at the Greyhound Bus Station, very young kids are getting off a bus. They are afraid of the big city, most running away from home. They are vulnerable and alone usually not used to a metropolitan inner-city life. They are hungry and scared. I have seen these children and I know what happens to them."

After about an hour of dialogue, I learned from this preacher a story that left an indelible impression in my heart and soul. Reverend Reimer told me about going to church on Sunday mornings ready to preach to his large, influential flock. He would go to the front door of the church and little children would be sitting on the steps staying out of the wind and rain, the cold in the winter. The first few Sundays, he would tell the children to leave and go find somewhere else to play. Then one Sunday, he engaged in a conversation with them. What exactly are you all doing here? Are you playing? Why would you be out here on the street in the middle of the winter in downtown Atlanta when most everything is closed on a Sunday morning? The children replied that they were waiting on the red light at the corner to make people in their cars stop. The church was a good location because it provided a little shelter on the stoop until the cars stopped. Then they would run out to a car and ask if the driver wanted something … sex. Sex for sale. Evidently it was a good location. A major thoroughfare. A famous street. As a matter of fact, one of the most famous streets in the world, Peachtree Street. A street that had hosted one of the most famous movies of all time, *Gone With the Wind*. A location that is iconic just blocks from the famous Fox Theatre. And here, small children as young as 12 years old were selling their soul in a transaction that is described in the Bible.

This particular Sunday, Reverend Reimer marched into his church throwing away his already prepared sermon for the day. He asked his flock … "What is wrong with us? What is wrong with our city? What is wrong with our society?" His flock was aghast. Was this preacher saying that older men were willing to pay to have sex with very young children? Well, we just can't talk about this. We have never heard of anything like this. The preacher could feel and sense the tension in his congregation. Of course, his parishioners had previously seen these children scattering about on the famous street. And then he proposed to his congregation, "Well, what are we going to do about this?" After they digested the scenario, and realized the depth of the problem they, along with him, were going to make a difference. Together they, would stand up and not tolerate the moral decay that was occurring every day in their beloved city, Atlanta. The commercial sexual exploitation of minors had finally hit home on the famous street and the wealthy congregation.

After researching the issue and defining the problem, Reverend Reimer discovered that child exploitation was predominant in Atlanta and, as it turns out, his church was just in a hot locale for the entertainment/convention trade. Atlanta was and remains one of the number-one locations in the United States for business conventions. And along with conventions and the mobility of people comes prostitution. People looking for a good time while away from home. Unfortunately, these same children were in the perfect place, in front of a church, to ply their goods. But to Reverend Reimer, it was also a perfect place to be saved, not just these children of the night, but future children who faced the same vulnerability.

As I listened to Reverend Reimer, I looked around my Capitol office in bewilderment. My office is filled with photos of famous people, awards for all kinds of humanitarian deeds, trips around the world, photos of my own children. And in a prophetic moment, it hit me a like a freight train ... of all the things I do, of all the great legislative accomplishments in my career, what on earth could be more important than helping just one child, just one helpless victim of the sex trade?

Senator Renee S. Unterman
Georgia

Foreword

This is not an easy book to read. Many of the images described in these pages will stay with the reader for weeks, but that is a small price to pay for an awareness of this new pandemic. It is critically important that we stop modern-day slavery. Although this phenomenon has been growing for more than a decade, there is little health care literature describing, explaining, or providing information on how to care for survivors.

Like many of my colleagues, I was simultaneously stunned and horrified to learn that slavery exists today. Not only "over there," but right here in our own communities. Earlier reports of human trafficking were distant and, while disturbing, those reports described a problem that would surely disappear on its own. Not only did it not disappear, it has been growing while we slept. We can no longer deny our complicity in this practice. To quote Pogo, "We have met the enemy ... and he is us" (Kelly & Crouch, 1982, p. 157). I do not mean to imply that health care providers are actively participating in modern slavery. We are made complicit by our ignorance and our unwillingness to see or know the stories of people who silently pass right by us. Dr. de Chesnay and her coauthors have presented an account of the modern slave trade that is compelling, informative, and an unmistakable "call to action."

The U.S. Department of State *Trafficking in Persons Report 2012* (2012) estimates there are 27 million people currently living in slavery. More than any other time in the history of the world, and the numbers of people enslaved are rising rapidly. There are many reasons proposed for this sudden increase in a practice long thought extinct. Probably, the most compelling reason is that criminal exploitation of people generates over $32 billion in profits for the traffickers each year, and is now the fastest growing criminal activity in the world (Polaris Project, 2010).

But there is more. All of us are involved, as consumers. In Chapter 2, Mark and Keisha Hoerrner explain the links between slavery and the supply chain. Insisting that the manufacturer of the goods you buy knows how the goods are produced and can prove that no slaves were involved in the manufacture will go a long way toward ending this practice. Go to http://slaveryfootprint.org to complete an assessment of how and where forced labor affects your life and how you can join the fight.

The most effective intervention to date has been the passage of laws that prevent traffickers from operating in a local jurisdiction; the United States has been actively writing legislation to address the many aspects of trafficking. However, laws are not enough. It is imperative to raise the veil of silence that hides slavery in our own neighborhoods. In the United States, there are 14,000 to 15,000 people trafficked across the border each year (American College of Obstetricians and Gynecologists, 2011). The organization, Not for Sale (2012), sponsors an interactive map with locations throughout the United States that have been sites of human trafficking http://www.slaverymap.org/. The first step toward ending slavery is recognition that it exists.

A variety of websites offer tools to help health care providers identify and assist survivors of trafficking. For example, The Polaris Project (2010) has created a Medical Assessment Tool, and other materials directed to educate nurses and other frontline health care providers (www.polarisproject.org/resources/tools-for-service-providers-and-law-enforcement) on how to recognize a survivor, and then who to contact and what to do. The United Nations Children's fund (UNICEF) has created the *Training Manual to Fight Trafficking in Children for Labour, Sexual and Other Forms of Exploitation* (2009). These manuals (a series of three, plus an exercise book and facilitators' manual) provide concrete information about how to identify, and help children who are being exploited. Another tool was created by experts in the field of trafficking survivors and the UN.GIFT/UNODC, in cooperation with the Austrian Criminal Intelligence Service and the Austrian NGO LEFOE-IB to create VITA, a Victim Translation Assistance Tool, www.ungift.org/knowledgehub/en/tools/vita.html. This free program can be downloaded to a laptop or smart phone. The audio tool has 35 basic phrases that were carefully designed to communicate with a suspected victim of trafficking. The phrases have been translated into 40 different languages. This very handy program was designed to assist law enforcement officers or victim service providers with victims who do not speak their language to increase the success rate in identifying and rescuing victims of trafficking.

Zimmerman, Hossain, and Watts (2011) call for a growing awareness of the health implications of trafficking. They have created a conceptual model that could be used to identify intervention points in the process of trafficking, to outline periods when health care providers should be involved in referrals and service planning, and/or provide a framework that could be used to develop research in this area. Although trafficking in people has been growing steadily for the past decade, the involvement of public health and health care providers is just beginning. Other disciplines have moved quickly to establish a variety of organizations dedicated to the abolition of slavery. So, there is hope, and we are not alone in the fight. There are already initiatives that have been showing promise in rescuing and recovering survivors. Health care is ready to join the chorus of disciplines focused on defeating this problem.

Melanie S. Percy, PhD, RN, CPNP, FAAN
University of Medicine & Dentistry of New Jersey
School of Nursing
Newark, New Jersey

REFERENCES

American College of Obstetricians and Gynecologists. (2011). Human trafficking. Committee Opinion No. 507. *Obstetrics and Gynecology, 118,* 767–770.

International Labour Office. (2009). *Training manual to fight trafficking in children for labour, sexual and other forms of exploitation.* Geneva, Switzerland: International Programme on the Elimination of Child Labour (IPEC). Available at: http://www.unicef.org/protection/57929_58022.html#CT

Kelly, W., & Crouch, B. (Eds.). (1982). *The best of Pogo* (157pp.). New York, NY: Simon & Schuster.

Not for Sale. (2012). *Slavery map.* Available at: http://www.slaverymap.org/

Polaris Project. (2010). *Human trafficking, international trafficking.* Available at: http://www.polarisproject.org/human-trafficking/international-trafficking

Polaris Project. (2010). *Medical assessment tool.* Available at: http://www.polarisproject.org/resources/tools-for-service-providers-and-law-enforcement

The Campaign to Rescue and Restore Victims of Human Trafficking. (2010). *Rescue & Restore Campaign Tool Kits, for Health Care Providers.* Washington, DC: US Department of Health and Human Services, Administration for Children and Families. Available at: http://www.acf.hhs.gov/trafficking/campaign_kits/index.html

United States Department of State. (2012). *2012 Trafficking in Persons Report—United States of America.* Available at: http://www.state.gov/j/tip/index.htm; http://www.unhcr.org/refworld/docid/4e12ee393c.html [accessed 19 July 2012].

Zimmerman, C., Hossain, M., & Watts, C. (2011). Human trafficking and health: A conceptual model to inform policy, intervention and research. *Social Science & Medicine, 73,* 327–335.

Preface

Like many Americans, I thought slavery ended with the Emancipation Proclamation. Nothing could be further from the truth. Today, millions of people live in misery, forced into agricultural labor, sweat shops, domestic servitude, child soldiering, or the sex trade. They live in appalling conditions of filth and deprivation, are routinely subjected to violence, and are largely invisible to health care professionals who should be able to recognize, treat, and refer them for long-term help in rebuilding their shattered lives. We see a "prostitute" instead of a victim of exploitation. We see a "bad kid" instead of a little child who was raped at home and then repeatedly on the street—exploited by a pimp she has come to believe is the only person in the world who cares about her.

This book is designed to raise awareness and provide helpful information to nurses with the hope that they will be better able to help one of the most vulnerable populations, women and children trapped in the global sex trade. Most of the case studies are derived from stories of real people whose privacy is protected by camouflaging their identifying information. My clinical practice over the past 40 years has been almost exclusively focused on survivors of family violence, including child sexual abuse, but I was unaware of the extent of the child sex trade until the mid-1970s, when I met an 11-year-old I will call Luisa, who presented with ectopic pregnancy. When asked who the father was, she thought carefully and replied: "Well, it could be my father . . . or one of my four brothers . . . or one of their friends." It seems her father and brothers used her at will and then rented her out on the weekends when they would hold open house and charge their friends to rape her. This had been going on since Luisa was eight.

A word of caution: this topic is painful to talk about and the stories of victims hard to hear. I remember working in the emergency room many years ago as the only night nurse and a number of people involved in a bad highway accident came in, bloody and broken, and in more pain than I had ever seen in my 20 years of life. I sat paralyzed in one of the exam rooms and started sobbing. The wonderful attendant pulled me aside and told me to "pull it together." He said those people needed me and this was not my time to fall apart. We got through the night and then he took me out for breakfast and talked soothingly about compassion and empathy and how necessary it was to compartmentalize—put our own feelings aside in order to do what was needed to care for others. His advice is particularly relevant here. Even if you never see a patient who has been trafficked, develop release valves to ease your own tension at reading this book. But do not lose your anger. Keep that and find a way to use it.

Mary de Chesnay, DSN, RN, PMHCNS-BC, FAAN

Acknowledgments

Many individuals generously contributed information, reviewed sections, or shared their time with the author to talk about sex trafficking and how we can help people caught in the vicious cycle of modern slavery. Some wish to remain anonymous, but to those and the following, I am deeply grateful for your help.

At Springer Publishing Company, the indispensable Margaret Zuccarini, my publisher, who answered numerous questions with encouragement, patience, and humor and Chris Teja, Christina Ferraro, Joanne Jay, Vice President, Production and Manufacturing, and Joseph Stubenrauch. Thanks also to Nick Barber, who formatted the manuscript into a real book.

Many service providers and other leaders in the effort to eliminate modern slavery generously shared their time talking with me about what they do or reviewed content related to their agencies: Randee Doe of Shared Hope International; Michael Klinkner of Streetlight, Phoenix; Dr. Kevin Ellington, pastor of Catalyst Church in Woodstock, GA; Janet Olson of Natalie's House, Phoenix; Julie Waters, director of Free the Captives; Heather McDaniel of the Georgia Governor's Office reviewed the section on the GCCO; and Pamela Perkins Carn, director of the Interfaith Children's Movement, Atlanta, a community leader and strong children's advocate in Georgia, who is dedicated to educating the public and professional community.

Students in my honors course on human trafficking helped with the research project on survivor stories as did my unpaid research assistant, Cheryse Chalk-Gaynor. Two of the doctoral students participated in the book project. Nancy Capponi prepared the policy and procedures for the Appendix and Katrina Embrey prepared the table of herbal remedies for the trauma chapter. Two of the honors students served as models for photographs for presentations of content in this book: Cherith Morgan and Alakea Woods. Another honors student, Toby Newcomer, is a professional photographer and helped design the photos.

Cynthia Elery, administrative assistant to the director of the School of Nursing took care of a number of details and made sure all the pages were there. Chadwick Brown, student assistant, prepared the table on resources.

Content reviewers for several chapters assured accuracy and improved the language: Janeen Amason; Dr. Melanie Percy; Natalie Overmann; Dr. Susan Y. Stevens, Donna Hunter, Dr. Jane Brannan, Dr. Patricia Hart, Dr. Anne White, Dr. Jackie Jones, and Chris Gisness.

Last but not least, I am deeply grateful to all the survivors who shared their stories and advice with me. You are anonymous here but not in my heart.

I

Theoretical Perspectives

CHAPTER 1

Sex Trafficking as a New Pandemic

MARY DE CHESNAY

*T*his book is written from the perspective of clinicians and researchers committed to addressing the global health issue of sex trafficking with the focus on best practices. The book consists of two parts: theoretical perspectives and interventions for practice. Part I presents the broad concepts, legislation, and population-based responses within communities. Part II is clinical, in which content experts in a variety of clinical specialties share their knowledge of best practices of treating the common health problems of people who have been trafficked. This chapter will lay the groundwork by presenting some key ideas that will hopefully lead to evidence-based research and subsequent treatment protocols for helping the vulnerable, often invisible, victims of sex trafficking.

The author hopes that readers of this book will become enraged and inspired: Angry that human trafficking exists today as the fastest-growing and one of the most lucrative crimes, and inspired to learn more about the lives these people endure in order to help them transcend their unbearable present and have a happier and healthier future. The resilience of the human spirit is proven time after time when we listen to the stories of survivors. Although it might seem impossible, the victims of sex trafficking can become survivors and beyond with help. Nurses are likely to be among the few outsiders they will approach. Yet we may not recognize them as being exploited. This book is an attempt to help us get ready to help them.

CONTEXT

Definitions

Some terms need to be defined in order to understand the complexity of trafficking. They are introduced here and discussed more fully in subsequent chapters.

3

Human Trafficking

"Article 3, paragraph (a) of the United Nations Protocol (2000) to Prevent, Suppress and Punish Trafficking in Persons defines Trafficking in Persons as the recruitment, transportation, transfer, harbouring, or receipt of persons, by means of the threat or use of force or other forms of coercion, of abduction, of fraud, of deception, of the abuse of power or of a position of vulnerability or of the giving or receiving of payments or benefits to achieve the consent of a person having control over another person, for the purpose of exploitation. Exploitation shall include, at a minimum, the exploitation of the prostitution of others or other forms of sexual exploitation, forced labour or services, slavery or practices similar to slavery, servitude or the removal of organs" (www.unodc.org/unodc/en/human-trafficking/what-is-human-trafficking.html#What_is_Human_Trafficking).

Precise statistics on the extent of the problem are hard to obtain. Bales estimated that 27 million people around the world live in slavery today (Bales, 2004; U.S. State Department, 2012). It is estimated that at any given time, there are about 2.5 million people worldwide who are victims of human trafficking with 40%–50% of those children (International Labor Office, 2005).

In the above definition, there are two forms of human trafficking: *forced labor* and *sex trafficking*. *Debt bondage* is a phenomenon common to both in which the traffickers create an increasing debt based on "expenses" for transporting the victims.

Forced Labor

Victims of forced labor might be migrant workers, other agricultural workers such as children who work in the African cocoa plantations, children who work the brick kilns in India, child soldiers (common in India and Africa), and sweatshop workers. The Restavek children of Haiti can be found in domestic servitude (Nicholas et al., 2012).

Sex Trafficking

Women and children comprise most of the sex trade around the world but adult men are also forced into the sex trade sometimes directly and sometimes through forced labor where they encounter torture and rape (Bales, 2005; Jones, 2010).

Commercial Sex Exploitation of Children (CSEC) or Domestic Minor Sex Trafficking (DMST)

These terms refer to sex trafficking of minors. The age of 18 is most commonly the age of majority in the United States and most countries (www.worldlawdirect.com/forum/law-wiki/27181-age-majority.html).

Pathways

In a landmark study for the Department of Justice, Bales and Lize (2005) reviewed cases from Florida, Chicago, and Washington, DC, and identified five stages of the process of human trafficking:

1. Vulnerability
2. Recruitment
3. Transportation
4. Exploitation
5. Exposure, discovery, liberation

People most **vulnerable** to trafficking tend to be young and fairly healthy, and are likely to be poor and powerless, but not necessarily from the poorest class of their societies. They may be educated and are rarely kidnapped. Traffickers are more likely to prey upon their dreams and aspirations because they know that cooperation by their victims eases the process. Traffickers favor victims from marginalized groups or who are women or children because these people are often looking for a better life for their families.

Selling the dream or **recruitment** is easier when traffickers are charismatic. They are expert at reading people and convincing victims that they can deliver on promises of golden opportunities in the destination country or city. They may use a woman or man, even a family member, who has been paid to recruit and who can be trusted to be loyal to the traffickers and lie to the victims about the opportunities. Once the victims arrive at the destination, the trafficker uses bait-and-switch techniques to keep the person. The rules change and threats and violence enforce the new rules.

Transportation might be simple, involving existing legal entities and legal visas or false documents. There might be a transporter who accompanies the victim and provides a safe house during transit. The next level of transportation is a segmented business operation in which the traffickers themselves transport and provide "stash houses." The third level and most difficult to identify and prosecute are complex integrated operations in which criminal networks with many resources control the transportation.

Exploitation is final when control is established. How control is established varies from debt bondage to confiscation of documents, threats of arrest or deportation, degradation, and violence. In many cases, traffickers wait until arrival at the destination to establish control because they need the victim's cooperation to pass borders. In the case of children, though, they have control as soon as they take custody of the child since children are more likely to do as they are told by an adult. Traffickers maintain a constant vigilance and may lock their victims in when not working and transport them to their place of work. Keeping victims isolated and disoriented is an effective control tactic.

The last stage is a progression of **exposure, discovery, and liberation**. Unfortunately, the rates of murder by traffickers and accidental death from injury and suicide are high for this population. Women and children in the sex trade are at risk for contracting HIV/AIDS. Relatively few victims are rescued by law enforcement and some manage to escape. The fortunate ones manage to be found by "good Samaritans" who may be of their own ethnicity or who are least able to recognize the signs of trafficking. If victims can connect with the right authorities they may be eligible for change of visa status, may be able to help authorities to arrest and prosecute their traffickers, and be eligible to receive services to reverse the effects of their enslavement.

Stages of Entrapment

While it is true that some children are kidnapped and others are sold by their parents, it is more common for children to be tricked by traffickers who present themselves as a friend, boyfriend, or protective employer. Barnardo's, a children's advocacy charity in the United Kingdom, identified four stages of entrapment into prostitution. These are presented in O'Connor and Healy (2006) and Hawthorne (2011) as the following:

- Stage 1 is *ensnaring,* in which the trafficker gains the child's trust by pretending to be her caring protector/boyfriend. He may buy her presents, give her shelter and food, and clothe her. He may be accepted by her parents as a "nice young man" if she is living at home.
- Stage 2 is *creating dependence,* in which he isolates her from family and friends, changes her name, and generally becomes more possessive. She interprets this possessiveness as his passionate love for her and, as proof that she loves him, she willingly distances herself from her family and friends and engages in prostitution to please him.
- Stage 3 is characterized by *taking control,* in which he exerts increasing control over her daily activities such as what she eats and wears and he may alternate violence with kindness in order to remain unpredictable. He usually becomes increasingly violent at this stage, but she still loves him and maintains hope that he will change. Because she is isolated from support systems and feels shame for her activities, she does not try to escape.
- Stage 4 is *total dominance,* in which he convinces her by force if necessary to have sex with whomever he directs. He may lock her in a room to ensure she does not try to escape and threaten to kill her or her family if she attempts to leave him.

Other authors (McClanahan, McClelland, Abram, & Teplin, 1999) have described pathways to child prostitution as running away and childhood sexual abuse. In a study of 1,142 female jail detainees, they found that running away in early adolescence had a dramatic effect on entry into prostitution, but little effect later in life. However, being sexually abused as a child nearly doubled the odds of entry throughout their lives. The role of drug abuse is inconclusive as some victims begin drug use after they enter the life and some are users beforehand.

Sex Tourism

Closely related to sex trafficking is sex tourism (de Chesnay, 2012). Sex tourism describes travel for sex, usually with partners who would be perceived as exotic (different race than the traveler) or with children who might be more accessible in destination countries in which the child sex trade is allowed to flourish. Thailand is so well known for sex tourism with both women and children, that *Fielding's Guide* devoted a section of its Thailand book to sex tourism (Dulles, 1996). Child sex tourism flourishes in impoverished areas of the world where parents can delude themselves that the traffickers to whom they sell their children will give them a better life. On the other hand, children who have no families and live on the street survive any way they can. Once the child is in the life, the benefits to the family of the sex trade and the options for leaving the life create a paradox for the child. The more he or she stays in the life, the more the child learns to tolerate the bad parts and becomes numb to any attempts to be rescued.

Scholars have studied cultural aspects of Thailand as a destination for the child sex trade. In an ethnographic study in which she interviewed children in Thailand, Montgomery (2008) concluded that the stereotype of the tourist visiting Thailand on organized sex tours was misleading and that some children did not define themselves as prostitutes, nor did they despise their "johns." Instead, they developed relationships with these men who helped support their families during times of severe economic stress (Montgomery, 2008). While definitely not making the case that sex with children is acceptable, Montgomery cautioned that the phenomenon of sex tourism is much more complex than tawdry advertisements would lead one to believe. Pedophiles succeed in seducing children and can be quite convincing that they love the children.

Solutions such as revoking passports of Americans who travel to Thailand for sex as suggested by some authors (Hall, 2011) might be effective at stopping the tourists from exploiting children in the destination countries but paradoxically might not be perceived as help by those we define as victims. If the police are corrupt, they will not cooperate with American authorities to detain or deport them because the sex tourists are a source of revenue for the police. Pedophiles flourish in places that allow sex with children. Who will step forward to protect these children if their own police look the other way? Unless governments find ways to reverse the poverty, violence, devaluation of women, and ignorance that underlie the sex trade, women and children, particularly in developing countries, will continue to have few alternatives.

The Caribbean is a destination for sex tourists of both genders. In the Dominican Republic, male sex workers specialize in male sex tourists from North America and Europe (Gigliotti, 2006; Padilla, 2008). Female sex tourists or "sugar mummies" as well as male tourists to Cuba and the Dominican Republic might define themselves as romance tourists and see themselves in long-term relationships with locals, sometimes leading to marriage and migration for the local to the tourist's home country (Aston, 2008; Cabezas, 2004).

The complexity of relationships in sex tourism masks the exploitation of children who are trafficked for the purpose of commerce. In an Organization of American States (OAS)-funded study of nine countries of Latin America and the Caribbean, researchers found that little has been done to implement the U.N. Protocol of 2000 that called for initiatives by member countries to halt human trafficking, prosecute traffickers, and provide services to victims (Langberg, 2005).

On a more positive note, though, the tourism industries in a number of countries have signed the *Code of Conduct for the Protection of Children from Sexual Exploitation in Travel and Tourism,* an industry-driven initiative funded by the Swiss government and private concerns and sponsored under the auspices of an international organization, End Child Prostitution and Trafficking (ECPAT). Notable signers of the Code are Delta Airlines, Hilton Hotels, and Wyndham Hotels (ECPAT, 2012). The criteria in the Code call for ethical commitment to end child trafficking with training for staff and screening of suppliers. One way to support efforts to abolish modern slavery is to patronize businesses that do not facilitate traffickers.

BEST PRACTICES AND EVIDENCE-BASED RESEARCH

There are no best practices for treating sex trafficking victims in the sense that research is sparse and clinical research almost nonexistent. The highest order of evidence is traditionally thought to be that derived from randomized clinical trials. However, evidence can also be based on nonrandomized trials, descriptive studies that build testable theory, case reports by clinicians, and qualitative studies that describe in rich detail the experience of members of the population of interest. In the case of sex-trafficked victims, who are difficult to identify and who do not have control of their own bodies or schedules, valid and reliable research data are difficult to acquire.

Several attempts by nurse scholars have been made to identify the key issues and barriers in working with this population. In this sense, Sabella (2011) and Crane (Crane & Moreno, 2011) are two nurses who have pioneered the process of identifying best practices of working with survivors of trafficking. Sabella is a Pennsylvania-based psychiatric-mental health nurse who teaches nurses and works with the population. She taught one of the first courses on human trafficking to assist health care providers to recognize and interact appropriately with victims. Crane (2011) is a forensic nurse who is instrumental in political advocacy for victims in Texas, one of the early states to pass legislation in the spirit of decriminalizing prostituted children. Both of these leaders in the field have published their work in the nursing literature so that other nurses may benefit from their experiences and they remain active and committed to this most vulnerable population.

Trout (2010) also has published on the need for nurses to identify these victims. McClain and Garrity (2011) addressed the need for nurses who work with adolescents to educate themselves about this growing problem. The American Nurses Association (ANA) and several states have passed resolutions opposing human trafficking (Alabama State Nurses Association, 2009; Kansas Nurses Association, 2008; Trossman, 2008). The American Academy of Nursing appointed a Task Force (chaired by Dr. Melanie Percy) under the Expert Panel on Global Health to prepare a white paper on human trafficking for presentation in 2012. In 2010, the National Student Nurses Association passed a resolution to increase awareness of human trafficking (NSNA, 2010). These efforts are a good start but need to be expanded.

Even though there is a great need for evidence-based research on human trafficking, there are best practices for treating a variety of health conditions that affect victims. For example, much work on posttraumatic stress disorder (PTSD) has been done to help soldiers re-adjust to civilian life (Bastien, 2010; Meis, Barry, Kehle, Erbes, & Polusney, 2010; Mulvaney, McLean, & De Leeuw, 2010). Although the issues for CSEC victims are different, some of the same treatments might be helpful. For example, pharmacologic management in concert with trauma-focused cognitive behavioral therapy can lead to better outcomes by alleviating at least one of the three symptom clusters of PTSD: reexperiencing, avoidance, and hyper arousal (Ipser, Seedat, & Stein, 2006). PTSD in child sexual abuse survivors, whether commercially exploited or not, is co-morbid with a host of other conditions, necessitating multiple methods of treatment.

Research on torture generated interventions to help victims of state-sponsored atrocities (Genefke, 2002; Glittenberg, 2003; Grodin & Annas, 2007; Levine, 2001; Moreno & Iacopino, 2008; Moreno & Grodin, 2002; Olsen, Montgomery, Bojholm, & Foldspong, 2006; Racine-Welch & Welch, 2000). Many of the signs of torture are similar to those of women or children who have been prostituted. They regularly endure beatings, fractures, sleep and food deprivation, sexually transmitted infections (STIs), and verbal messages that they are worthless. Like torture victims, they live with chronic pain from the many types of injuries suffered during torture and they suffer the effects of malnutrition from being deprived of food and water for long periods. Certainly there are best practices for the health conditions of pregnancy, STIs, physical trauma, and so on and these will be discussed in more detail in Part II.

Primary prevention is one of the most important concepts when discussing best practices in health care. In the United States, great attention is given to teaching people how to stay healthy and prevent illness and injury. However, for the population of trafficked victims who are still "in the life," prevention is not only irrelevant but impossible, and trying to teach about prevention could have the paradoxical effect of reinforcing the victim's view that we really have no idea what she is going through. For example, the best prevention practice for vesico-vaginal fistula is not to bear children until beyond adolescence. Wearing condoms goes a long way toward preventing AIDS and STIs and, of course, early pregnancies. How is a prostituted child supposed to follow that advice when she does not get to decide with whom and when she will engage in sex?

Prevention means being able to avoid activities that place one at risk for specific health problems or generalized poor health. However, vulnerability due to poor family resources creates risks for girls who connect with traffickers who promise them or their families a better life. "Romeo pimps" in the United States (men who pretend to be in love with their victims) sometimes deliberately impregnate the girls in order to control them (Anonymous, personal communication, 2011). Once the baby comes, they can then alternately hold out the hope that they will be a "real family" or that they will sell the baby if the girl does not stay in line.

Alternatively, some traffickers, particularly in Eastern Europe take children for organ harvesting (Kambayashi, 2004; Lita, 2007). Yea (2010) reports on two additional ways children are trafficked in addition to sex trafficking. Some children are taken for begging assignments and these children may be deliberately disabled to create sympathy or they might be disabled already and then forced to beg for the traffickers. Deaf children are particularly attractive to the traffickers because they are less able to communicate with people who might help them. A second way children are used is to train them as camel jockeys. Male children who are preferably around age 5 are taken from India, Pakistan, and Bangladesh to the Arab Emirates to be camel jockeys for the racing industry. Their parents are told the boys will earn much money to send home, but in reality, the children are sent to desert camps where they undergo brutal training and punishment with electric shocks and food deprivation. They are contained within complexes where they sleep in cardboard boxes making them prone to scorpion bites. They arise at 4 a.m. to exercise the camels and then must care for the camels before the afternoon-to-nightfall exercise periods.

Given the limited outcomes research on sex trafficking, this book is an attempt to present the best practices to date with the hope that those working with victims will have some basis on which to set priorities and provide the best care possible under limited conditions. Human trafficking is receiving wide attention from the media, legislators, and prosecutors. Health care professionals need to partner with others in their communities to address the medical and psychological needs of victims holistically. It is hoped that nurses who practice in settings in which victims are likely to appear will recognize their need for help, define them as victims and not criminals, and, in working with them, improve upon the ideas presented here.

CULTURAL ASPECTS OF SEX TRAFFICKING

The Culture of the Street

Culture is a set of life-ways, rituals, values, language, and behaviors that are held in common by a people who may or may not live in proximity to one another. Traditionally, culture is discussed in connection with geographic home but culture can also describe the shared values and life-ways of people who share other common characteristics. Nurses are a good example of a group of people who live in many areas of the world but who share a common culture. Whatever our education and wherever in the world we practice, we share that our lives are dedicated to helping our people improve their health. We use both the science and art of intervention to help our patients attain a higher level of health. We have rituals such as pinning ceremonies and protocols such as best practices to guide our work.

Language defines where we live (New Yorkers, Californians); our nationality (Cambodians, Canadians, Australians); what kind of work we do (nurses, police officers, dog groomers, teachers, social workers, carpenters, postal workers); or how we see ourselves in relation to others (child advocates, leaders, advisors, Republicans, retirees). Language is shared by a cultural group, not only in terms of the primary language of English, French, Japanese, or Swahili, but also in terms of dialects and jargon.

Language expresses power and can be used to exclude or include individuals from a group. For example, jargon is sometimes used to prevent nongroup members from fully understanding in-group members. The language of the street provides a way for people who live "on the street" to exclude members of the "establishment" and to make themselves feel more powerful in relation to powerful people around them.

Similarly, street language of whore, "ho," "hooker," or prostitute—even euphemisms such as "sex workers," "call girls," and "ladies of the night"—are negative labels used to stereotype those who sell their bodies for sex. There is even controversy over the term "selling" since that implies choice on the part of the girl. Linda Smith, a former Congresswoman and the founder of Shared Hope International, tells the story of her husband mentioning to her that what really happens is that the pimp rents the child to others for money (Smith, webcast 12/1/2011). Renting is a more descriptive term since it connotes the involvement of the person usually in control of the process. Shared Hope International (2011) sponsors a billboard campaign to fight trafficking in which one billboard shows a picture of a man's torso with his hands (showing a wedding ring) in the process of removing his jacket and with his belt partially undone. The caption is: "This man wants to rent your daughter."

Another example of how language is used is particularly relevant for those who would help commercially sexually exploited people. For the purposes of this book, we will sometimes refer to these women and children as victims (almost all are women and children of both sexes) but with the caution that they not only do not always see themselves as victims and, in fact, might become angry at the thought of anyone else calling them victims. Anger at being labeled a victim could be a defense mechanism to exaggerate what little control they have in their lives. The reality is that no matter how demoralized they are, they are all survivors. The term "survivor" is preferred but it is critical to use the term "victim" as well to convey that these children do not choose a life of exploitation, rape, and torture. They may choose to go with a Romeo pimp because they are conned or coerced, but their choice quickly becomes, "Comply or die." Those who would label them as criminals need to understand the lengths to which these women and children must go in order to survive.

When Rachel Lloyd (2011) founded the Girls' Education and Mentoring Services (GEMS) to assist prostitutes to make the transition out of "the life," she constructed a language model from victim to survivor to leader to capture a sense of hope for these women. Whether they are called victims, survivors, or leaders, and whether we as nurses call them patients or clients, it is critical to understand that they are human beings forced into a life in which their choice is usually to comply or die.

Life-ways and rituals are also part of life on the street and define rules and how they are to be followed for survival. The rules about appropriate behavior for girls "in the life" are designed by pimps to control every aspect of the girl's life in order to minimize the chance that she will leave. The trafficker or pimp makes rules about where she sleeps, how much she eats, how she obtains basics such as tampons, and how much toilet paper she can use. Rules are enforced brutally with beatings with fists or a pimp stick. A pimp stick can be a cane or coat hanger doubled over itself to form a thin rod. Other common forms of torture are cigarette burns, dragging by the hair until clumps come out, submersing the face in a toilet, and gang rape.

Pimps are businessmen and their goal is to make money for themselves by sexually exploiting women and children. They may work in apparent isolation and competition with each other, but they have informal networks with other pimps. For example, they will trade or sell girls to each other. A girl who looks at or talks to another pimp is likely to be beaten by her pimp, but the pimp may initiate deals to obtain a younger model or a girl may negotiate to be traded. It would be reasonable to assume that pimps would want to protect their investment and protect the girls rather than torture them, but control trumps caring and keeping the girls malnourished, sleep-deprived, and in pain maintains dominance.

Pimps celebrate their accomplishments at exploiting women and children by dressing in their finery and holding an annual convention called the Players' Ball, which is an opportunity to buy and sell women and children (The World Famous Players' Ball, 2005). They give an award to the pimp who has made the most money during the year. The author deliberated long and hard about including mention of the Players' Ball here, which might be viewed by some as helping to glorify pimps, but decided to do so in the hope that residents of the cities to which they apply to hold their convention will follow the lead of Mayor Shirley Franklin of Atlanta, who refused to support the convention in Atlanta in 2003. It was moved to a private club outside the city (Interfaith Children's Movement, 2009).

Culturally Competent Care

Cultural competence is a trendy term that has been widely used in nursing, education, and social work to convey the importance of understanding cultural differences when working with diverse groups of people. It can be confusing, though, because some practitioners assume cultural competence means to become proficient in another's cultural behavior. However, trying to be something one is not is more likely to be viewed as insincere and disrespectful, particularly with sex trafficked victims who are likely to have little reason to trust anyone.

For the purposes of this book, cultural competence will be defined as the ability to use information about another's culture to provide care that the person can accept comfortably while remaining authentic to one's own culture.

For example, in providing care to a Navajo man whose culture teaches that it is rude to look people directly in the eyes, an Anglo nurse who might have been taught that it is rude not to look directly at others when conversing would not interpret his behavior as rude but rather as respectful according to the norms of his culture. Similarly, when treating a young prostituted girl in the emergency department, it would be helpful to understand the culture of sex trafficking and not be frustrated by the patient's fearful or angry resistance to being rescued.

HOW SURVIVORS PRESENT

The following cases were drawn from real people but the identifying information has been changed to protect their privacy. The people represented here are examples of the variety of ways girls enter the life and show the systematic pattern of abuse that destroys their sense of self. The presenting behavior when seeking medical help shows some of the issues that we might expect to encounter with this population.

CASE STUDY: ANGEL

Angel is a 14-year-old African American girl who has been in "the life" for 3 years. At the age of 11, she met a 22-year-old White man named Johnny who was the first person to make her feel special. He listened to her talk about the abuse she endured at home and comforted her by telling her she was pretty and buying her small presents. Johnny told Angel he would help her escape her violent home situation. Her mother worked nights in a bar, often came home drunk, and had a variety of boyfriends all of whom regularly raped Angel while her mother was at work. Her first sexual encounter was with her stepfather when she was 5 years old but when she told her mother, she was accused of lying, so she never told anyone else about the later abuse until she met Johnny. He said all the right things, comforted her in a tender way, and she immediately fell in love with him. He took her away to another city where they lived together in what was to be a short period of happiness in Angel's life. For 2 weeks, Angel and Johnny lived together in his apartment and gradually Angel realized she was not the only girl in his life. However, she loved him and when he asked her to go on "dates" with his friends she complied in the belief that they were building a future together. When some of his friends got too rough, well, that was nothing new to her and she would do anything to please Johnny. It was almost a month before he seemed to undergo a personality change and started beating her if she did not bring home her quota. He called it his 25/25 rule: $25 a trick at a rate of 25 men a night.

(continued)

She presented in the emergency department with a fractured rib, multiple hematomas and abrasions, clumps of hair missing, and two broken teeth. She was accompanied by an older woman who said she was Angel's aunt and who insisted on speaking for her. The nurse did not separate the two when conducting the assessment interview and exam, but when she asked the appropriate questions about whether Angel felt safe in her home and whether she had been beaten, Angel lied and insisted she had been hit by a car. The emergency department team decided there was nothing they could do for her if she did not tell the truth, so they treated her for the fractured rib and sent her home with no report to protective services even though they believed she was younger than the 18 years she claimed.

CASE STUDY: STARR

Starr is a 15-year-old White girl whose father sold her at the age of 12 to a pimp to pay off his gambling debt. She was violently beaten on a regular basis by this man who eventually sold her to another pimp. At the time of admission to the emergency department, she had been trafficked around the country from East coast to West coast and looked emaciated, depressed, had bloody urine, rectal bleeding, and had one eye closed. When asked about the reason for coming to the emergency department, she said she had been gang raped. The intake person laughed about this and asked how a whore could possibly have been raped. Starr tried to explain that when a customer takes her by force, that is the same as what happens to women who are not whores. The intake person answered the phone and when she looked up Starr had gone.

CASE STUDY: BOTUM

Botum, whose name means "princess" is a 14-year-old Cambodian refugee who was married at the age of 6 in Cambodia at the insistence of her parents who struggled to support their family of 10 children and older parents. Her husband sold her to a brothel at the age of 9 when he tired of her and arranged for the brothel owner to send small amounts of money from her earnings back to her parents. Botum experienced many sexually transmitted diseases and has had two pregnancies that were terminated via coat hanger by a woman employed by the brothel. However, she has only had to endure beatings by occasional violent customers and not the brothel owner because Botum quickly understood that if she cooperated she was helping her family, a strong Cambodian cultural value. She came to the United States as part of a container shipment of illegals from Singapore to work in American massage parlors owned by a Chinese gang. The gang

(continued)

tells the girls they will send money home to their families but first they have to repay their expenses to come to America.

Botum was arrested in a raid on a massage parlor and brought for medical treatment, but she refuses help escaping "the life" because she would have no way to help her family. In a paradoxical situation, she insists she is ruined and can never go home because she would be shunned for shaming her family by working as a prostitute. Yet, if she stops working as a prostitute she will have no way to earn money to send home. In her culture, the value of helping family trumps individual freedom.

Analysis

These three young women exemplify several difficult issues in trying to help women leave the life. Angel was first sexually abused within her family and had a dysfunctional mother who did not protect her. She came to the life with a desperate hope in the stranger Johnny whom she decided she loved and whom she believed was her protector. As bad as life with Johnny was, it was better than going home. In the emergency department, the staff failed to separate Angel from her "aunt" (often pimps send a trusted accomplice, called a "bottom girl" with the injured girl), and seemed to expect Angel to trust them immediately although they had given her no reason to do so. The staff not only failed to provide safety, but they failed to follow up. They chose to ignore their own instincts about her age and did not report the situation to protective services as they are mandated to do in cases of child abuse.

What should have happened for Angel is simple: Provide safety for her immediately by separating her from the accompanying person and report the situation to protective services regardless of how old she claimed to be. It would then be the responsibility of protective services to investigate since they employ social workers trained to sort out the truth.

Starr and Botum entered the life as many do—at the hands of their parents. In Starr's case, she endured long-term torture and was trafficked around the United States in such a way that she was disoriented as to where she was at any given point in time. When she sought help in the emergency department, she was treated with cruelty instead of the caring attitude toward all patients that we in health care like to hold as a cherished delusion.

Botum's cultural value of family was much stronger than her need for personal safety and freedom. Without concentrated services, there would be little hope of convincing her she could be trained to earn money she could send home by other means. In her situation it is critical to show her that she would have options. Under the Trafficking Victims Protection Act (TVPA), she would be eligible for a T-visa, one given to victims of trafficking who find themselves in the United States without immigration documents (United States Citizenship and Immigration Services, 2012).

USEFUL INTERVENTION MODELS

In Part II, the best practices for specific conditions will be presented, but it is helpful to gain a sense of the theoretical support for applying best practices to victims of human trafficking. The models are mentioned here but will be discussed in later chapters.

Stages of Change Model

The Stages of Change Model (Prochaska & DiClemente, 1983) was developed for substance abuse cessation but has relevance to the psychotherapeutic process and can be useful in helping the therapist identify the receptivity for change of the client. The original stages are precontemplation, contemplation, action, maintenance, and relapse. Knowing that relapse is normal and to be expected assuages the guilt of the client for not improving because it takes the pressure off the therapist to move the client forward too quickly.

   While considering the stage that patient is currently in when she seeks help is critical, it is equally important to conduct a thorough assessment in order to address malnutrition, sleep deprivation, physical injuries, and comorbid diseases. Trauma-focused cognitive behavior therapy and dialectical cognitive behavior therapy are two treatment methods that are evidence-based with survivors of child sexual abuse and PTSD. Eye movement desensitization and reprocessing (EMDR) is a technique that has efficacy in PTSD and can produce results in a short time.

   Family therapy is appropriate if the person can be returned to a family or if the person wishes to work on underlying family issues. Reintegrating into the family of origin would not be advisable when the parents have served as the traffickers. Substance abuse treatment will be necessary for a large percentage of victims of trafficking. Traffickers often use drugs to control the victim, making her less likely to run and more likely to do whatever the pimp requires in order to obtain more drugs. Group therapy, particularly the peer support model described by Lloyd (2011), provides a chance for survivors to benefit from the therapeutic relationship with other survivors. Finally, medications can take the edge off symptoms, but should not be used long term or as a substitute for comprehensive services.

ASSUMPTIONS AND EXPECTATIONS

Expect the Unexpected

We might expect trafficking victims to welcome our help with open arms, but the reverse is often true for a variety of reasons. These women and children have been conditioned, often from an early age and certainly by their pimps, to mistrust everyone. As nurses, we are usually thanked profusely for our help not only from our patients, but also from their families and friends. Trafficked victims do not have family and friends they can count on. The person they are closest to is their exploiter, who will certainly not cooperate with us for interfering in his business. Victims bond with their abusers and will defend their abusers to outsiders because they have been conditioned to be totally dependent upon them and to mistrust anyone else. The devil one knows is less frightening than the devil one does not know. Victims sometimes exhibit the Stockholm Syndrome and will go to great lengths to protect their pimps (Jameson, 2010).

Relapse Is Normal

The Stages of Change Model is useful in understanding this process. With a high rate of physical and psychological abuse by pimps and customers, these women and children become numbed. They usually live with chronic pain from the beatings and rapes. One of their coping mechanisms is denial. They do not have a way to earn money any other way and they cannot save money since the pimp controls the money they earn. If they could scrape together enough for a bus ticket, where would they go? Their original homes are not likely to be seen as a refuge. Even when excellent services are provided, they often have such a poor self-image that they mistrust their ability to do anything else. So they return again and again to the exploiter. The known is less fearful than the unknown.

Respect Their Right to Self-Determination

Sex-trafficked children and women most likely receive continuous messages from their pimps that they are worthless. They are literally slaves. They do not control their own money, are often disoriented by being moved from city to city and forced to work nights, with the result that they are sleep deprived and malnourished. The health care system is designed for compliance—or as now fashionable to say—adherence. We are the experts, we care deeply about our patients, and we know how to help people if they will only do as we say and not fight us or argue with us. This approach is a guaranteed way to fail with victims of sex trafficking. What little self-control they have over their bodies they are not likely to relinquish to us if they do not see immediate positive results. And how many medical interventions are that dramatically successful? It is critical to approach these patients in a radically different way than the usual. We need to look for opportunities to demonstrate that we respect their right to self-determination. We need to explain medical procedures thoroughly and ask for their permission to proceed at every step rather than assume they will trust us to do what is necessary to help them. This takes time and patience.

Assume That the First Visit Is the Last

Many health conditions and treatments require follow up. A broken arm requires a cast, monitoring circulation, and removal of the cast. STIs require a course of medication. Antibiotics usually need to be administered for 10 days. Pregnancy requires prenatal care for months, safe delivery, and follow-up. None of these conditions can be met if the traffickers feel threatened and if the girls cannot be rescued during the first visit. As seen in the case examples, the girls will often resist being rescued. The traffickers will move girls around from city to city to avoid detection. They know they cannot be prosecuted if the victims cannot be found to testify. We must do what we can during the brief time we see these victims. One example is using a single dose of Gardesil rather than the customary three doses to treat HPV (Anne Nichols, personal communication, 2012). Another strategy is to leave the door open by making the patient feel so comfortable that she will return if she can.

SUMMARY

This chapter serves as an introduction to the problem of sex trafficking. The culture of the street serves as a framework for how nurses might interact with victims and survivors. Some of the basic concepts have been introduced and will be expanded upon in subsequent chapters.

REFERENCES

Alabama State Nurses' Association. (2009). Human trafficking: 21st century slavery. *The Alabama Nurse, 36*(1), 1 and 7.

Aston, E. (2008). A fair trade? Staging female sex tourism and trade. *Contemporary Theatre Review, 18*(2), 180–192.

Bales, K. (2004). *Disposable people: New slavery in the global economy.* Berkeley, CA: University of California Press.

Bales, K. (2005). *Understanding global slavery.* Berkeley, CA: University of California Press.

Bales, K., & Lize, S. (2005). *Trafficking in persons in the United States: A report to the National Institute of Justice.* Retrieved May 16, 2012, from http://www.ncjrs.gov/pdffiles1/nij/grants/211980.pdf

Bastien, D. L. (2010). Pharmacologic treatment of combat-induced PTSD. *British Journal of Nursing, 19*(5), 318–321.

Cabezas, A. (2004). Between love and money: Sex, tourism, and citizenship in Cuba and the Dominican Republic. *Signs: Journal of Women in Culture and Society, 29*(4), 987–1015.

Crane, P., & Moreno, M. (2011). Human trafficking: What is the role of the health care provider? *Journal of Applied Research on Children: Informing Policy for Children at Risk, 2*(1), 1–27.

de Chesnay, M. (2012). Sex trafficking and sex tourism. In M. de Chesnay & B. Anderson (Eds.), *Caring for the vulnerable: Perspectives in nursing theory, practice and research* (pp. 385–392). Sudbury, MA: Jones and Bartlett, Inc.

Dulles, W. (1996). *Fielding's guide to Thailand: Including Cambodia, Laos, and Myanmar.* Redondo Beach, CA: Fielding Worldwide.

ECPAT. (2012). *Code of conduct for the protection of children from sexual exploitation in travel and tourism.* Retrieved May 12, 2012, from http://www.ecpat.net/ei/Publi cations/CST/Code_of_Conduct_ENG.pdf

Genefke, I. (2002). Chronic persistent pain in victims of torture. *Journal of Musculoskeletal Pain, 10*(1/2), 229–259.

Gigliotti, S. (2006). "Acapulco in the Atlantic": Revisiting Sosúa, a Jewish refugee colony in the Caribbean. *Immigrants & Minorities, 24*(1), 22–50.

Glittenberg, J. (2003). The tragedy of torture. *Issues in Mental Health Nursing, 24,* 627–638.

Grodin, M., & Annas, G. (2007). Physicians and torture: Lessons from the Nazi doctors. *International Review of the Red Cross, 89*(867), 635–654.

Hall, J. (2011). Sex offenders and child sex tourism: The case for passport revocation. *Virginia Journal for Social Policy and the Law, 18*(2), 153–202.

Hawthorne, E. (2011). Women in Northern Ireland involved in prostitution. *Irish Probation Journal, 8,* 142–164.

Interfaith Children's Movement. (2009). *Child exploitation and trafficking in Georgia.* Atlanta: Interfaith Children's Movement.

International Labor Office. (2005). *A global alliance against forced labor global report under the follow-up to the ILO Declaration on Fundamental Principles and Rights at Work 2005.* Retrieved June 4, 2012, from http://www.ilo.org/wcmsp5/groups/ public/@ed_norm/@declaration/documents/publication/wcms_081882.pdf

Ipser, J., Seedat, S., & Stein, D. (2006). Pharmacotherapy for post-traumatic stress disorder: A systematic review and meta-analysis. *South African Medical Journal, 96*(10), 1088–1096.

Jameson, C. (2010). The short step from love to hypnosis: A reconsideration of the Stockholm Syndrome. *Journal for Cultural Research, 14*(4), 337–355.

Jones, S. (2010). The invisible man: The conscious neglect of men in the war on human trafficking. *Utah Law Review, 2010*(4), 1143–1188.

Kambayashi, T. (2004). *Human trafficking plagues vulnerable Moldovans.* Interview with Agnes Chan in *Washington Times,* 6/18/2004, p. A17.

Kansas State Nurses' Association. (2008). Human trafficking. *The Kansas Nurse, 83*(8), 22–23.

Langberg, L. (2005). A review of recent OAS research on human trafficking in the Latin American and Caribbean region. *International Migration, 43*(1), 129–139.

Levine, J. (2001). Working with victims of persecution: Lessons from Holocaust Survivors. *Social Work, 46*(4), 350–360.

Lita, A. (2007). *Organ trafficking in Eastern Europe.* Retrieved April 23, 2012, from http://www.americanhumanist.org/hnn/archives/index.php?id=319&article=6

Lloyd, R. (2011). *Girls like us.* NY: Harper Collins.

McClain, N., & Garrity, S. (2011). Sex trafficking and the exploitation of adolescents. *Journal of Obstetric, Gynecologic & Neonatal Nursing, 40,* 243–252.

McClanahan, S., McClelland, G., Abram, K., & Teplin, L. (1999). Pathways into prostitution among female jail detainees and their implications for mental health services. *Psychiatric Services.* Retrieved May 15, 2012, from http://ajp.[psychiatryonline.org/ article.aspx?articleid=83780&RelatedWidgetarticles=true.

Meis, L., Barry, R., Kehle, S., Erbes, C., & Polusney, M. (2010). Relationship adjustment, PTSD symptoms, and treatment utilization among coupled National Guard soldiers deployed to Iraq. *Journal of Family Psychology, 24*(5), 560–567.

Montgomery, H. (2008). Buying innocence: Child sex tourists in Thailand. *Third World Quarterly, 29*(5), 903–917.

Moreno, A., & Grodin, M. A. (2002). Torture and its neurological sequelae. *Spinal Cord, 40*, 213–223.

Moreno, A., & Iacopino, V. (2008). Forensic investigations of torture and ill-treatment in Mexico. *The Journal of Legal Medicine, 29*, 443–478.

Mulvaney, S., McLean, B., & De Leeuw, J. (2010). The Use of stellate ganglion block in the treatment of panic/anxiety symptoms with combat-related post-traumatic stress disorder; preliminary results of long-term follow-up: A case series. *Pain Practice, 10*(4), 359–365.

Nicholas, P., George, E., Raymond, N., Lewis-O'Connor, A., Victoria, S., Lucien, S. et al. (2012). Orphans and at-risk children in Haiti. *Advances in Nursing Science, 35*(2), 182–189.

NSNA. (2010). *In support of increasing awareness of human trafficking.* Retrieved January 11, 2012, from http://www.nsna.org/Portals/0/Skins/NSNA/pdf/Final%20 Resolutions%202010_revised %205-05-10.pdf

O'Connor, M., & Healy, G. (2006). *The links between prostitution and sex trafficking: A briefing handbook.* Retrieved May 15, from http://www.catwinternational. org.

Olsen, D., Montgomery, E., Bojholm, S., & Foldspong, A. (2006). Prevalent musculoskeletal pain as a correlate of previous exposure to torture. *Scandinavian Journal of Public Health, 34*, 496–503.

Padilla, M. (2008). The embodiment of tourism among bisexually behaving Dominican male sex workers. *Archives of Sexual Behavior, 37*, 783–793.

Prochaska, J., & DiClemente, C. (1983). Stages and processes of self-change of smoking: Toward an integrative model of change. *Journal of Consulting and Clinical Psychology, 51*(3), 390–395.

Racine-Welch, T., & Welch, M. (2000). Listening for the sounds of silence: A nursing consideration of caring for the politically tortured. *Nursing Inquiry, 7*, 136–141.

Sabella, D. (2011). The role of the nurse in combating human trafficking. *American Journal of Nursing, 111*(2), 28–39.

Shared Hope International. (2011). *"This man wants to rent your daughter."* Vancouver, WA: Shared Hope International.

Smith, L. (webcast, 2011, Dec.). *Report of the state report cards.* Vancouver, WA: Shared Hope International.

The World Famous Players Ball: A Briefing Document Based on Online Research and General Knowledge. (2005). Retrieved June 6, 2012 from http://www.crisisconnectio ninc.org/pdf/Players_Ball.pdf.

Trossman, S. (2008). The costly business of human trafficking. *Amercian Nurse Today, 3*(12). Retrieved November 4, 2011 from http://www.americannursetoday.com/ article.aspx?id=4134&fid=4104.

Trout, K. (2010). The role of nurses in identifying and helping victims. *Pennsylvania Nurse, 65*(4), 18–20.

United Nations Protocol on Human Trafficking. (2000). Retrieved May 12, 2012, from http://www.unodc.org/unodc/en/human-trafficking/what-is-human-trafficking.html#What_is_Human_Trafficking).

United States Citizenship and Immigration Services. (2012). Victims of human trafficking: T nonimmigrant status. Retrieved June 6, from http://www.uscis.gov/portal/site/uscis/menuitem.eb1d4c2a3e5b9ac89243c6a7543f6d1a/?vgnextoid=02ed3e4d77d73210VgnVCM100000082ca60aRCRD&vgnextchannel=02ed3e4d77d73210VgnVCM100000082ca60aRCRD

United States State Department. (2012). *Trafficking in persons report—2012*. Retrieved June 1, 2012, from http://www.state.gov/j/tip/rls/tiprpt/2012/

World Law Direct. (2012). Retrieved June 20, 2012, from http://www.worldlawdirect.com/forum/law-wiki/27181-age-majority.html

Yea, S. (2010). Human trafficking: A geographical perspective. *Geodate, 23*(3), 2–6.

CHAPTER 2

Human Trafficking

MARK HOERRNER AND KEISHA HOERRNER

It's a frosty 3 a.m. in Georgia as Tanya (pseudonym) pulls her coat tighter around her, though the garment covers only a small part of her body. She walks briskly to try to generate some heat to stay warm knowing that she will be walking Fulton Industrial Boulevard until dawn unless she can find a way to meet the quota set by her controller. Unlike many of the other 6 million people in the city of Atlanta, Tanya lives from day to day selling sex on the street, at truck stops, and via online ads. She is not out on "the track"—a typical street name for working the street—because she chooses to be; she works as one of Demetrius's girls. He will keep her out this morning until she manages to collect whatever his nightly goal for the girls working in his "family" are charged with earning to stay in his good graces. Doing so means he might buy them a gift, let them eat, or give them a warm place to sleep. Failing him could mean anything from a lack of food to a severe beating. It's not about love, relationships, or care for the human condition. To Demetrius, Tanya is money, pure and simple. And if she fails to make her goal, well, he will just have to make sure that does not happen again. This was Tanya's 16th birthday.

*T*anya, in the above account taken from a Fulton County police officer, is a victim of domestic minor trafficking in the United States. The crime is a growing problem in the country. Such victims have an average age of 15.1 years, according to the national nonprofit organization A Future, Not A Past (Hoerrner, personal conversation, 2009a, b; McCullough, personal communication, 2010).

Tanya is part of a larger population, however, that claims somewhere between 27 and 40 million victims worldwide (Bales, 1999; Skinner, 2008). These victims represent a vast tide of individuals whose futures are not their own. The crime takes many forms across national borders but worldwide is known by a simple collective term: human trafficking. It is a growing criminal activity not only in the United States but across the globe.

When justice systems refer to a "crime," it is usually just that—a single crime. A burglar who breaks into a house may be charged with "breaking and entering" but is more likely to be charged with burglary if caught in the act. After the fact, a burglar is likely to be charged with possession of and/or sale of stolen goods. In each case, the crime is one specific act. Human trafficking, however, is a criminal incident that often involves a multitude of offenses committed in a series of criminal acts. Crimes such as involuntary servitude, false imprisonment, rape, sexual assault, forced sex, assault, battery, terroristic threats—and even murder—can be part of a human trafficking scenario. When studying human trafficking as a social event, it is important to keep this fact in mind: While rape, by itself, is a traumatic experience, human trafficking is a *series* of traumatic events.

THE POWER OF TERMINOLOGY

While the term "human trafficking" is used as a general descriptor for the process of the sale of people, it should be noted that the term is often misunderstood. "Trafficking" implies movement, but victims do not have to be moved across physical or political borders to be "trafficked." Victims can be trafficked out of the house they are currently living in by parents or relatives, or victims can be kidnapped and trafficked just a couple of miles from their home, as was the case with two Ohio teens walking to a fast food restaurant (Strauss, 2008).

Popular movies such as *Taken* have led to the idea that most human trafficking is something that happens in the metaphorical "over there," whatever foreign location that might be perceived to be. It probably comes as a shock that the United States has a significant human trafficking problem made up entirely of domestic victims. While foreign nationals are trafficked into the United States for the purposes of both labor and sex, there are a growing number of U.S. citizens who have fallen victim to traffickers in their own backyard.

The pop culture lexicon of the current age includes a number of terms that have become commonly used phrasing. For example, in recent years, the term "pimp" has become synonymous with wealth and sexual power. Society refers to heavily customized cars as "pimped out," and some refer to persons who flash around large sums of money or wear lavish clothing as "pimpin" or "big pimping." In the scholarly pursuit of studying perpetrators of sexual trauma, it is critical that these terms are sterilized and returned to nomenclature that indicates the true nature of the thing. A pimp is an offender, human trafficker, or controller.

Additionally, as victims are described, popular media has a tendency to describe events with phrasing such as "they lived in slave-like conditions" or "the people at this business were treated like slaves." Though there are times when people use hyperbole to describe their condition, especially when it comes to the world of work such as "working like a slave"—the truth is usually very different. Slaves are robbed of their personhood, are completely denied freedom, segregated from society, mentally and physically abused, and, often, sexually tortured. When describing actual victims of slavery, it should be that simple; the victims were either slaves or they were not. Many researchers utilize the term "modern-day slavery" to describe human trafficking. For the purposes of this chapter, the terms slave, modern-day slave, and trafficking victim are synonymous.

UNDERSTANDING HUMAN TRAFFICKING

At the core, human trafficking is the sale or rental of one human to another for exploitation. It is not exclusively gender- or age specific, though of the estimated number of slaves in the world, 80% are female individuals and 50% are children. This means that the typical slave is a girl between the ages of 12 and 16 years old (Bales & Soodalter, 2010).

Europol, the European Union's largest law enforcement agency, described human trafficking:

> Essentially, trafficking consists of actions in which offenders gain control of victims by coercive or deceptive means or by exploiting relationships, like those between parents and children, in which one party has relatively little power or influence and is therefore vulnerable to trafficking. Once initial control is gained, victims are moved to a place where there is a market for their services and where they often lack language skills and other basic knowledge that would enable them to find help. Destinations are commonly in foreign countries, but that is not always the case—international borders do not have to be crossed. Upon arrival at their destination, victims are forced to work in difficult, dangerous and usually unpleasant occupations, such as prostitution, the production of child pornography or general labour, in order to earn profits for the traffickers. Sometimes, victims are simply sold from one criminal group to another, but unlike other commodities, they can be made to work for long periods after arrival at their final destination, generating far greater profits for traffickers at all stages of the process.
> —*Europol, 2005, p. 9*

Source, Transit, and Destination

While the term "human trafficking" implies movement of goods, individuals can be trafficked within the borders of their own country. However, the movement of persons from one country to another happens in staggering numbers. Anti-Slavery International, the world's oldest abolitionist organization, estimates that 800,000–900,000 people are trafficked across international borders each year (Bales, 2007). The United Nations Children's Fund contends that 1.2 million children alone are moved across national borders (UN GIFT, n.d.), and the United Nations High Commissioner for Refugees estimates a much higher number of persons—between 700,000 and 4 million—are trafficked worldwide each year (United Nations High Commissioner for Refugees, 2007).

While the numbers do not often seem to mesh, they point to the core of the problem: Regardless of whose numbers are the most accurate, hundreds of thousands of slaves are being moved across international borders to be sold for sex or labor. All countries fall into at least one of three categories—source, transit, and destination—but are frequently classified as existing in multiple categories. While each trafficking case is unique, many victims see the same patterns emerge in their treatment: They are procured in a source country, moved through a transit nation, and end up in destination venue. Again, making a generalization about global movement is to tread upon treacherous footing as the process can be interrupted at any point by the victim being exploited in a transit nation rather than the intended destination, or more optimistically, by virtue of the victim being rescued by law enforcement or social services organizations.

Source Countries

Nations whose populace tends to be highly exploited, providing the fuel for human trafficking—are numerous. More than 160 nations are classified by the United Nations Office on Drugs and Crime (UNODC) as being countries of origin for modern-day slaves. Leading this group are Mexico, Russia, Brazil, India, China, and a host of African nations. Many Southeast Asian and Eastern European countries also rank near the top of this list (Kangaspunta, 2006).

Transit Countries

These are nations through which victims are transported on the way to destination countries. Victims may be temporarily exploited while in these countries to increase the overall profitability of transporting the victims to their destination, or "recruiters" may hand off victims to transporting groups or to the end recipient or their agents for removal to the victim's final destination. More than 100 countries are considered transit venues for victims, including Albania, Belgium, Poland, Thailand, Bulgaria, Hungary, Bosnia, France, Germany, Romania, Turkey, Italy, Benin, Egypt, and the United Kingdom (Kangaspunta, 2006).

Destination Countries

These nations are the end of the journey for many victims. The goal of transporting a victim to a destination country is usually pure economics: Sourced from poorer nations, victims are taken to a destination that will result in the highest possible prices for their labor or other exploitation (Malarek, 2003). Of the more than 140 destination countries, the highest reporting nations are Belgium, Germany, Greece, Israel, Italy, Japan, Netherlands, Thailand, Turkey, and the United States (Kangaspunta, 2006).

Law Enforcement in the United States

While a number of code sections in U.S. federal law are related to the act of human trafficking, most offenses were prosecuted under a relatively narrow code description until 2000, when President William J. Clinton signed the

Trafficking Victims Protection Act (TVPA) into law. The TVPA was the first truly comprehensive antihuman trafficking law passed in the United States, and it mirrored several international protocols. In the TVPA, "severe forms of trafficking in persons" includes both sex and labor trafficking:

> **Sex trafficking** is the recruitment, harboring, transportation, provision, or obtaining of a person for the purposes of a commercial sex act, in which the commercial sex act is induced by force, fraud, or coercion, or in which the person induced to perform such an act has not attained 18 years of age. (22 USC § 7102; 8 CFR § 214.11(a))

> **Labor trafficking** is the recruitment, harboring, transportation, provision, or obtaining of a person for labor or services, through the use of force, fraud, or coercion for the purposes of subjection to involuntary servitude, peonage, debt bondage, or slavery. (22 USC § 7102) (Polaris Project, 2012)

Global Law Enforcement

At the same time in 2000, the United Nations developed an international protocol for dealing with slavery commonly known as the "Palermo Protocol," though the full title is the *UN Protocol to Prevent, Suppress and Punish Trafficking in Persons, especially Women and Children*. While the two governmental entities were clearly collaborating, the two reached slightly different language on how to define the crime. The Palermo Protocol included a definition of human trafficking as follows:

> Trafficking in persons shall mean the recruitment, transportation, transfer, harboring or receipt of persons, by means of the threat or force or other forms of coercion, of abduction, of fraud, of deception, of the abuse of power, or of a position of vulnerability or of the giving or receiving of payments or benefits to achieve the consent of a person having control over another person, for the purpose of exploitation. Exploitation shall include, at a minimum, the exploitation of the prostitution of others or other forms of sexual exploitation, forced labor or services, slavery or practices similar to slavery, servitude or the removal of organs. (*Europol, 2005, p. 10*)

U.S. Interaction With Global Governments

As a result of the TVPA, the U.S. Department of State began publishing an annual report called the *U.S. Trafficking In Persons Report,* in which countries were rated based on their internal efforts to combat human trafficking. It should be noted that while this is a global report, countries categorized within the report are rated not based on Palermo but on the TVPA minimum standards (U.S.

Department of State, 2011). In the report, countries are rated on three tiers of progress, with an extra Tier 2 "Watch List" designation that acts as a warning to countries the United States deems as on the brink of not doing enough to combat human trafficking. Tier 1 nations are those that are in full compliance with U.S. guidelines; Tier 2 countries are not in complete compliance but are making significant inroads toward curbing the growth of human trafficking within national borders; and Tier 3 countries are regarded as failing the majority of criteria and are not actively seeking change. Until 2010, the United States did not include itself in the report. In its debut, it ranked itself Tier 1 (U.S. Department of State, 2010).

Countries with Tier 3 rankings in the report are subject to sanctions and other economic restrictions. These restrictions are decided on a case-by-case basis and can be altered by promises from governments toward future development of antihuman trafficking laws, promises of greater enforcement, and/or developing internal policies that might make trafficking of persons harder to conduct within national borders.

While the plight of the victims is first responded to by law enforcement agencies, there are quite a few nongovernmental organizations dedicated to the rescue and restoration of such victims. Organizations like Transitions Global (www.transitionsglobal.org), headquartered in Cincinnati, Ohio, but operating in multiple venues around the world such as Mumbai, India, and Phnom Penh, Cambodia, utilize unique treatment strategies at safe house facilities to respond to a growing tide of victims uncovered by exposing human trafficking syndicates. Girls Education and Mentoring Services (GEMS; www.gems-girls.org) is a New York-based organization that deals specifically with domestic minor trafficking victims. The organization provides medical and psychological services, as well as providing education, job training, and group support for teens who have been trafficked for sex.

In 2011, the Cable News Network (CNN) chose Anuradha Koirala as its 2010 CNN Hero of the Year (Ruffins, 2010). Koirala is the founder and executive director of Maiti Nepal, an antitrafficking organization with more than two decades of experience in not only rescuing and restoring victims of human trafficking but also putting traffickers behind bars. As of 2011, Maiti had participated in the convictions of more than 700 offenders (Hoerrner, personal conversation: Joe Collins, 2011).

The Maiti strategy is unique and specific to the geographic region that includes the Nepal/India border. Traffickers recruit women and girls in Nepal for sale to brothels in India where the demand for sex slaves is high. Maiti staffs "border crossings" in partnership with Nepalese soldiers. Together, Maiti representatives (some of whom are former victims) and soldiers board vehicles bound for and coming from India at the Nepal side of the border. The teams are looking for anything that might be a red flag—young girls in new clothing, women or girls traveling with older men—indicating a possible trafficking situation. The Maiti personnel and soldiers separate the individuals and question them thoroughly (Maiti Nepal, 2012). It's a program that works.

Joe Collins, head of Friends of Maiti Nepal, notes that Maiti has been successful in rescuing more than 20,000 women and girls during its history (Hoerrner, personal conversation: Joe Collins, 2011). These organizations are examples of many dedicated nongovernmental entities around the world serving victims of human trafficking.

A HISTORY IN CHAINS

Most of the common perceptions of contemporary slavery are derived from the historical knowledge of the Trans-Atlantic slave trade. During this 400-year period, African tribes would hunt other African tribes and sell them to slave ships docked along the western coast. Slavery fueled the agricultural boom in early America. These were ethnic Africans, or Africans who had been imported directly from Africa and had yet to begin generations of births while in captivity on plantations in the pre–Civil War Southern United States (Thomas, 1997). Unlike that period, modern-day slavery knows no ethnic or geographic boundaries. Slaves from Africa end up in Europe; those from Australia find themselves in Japan; and Eastern Europeans show up in brothels in Israel. The modern market for slaves is limited only by the means available to transport a person from one place to another; buyers exist in all parts of the world. While slavery is now illegal in every single country in the world, there are documented cases in almost every one of those nations. Slaves do not often appear on the public auction block in the 21st century but are still held in bondage (Nazer & Lewis, 2003).

Slavery has existed in one form or another for at least 8,000 years. In his book, *Woman, Child for Sale*, author Gilbert King (2004) notes that a find of grave sites indicates that early Egyptians may have been enslaving people from several different ethnic groups in Africa. These slaves were likely builders of the Egyptian pyramids. In the culture of Ancient Rome, slaves were prevalent as the Empire stretched across most of Europe, Asia, and Africa and the middle- and high-income estates demanded more and more servants and laborers. Recent television series such as *Rome* and *Spartacus: Blood and Sand* have taken creative license in looking at slavery in the Roman Empire and profiling both the numerous cultures from which slaves were taken as well as the complete domination of the slaves by their masters.

As the world progressed into the Middle Ages, slavery simply transformed itself into a form of economic bondage. While a man might "own" a piece of land, that land and the labor used on it belonged to the man's liege lord. Feudalism, then, became the new form of slavery (King, 2004). The slaves, known as serfs, represented the poorest of the poor. These slaves were brought from countries all over Europe, and it was not unusual to prey on various groups because of their ethnic or religious background.

Several attempts were made to end slavery in Europe, though not always for humanitarian reasons. In 1556, Genoa, Italy, banned the slave trade, although the move was primarily to lessen the number of Africans found in the city. France, in 1571, declared all slaves, including Africans and Moors, to be free and outlawed the practice. General James Oglethorpe, chartered by England's King George II, founded the city of Savannah in the colony of Georgia. As one of four founding tenets for the colony, Oglethorpe banned the practice of slavery (King-Tisdell Cottage Foundation, n.d.). Throughout history, humanity has been in a battle with itself over the concept of enslavement. Many individuals, such as Fernao de Oliveira, author of *The Art of War at Sea*, denounced the slave trade as an evil construct. But the economic power of slavery drowned out many of those voices (King, 2004). Though slavery is now criminalized in every country on the planet, the trade itself has simply gone underground, not ceased. In fact, all evidence points to the fact that the trade in humans is not only much larger than it was in earlier times, but that it continues to grow at an alarming rate.

TYPES OF MODERN-DAY SLAVERY

Human trafficking victims typically fall into one of two super categories: forced labor or sexual servitude. There are situations where one can be a victim of both. Falling within these two super categories is a host of subcategories that detail the type of slavery visited upon the victim.

Sexual Servitude

A person is a victim of sexual servitude when he/she is forced to have sex against his/her will for the material gain of another. Both United States and international law contain similar language on this issue. Victims of sexual servitude may be child or adult, male or female, and may or may not work in a brothel (McGill, 2003). A person who voluntarily—and who has no controller—sells his/her own body for sex is *not a victim of sexual slavery*. Thus, a prostitute is not automatically a victim of sexual servitude. This is an important distinction. It should be noted, however, that individuals who, in their adult ages, work as independent prostitutes were likely introduced to prostitution by a controller in their earlier years given that the average age for entry into prostitution is in the early teen years. Social autopsies conducted on such victims have revealed this connection (National Center for Missing and Exploited Children, 2009).

U.S. Secretary of State Hillary Rodham Clinton has been quite outspoken on the subject of human trafficking, most specifically on the trafficking of women for sexual purposes. In an interview while she was a U.S. senator, she told PBS's *Wide Angle* news program: "It's just heartbreaking and outrageous that, in the 21st century, we would see anyone treated like [a slave]. But it particularly reflects the continuing disregard for women's rights and the way women are considered somehow less than human in many parts of the world and how they are used for sexual purposes without any regard to their human dignity and rights" (Rubin, Dying to Leave, 2003, n.p.).

Forced Prostitution

Perhaps the broadest subcategory of sexual slavery, forced prostitution is exactly what it sounds like—a relationship in which a controller rents the body of another person for material gain. Though that description is highly antiseptic compared to the actual act of being forcibly raped for commercial gain, it underscores the primary factor in driving human sexual commerce: economics. The practice generates billions annually in untaxed profits (Kara, 2009). According to the National Center for Missing and Exploited Children (2009), types of forced prostitution include the following:

- Crack (or related drugs) Prostitution—Individuals forced into prostitution through manipulation of the victim's drug habit.
- Street-Level Prostitution—Traditional form of street solicitation of sex acts, usually overseen by a street-level controller, though not necessarily the primary offender.
- Computer-Assisted Family Prostitution—Use of the Internet to sell sex with a family member, often children.
- Call Operation—Prostitution managed through regional call centers found through ads usually in newspapers or online; victims are dispatched to a buyer's location (outcall) or the buyer is invited to the victim's residence or a hotel (incall).
- Brothel Operation—A "house" of prostitution, usually managed by a single controller or syndicate of controllers in which buyers come to the location to purchase sex with victims. In Nevada where prostitution is legal in certain areas, these are moderately upscale operations. A brothel may also be housed in a subdivision, a farm, a traveling vehicle, a massage parlor, or similar facility.
- Gang-Related Prostitution—Victims are often used as "perks" by gang members, forced to provide sexual services on demand to any member of the gang and often prostituted outside of the gang itself to generate money.
- Male Prostitution—Any of the preceding elements, simply involving men instead of women as the victims.
- Ethnic Prostitution—Forced prostitution, but the victim is of the same ethnic group as the buyers and controller.
- Cab Operation—Usually found within an immigrant population, victims are driven by "taxi" or "cab" drivers to appointments with buyers; victims typically see 40–50 buyers a day.
- Generational Prostitution—Victims are born into a family that already operates or exists as part of a prostitution syndicate; often, victims are auctioned off while still virginal (sometimes several times) before beginning a life of forced sex.

Massage Parlors

In 2008, there were 4,815 massage parlors nationwide in the United States identified by theeroticmp.com as possible settings for the sale of sexual services. In Atlanta, a nonprofit organization conducted surveillance on 12 suspected brothels disguised as specifically Asian massage parlors (Hoerrner, 2008). Eleven of the 12 parlors, including several with multiple locations, were allegedly found to be sellers of sexual services. The majority were suspected of either using victims smuggled illegally into the country or of having human trafficking victims on the premises.

As would be imagined, the price of sexual slaves varies by geographic region. Whereas many massage parlors in the United States charge anywhere from $60 to $180 per hour (for full intercourse), a typical Bangkok, Thailand, facility might only charge about $4 to $6 for the same time allotment or act (Kara, 2009). Translated into profit, that Bangkok massage parlor will generate an annual profit of about $60,000 per year from the sale of sex. American massage parlors will generate profits in much greater amounts—anywhere from $170,000 to nearly $1 million. All of this illegal, untaxed profit is generated with an average of only four to six women or girls on the premises.

Ironically, most of these massage parlors operate in the open, despite the fact that the sale of erotic services is expressly prohibited by law. While parts of their business might be concealed, the establishments are advertised in local newspapers and magazines as well as in online communities. There are significant law enforcement challenges to shutting down massage parlors. Some brothel owners are particularly adept at foiling police attempts to catch massage parlor personnel in an illegal act, utilizing everything from consistently altering public records to throw investigators off a paper trail to the strategic placement of devices that signal criminals when someone enters the massage parlor with audio or video recording equipment (Hoerrner, personal conversation with law enforcement, 2009a). Some of these victims may be seen by health care workers, however, which can lead to the exposition of a human trafficking scenario.

Mail-Order Brides

The practice of seeking a bride online or through a published catalog of available women has been a growing one. Typically, Westerners are seeking brides from Europe (predominantly Eastern Europe), Russia, the Balkans, or Asia. In a *Washington Post* article, journalist Lena Sun noted, "In the United States, mail-order-bride agencies are developing everywhere. One business, A Foreign Affair, has had more than 15,000 male buyers since it began 3 years ago. Now there are 200 to 250 of these companies in the United States, a third of which started in 1997. At least 80 of these focus exclusively on Russian and Eastern European women. A Foreign Affair has about 3,500 women from Russia, Eastern Europe, Asia and Latin America. The business claims they are responsible for an engagement or marriage every week" (Sun, 1998, n.p.).

In some cases, these bridal organizations are well-regulated and scrupulous, exacting a fee for putting eligible women and men together. In a growing number of cases, however, this is an excellent way to legally shroud the practice of selling sex slaves. In a typical mail order bride scam, a woman is courted by her prospective husband and all seems normal until she arrives in the destination country. It is then that the "husband" reveals himself to be a controller and introduces the woman to a life of sexual enslavement. In other cases, such brides become domestic servants, taking on a harrowing 24/7 life of providing for another individual with no compensation, frequent abuse, rape, and little hope of escape (United States Congress, Committee on Foreign Relations, 2004).

The Internet has spawned considerable growth for mail-order bride operations. Researcher Jen Marchbank of Simon Fraser University issued a study that noted the rise in the use of electronic resources. "The growth of the business can be traced to the explosion of the Internet in recent years—and the cost-effectiveness of running a website. They're cheap to keep updated and simpler to manage than paper catalogues. It's estimated there could be as many as 10,000 Internet sites worldwide offering mail-order brides. One such site listed 128 countries" (Hainsworth, 2006, n.p.). Marchbank herself said, "This is about women as a commodity to be purchased. This is to me very much about international inequalities in economics" (Hainsworth, 2006, n.p.).

Child Sexual Exploitation

Child sexual exploitation, often referred to as CSEC (commercial sexual exploitation of children), is a growing problem in many large urban areas, according to experts at the Federal Bureau of Investigation. Large metropolitan areas attract child predators and tend to be hubs for the sale of sex with children. Ease of access—train stations, major highways, airports, bus depots—contributes to the exploitation with children because buyers of sex can easily reach the city and traffickers can easily move victims around. A child, as classified by both U.S. federal law and international law, is any person under the age of 18 years.

The International Labour Organization (ILO) (2012) classifies CSEC as existing in one of the following situations:

- The use of girls and boys in sexual activities remunerated in cash or in kind (commonly known as child prostitution) in the streets or indoors, in such places as brothels, discotheques, massage parlors, bars, hotels, restaurants, and so on.
- The trafficking of girls and boys and adolescents for the sex trade
- Child sex tourism
- The production, promotion, and distribution of pornography involving children
- The use of children in sex shows (public or private)

The ILO is a specialized agency housed in the United Nations. Fighting CSEC is part of its *International Programme on the Elimination of Child Labour* (IPEC).

CSEC within in the United States can take a number of forms, but the most common is the single controller–victim relationship commonly known as "pimping." According to law enforcement, child victims bring higher prices: the younger the child, the more exclusive the clientele and the higher the price for the trafficker. Outside the United States, this is not necessarily true. Children are sold in illegal sex practices in many countries, especially those with developing economies or high poverty rates, for pennies on the dollar compared to prices within the United States (Kangaspunta, 2006).

The Polaris Project is a nongovernmental entity that operates the National Human Trafficking Resource Center as well as several shelters for victims. In their work with victims, it is not unusual for Polaris personnel to encounter domestic minors engaged in the sex trade. Keisha was one of those children found through outreach efforts conducted at street level. Exploited since age 14, Keisha was the victim of a master predator.

CASE STUDY: KEISHA

Keisha (pseudonym) is a 16-year-old African American female originally from Florida. She was raised by an aunt until she was 10 years old and then placed in the foster care system. At the age of 14, Keisha first ran away from her foster family to avoid sexual harassment from one of her foster family's relatives. During that time, she met "Mastur D," a 26-year-old man who offered to help her get back to her biological family. He said he would be able to pay for some of the expenses to get them there, but that she needed to help support them financially by engaging in commercial sex with some of his friends. With no money or other options Keisha took him up on his offer. He drove her back to Florida but insisted when they arrived that she had not earned enough money to cover their hotel and gas costs. He physically assaulted her and told her she would never see anyone else in her family if she did not engage in sex with other men of his choosing. She felt she had no other choice and continued to earn money for Mastur D to pay him back for the money he paid for her to get back to Florida. Keisha was arrested for solicitation in Florida and, after serving time in a juvenile detention center, was returned to her foster family and was, therefore, returned to sexual harassment by her foster family's relative. Keisha ran away again a year later and called Mastur D to help her get back to Florida. He agreed to help again. She was arrested again.

While participating in an outreach group at a detention center, Keisha reached out to a Polaris Project social worker and told her parts of her story. The Polaris Project immediately stepped in to provide emotional support and additional social services. The social worker helped Keisha talk to her case manager at the detention center about what happened and helped Keisha's probation officer understand other options for support instead of a detention center and returning to her foster family. Keisha now has an order of protection against Mastur D and was able to leave the detention center and go to an out-of-state residential program for young girls who were victims of sex trafficking. Keisha is doing well in her program and is almost finished with her GED. (Polaris Project, 2012, n.p.)

Military Prostitution

The militaries of the world are some of the largest consumers of sex for hire in history, often with the direct consent of governments or military commands. While this might seem a likely practice relegated to ragtag militias or rebel movements where discipline is, at best, tenuous, the truth is stark: Considerable evidence links most modern militaries, including those of the United States and the United Nations, with promoting and, in some cases, directly building and populating brothels for the use of soldiers (Jeffreys, 2009).

UN Peacekeepers, specifically, have been identified as driving sexual slavery in multiple countries. When Peacekeepers arrived on mission in Cambodia in 1990, the number of prostituted women and girls in Phnom Penh rose from just 1,500 to over 20,000 victims. Later, when the UN Transitional Authority in Cambodia (UNTAC) was criticized over the Peacekeeper-created prostitution industry, the representative there defended operations, citing that "boys will be boys" (Jeffreys, 2009, p. 120).

Just 2 years later, UN Peacekeeper presence in Mozambique necessitated the appointment of a special UN military liaison officer to "mediate between troops and prostitutes and traffickers" (Jeffreys, 2009, p. 120). Africa and its many conflicts created fertile ground for trafficking operations. UN presence in Rwanda, Sierra Leone, Liberia, and Guinea created large-scale prostitution of women and girls, often by third parties, in exchange for medicine and food (Jeffreys, 2009).

During the periods of ethnic cleansing in Bosnia, "rape camps" were set up to service Serbian militias. These rape camps were often fatal for the women kidnapped to serve the soldiers, save for cases when the women became pregnant. Because the Serbians wanted to dilute the purity of the Bosnian ethnic groups, these women would often be sent home carrying the children of the troops as a point of humiliation (Jeffreys, 2009). In investigations since the atrocities during the Bosnian genocide, the Federal Bureau of Investigation has sent multiple teams to Bosnia to determine the extent of the genocidal actions there and has noted the countless stories of rape and kidnapping for the purposes of sexual servitude (Whitcomb, 2001).

JAPAN'S DEVELOPMENT OF INSTITUTIONAL SEX SLAVERY: A CASE STUDY

"Camp followers," a term for women who trailed behind the various militaries of the world living off the scraps of plunder and supplies, were often either voluntary prostitutes or ended up raped, often by multiple individuals, in times of war and peace. These were not women who were technically co-opted into the military machine, but certainly, military leaders the

(continued)

world over did not discourage the practice in order to keep soldiers, especially those on long marches far from home, entertained (Tanaka, 2002, p. 92).

Institutionally, one of the earliest and most comprehensive programs featuring women sold as sex slaves began in Japan. The country already had an extensive brothel industry into which many women were sold by parents and guardians more interested in cash than raising another child. From this system of brothels came nearly 200,000 victims indoctrinated into Japan's (and Korea's) institutional "comfort women" system (Tanaka, 2002, p. 94). This occurred at a time when Japan was struggling with an uneasy shift from a deeply patriarchal feudal system to a capitalist society.

> The first military brothels were set up exclusively for the military in Shanghai in 1932 as Japan's colonial expansion into Asia began to accelerate. Previously, Japanese brothels were privately run and not just for troops. Women in military brothels were examined twice weekly for venereal disease and the provision of brothels was expected to deter the rape of civilians, which had the unfortunate effect of alienating subject populations and creating "anti-Japanese sentiment." The "comfort women" selected were mainly Japanese at first, drawn from the women and girls sold to the brothels by their families. In some areas of China women were requisitioned by requiring local Chinese security councils to provide women for the purpose. By 1938 there was a full-scale mobilization of Korean women. Japanese pimps and procurers were employed too, being asked to come to China to set up private brothels stocked with Japanese women.
>
> —*Jeffreys, 2009, p. 111*

While the Japanese government recognized the likelihood of their own troops seeking to rape women in times of war, it espoused the same opinion about U.S. troops during Japan's occupation at the end of World War II. The government ordered that "comfort stations" be set up for the patronage of U.S. troops, staffed by women from existing brothels, but also extending the mandate to "geisha ... waitresses, barmaids, habitual prostitutes and the like ..." (Jeffreys, 2009, p. 114). Some of the victims were actually high-school students working in munitions factories.

Most of these students had lost their families in the war and were targeted directly by recruiters looking for young faces for the brothels. Many were introduced to the sex trade through gang rapes by groups of American soldiers (Tanaka, 2002). Postwar research suggests that the U.S. military and Allied commands had already planned to set up brothels as they secured various regions in Japan. In fact, some of these brothels were so

(continued)

large that they likely set the stage for the global industrialization of prostitution, employing as many as 400 women at a single location. By the end of 1945, an estimated 10,000 women in Tokyo alone were being used by occupation troops. This led to the development of the state-run Recreation and Amusement Association (RAA), the largest White slavery operation in history. The Japanese government funded and owned more than 60% of the RAA, which saw nearly 70,000 women in brothels throughout the country almost exclusively for the use of American soldiers (Jeffreys, 2009).

In 2003, the UN developed a zero-tolerance policy for the 99,000 uniformed personnel serving in Peacekeeping operations. According to the 2011 TIP Report, "The UN requires peacekeeping personnel (civilian, police, and military) to sign a code of conduct on sexual exploitation and abuse that forbids sex with minors regardless of the local age of consent, sex with persons in prostitution, and offering favors or goods in exchange for sexual favors. The UN's model memorandum of understanding (MOU) (GA resolution 61/267 B) includes provisions for addressing sexual exploitation and abuse by uniformed personnel … many UN peacekeeping missions have prevention measures such as 'off-limits premises and areas,' curfews, and telephone hotlines, and require mission personnel to wear uniforms at all times" (n.p.).

The UN has also endeavored to encourage countries to increase the number of women assigned to peacekeeping missions in order to facilitate a greater outreach to women in the areas where operations are taking place. While the UN has increased the number of investigations into suspected trafficking operations since 2003, in 2010 it completed only 44 investigations with only half of those deemed as credible allegations of improper actions by peacekeepers (U.S. Department of State, 2011).

Forced Labor

If a victim is forced to work for little or no pay without the possibility of voluntarily leaving a job and that work creates a materiel benefit for another, it is generally considered to be "forced labor." Forced labor is not inequality in working conditions; some people consider "sweat shops" to be examples of forced labor, but they are simply a matter of labor exploitation, not true slavery. Nor is a tyrannical boss at a corporation who wants his employees to work weekends a "slave driver," or perpetrator of forced labor. Those are colloquialisms that have become staples of popular language. Victims of forced labor may not leave their job, are usually trapped into debt bondage, and can suffer significant abuse at the hands of their captors.

The force and coercion used to control victims of forced labor may take the form of physical aggression, implied aggressive acts, or forceful threats. Individuals may be defrauded, having been promised a paying job in a new city or country only to find themselves enslaved once they arrive for work. In Russia, at the height of the late 1990s building boom, men were travelling from all over Europe to get a shot at working on construction crews. They were literally recruited right off the trains that brought them into the country as recruiters would man the platforms looking for laborers. Upon arriving at a job site, many of these men were told that they would be paid little or nothing for their labor, were threatened if they did not do the work, and were at the mercy of the hiring contractor. In other countries, prisons may be used as forced labor facilities.

CHINESE LAOGAI: A CASE STUDY

Laogai—a term for Chinese "reform-through-labor camps" —are spread out in some 1,100 locations throughout Mainland China. These camps often include practitioners of Falun Gong, a peace movement outlawed in 1999 by the communist government. Other prisoners include Tibetan dissidents, Catholics, Protestants, and ethnic minorities. According to the Laogai Research Foundation, between 4 and 6 million people are incarcerated in these camps (Bales & Trodd, 2008). The camps often share the names of companies or corporations as these camps produce a large number of goods utilizing the prisoners as slave labor. These prisoners, who are mostly low-level, nonviolent offenders or government dissidents, often face many of the challenges of being incarcerated in maximum security prisons: 16-hour workdays, torture, solitary confinement, gang rape, malnutrition, drugging, and rampant disease (Bales & Trodd, 2008).

Ying, a prisoner at the Tuanhe Prisoner Dispatch Center, recounted the conditions of her incarceration:

I was locked up with over a dozen Falun Gong practitioners in a cell that was twelve square meters (130 square feet) in size. There were only eight bunk beds in the room; thus, some of us had to sleep on the floor. While we were sleeping, we had to keep our heads visible to the guards. We did everything in this cell including working, eating, drinking, and using the toilet; therefore, there were many flies and mosquitoes. At the dispatch center, we were only allowed to eat at certain times. Water was rationed; drinking water was limited. The prison guards never allowed us to wash our hands before meals . . . . Twice a day we were given five minutes for personal hygiene . . . . If we could not finish the work assigned to us, we were not allowed to clean ourselves.

We were allowed very little sleep each day; we were forced to start working the moment we opened our eyes. My hands had blisters and

(continued)

calluses from working long hours to finish the assigned quota of packaging disposable chopsticks.

We were forced to work 16 hours every day.
—Bales & Trodd, 2008, pp. 23-24

Ying was later transferred to the Xin'an Female Labor Camp where her conditions worsened. She was forced to manufacture massive quantities of goods, including knitted sweaters, slippers, crocheted hats, woolen gloves, and a host of stuffed animals. Based on her experience, she believed that many of these goods were being sent to European outlets for sale (Bales & Trodd, 2008). Stephen Mosher, president of the Population Research Institute, said that the laogai system has a considerable impact on the Chinese economy, noting that in 1998, it generated nearly $800,000,000 in revenues (Ax & Fagan, 2007).

Forced Labor in the United States

The Southern United States has a significant amount of agricultural enterprise as well as documented cases of forced labor. The Coalition of Immokalee Workers (CIW) is an organization dedicated to rooting out forced labor in immigrant and migrant populations. In 2008, CIW participated in the uncovering of one of the largest agricultural slavery cases prosecuted in the nation.

Guatemalan and Mexican workers were hired by five family members, Cesar, Geovanni, Jose, Villhina, and Ismael Navarrete, and their associate, Antonia Vargas, to pick tomatoes on farms in southwest Florida. The workers claimed to have been locked in U-Haul trucks overnight in 100-plus degree heat, to have been charged for showers and food, and to have received no compensation for their labor. The Navarrete operation ranged from South Carolina to Florida and involved dozens of victims. If the workers tried to leave, they were threatened with physical harm and/or beaten.

Law enforcement officers described the workers' environment:

Workers' living conditions were substandard. In Immokalee, Florida, workers slept outside, in vans, or in a shack on the Navarrete property. In northern Florida, and North and South Carolina, workers slept in crowded trailers for which the Navarretes deducted $40 a week from their earnings for housing. Fifty dollars a week was deducted for two basic meals a day. No food was provided on Sundays. Workers were charged for everything—including beverages, showers, and laundry. These expenses were deducted from unpaid earnings.

Cesar, Geovanni, and "Trompas" [a juvenile who was not charged] locked five workers in the back of a box truck. After about 7 hours, one of the men noticed light at the top back corner of the truck and with his head he pushed loose some of the sheet metal roof. Eventually, two of the men squeezed their way out of the truck and jumped to the ground. They observed that the truck was pad-locked on the outside so they could not open it and release the other men. They located a wooden ladder and rescued the remaining confined men. One of the men later returned to the subjects' compound for his property. Cesar beat him and cut his arm with a sharp object. Cesar told the man that he would work for him in the morning. Cesar again locked the man in the same box truck. After a few hours someone, he does not know who, unlocked the truck, and he ran away.

The men reported the lock in to the Collier County Sheriff's Department and other workers notified a frequent NGO partner, the Coalition of Immokalee Workers.

—Human Trafficking and Smuggling Center, 2008, p. 12

Deputies from the Collier County Sheriff's Department contacted ICE agents and arrests of more than a dozen people were made. All of the victims and their controllers were found to be in the United States illegally. Cesar and Giovanni eventually pled guilty to charges of conspiracy, involuntary servitude, and peonage. The brothers each received 12 years in federal prison. Jose "Pepe" Navarrete received 51 months and Ismael, 46 months. Villhina, because she was of advanced age, was sentenced to time served and deported. The family was ordered to pay more than $200,000 in restitution to the workers. Once their sentences were served, Jose, Villhina, and Ismael were deported. The rest of the defendants will be returned to their home country upon completion of their jail terms (Coalition of Immokalee Workers, 2012).

Bonded Labor

The practice of bonded labor is similar to the practice of debt peonage, described below. In bonded labor, an individual seeking a loan promises to pay for the loan with a specified amount of labor, usually for a certain length of time. The two parties typically sign a contract and in most cases, these loans are for very small amounts of money. Unscrupulous loan makers then exploit the workers, either by drawing out the length of the contract beyond the specified guidelines or by adding minor "incidental" charges to the loan, such as housing, medical aid, tool rental, clothing needs, family needs, food provision, or other fees to increase the amount of the loan, thereby increasing the amount of free labor. Because of the prevalence of this practice and the ease of extending the life of the loan, many debt bondage situations become generational, with the children of a loan grantee assuming the mantle of the debt as it grows over time. This practice also has an effect on migrant populations, which are highly vulnerable to exploitation (Bales, 1999).

Involuntary Domestic Servitude

In Brookfield, Wisconsin, a young Filipino woman was discovered in a home in a lavish suburb. She had been in the home for 20 years, serving as the household cook and maid. She had been promised that compensation was being kept for her in a "special" account, though the woman had no access to such an account. She had been lured into the situation by the homeowners who had brought her from her home country under false pretenses. Forced to work exceedingly long days, she catered to every whim of the family (Kouri, 2006).

Situations like this where individuals are forced into domestic labor in a home are extremely hard to identify because most of these slaves are never allowed into a situation where the general public might identify them, and those who are rescued are generally discovered by "accident." In Kevin Bales' *The Slave Next Door*, he relates the story of a young Mexican girl who was lured from her parents and home to work as a nanny and maid for a Texas homeowner. She was promised an education and the greatest of care but found a dark reality of beatings, abuse, and torture. When not serving the family, the girl was chained to a pole in the back yard. Luckily, a neighbor who had to climb on top of his house to examine a roof issue saw the young girl and called the police.

The victims in these scenarios are often lured with the promise of being a child's caretaker, a maid, a cook, or similar household worker. The truth is that many of these situations result in the enslavement of the unsuspecting, sometimes accompanied by rape or sexual abuse.

THE NANNY NIGHTMARE: *U.S. GOVERNMENT V. GARRETT*: A CASE STUDY

Soumya (pseudonym) is a young, vibrant woman who is married and lives in the United States with her husband. She often makes and sells her own jewelry in addition to working a full-time job. Her life was not always this prosperous, however. She was brought to the United States by the Garretts, a family looking for a full-time caretaker for their two children. The mother of the children, Malika Garrett, also a native of India like Soumya, had desired to bring someone from her homeland so that her children would have some cultural continuity. Soumya came to the United States on a visa sponsored by Russell Garrett's father, a former magistrate court judge. For the first couple of months, Soumya was worked hard but paid for what she did. Soon, however, the Garretts devised a different plan: They would save a great deal of money if they stopped paying Soumya. But they didn't want to lose her, so the Garretts decided that they would issue three threats to Soumya to keep her on the job. First, Malika threatened to call Soumya's conservative Muslim family back in India and tell

(continued)

them that Soumya had actually been engaging in prostitution and had become pregnant by one of her "johns." Second, Malika would call the Department of Homeland Security and report Soumya as a terrorist. Third, Malika would call Immigration and Customs Enforcement and report Soumya as an illegal alien. The Garretts had taken Soumya's passport and visa, so she would have no way to prove her immigration status.

The Garretts then forced Soumya to work 16-hour days, nearly every day. She was not only in charge of the children but forced to do housework, cooking, and any other tasks the Garretts directed her to do. Soumya was emotionally and physically tired and began to drastically lose weight from the stress. But Soumya had not gone unnoticed. Hope came in the form of a nearby neighbor who had seen Soumya walking the Garrett's children around their neighborhood. The woman, in her 60s at the time, was a devout Christian and approached Soumya about the possibility of going with her to church. Soumya was highly resistant, afraid of what the Garretts might say. She hungered for friendship, having lived her nightmare in silence and alone at the Garrett residence. Undaunted, the neighbor approached Malika Garrett repeatedly about taking Soumya to church with her. Eventually, the Garretts relented, and Soumya was allowed to leave the house to attend church with the neighbor for short periods. Their friendship grew to the point at which Soumya finally broke down and confessed to the neighbor everything that had taken place at the Garrett home. Infuriated by what she heard, the neighbor went to the Garretts' house and demanded that Soumya be allowed to pack her bags and come with her; she told Malika Garrett that she had already notified the FBI. Soumya was allowed to leave, though Malika told Soumya that her husband, Russell, would come get her. Russell Garrett, at the time of the case, was employed full-time as a Sheriff's Deputy. He showed up at the neighbor's home in uniform and armed, demanding that they return his slave. Luckily for Soumya, the neighbor and her husband refused. Frustrated, Malika Garrett made good on her previous threats, calling Soumya's family and the government agencies.

The Garretts were arrested on human trafficking charges but would later seek a plea deal on charges of harboring an illegal alien. William Garrett, Russell's father, who had arranged Soumya's work visa, was also arrested on charges of falsifying government documents. Ultimately, only Malika Garrett would serve jail time, though not for human trafficking. She was charged by agents of the Department of Homeland Security for making false reports related to terrorism and was sentenced to 18 months in federal prison. Russell Garrett was fired from his law enforcement position and given 22 months' probation for his alien harboring conviction. Soumya received thousands of dollars in restitution for her ordeal and was granted a specialized visa that allowed her to remain in the United States (Hoerrner, personal conversation: U.S. Asst. District Attorney Susan Coppedge, 2009b). Aspects of her story—including the traffickers taking vital documents and using threats—are found in numerous domestic servitude cases.

Child Labor

Many countries survive based on the economic output of the agricultural industry. While many large corporations and businesses operate these farms, the vast majority of subsistence farming is still done by families. These families often utilize their children as laborers as a normal practice. Almost every government has a law covering when, where, and how a child may be put to work. Sadly, these laws are often ignored by slavers who seek vulnerable populations to exploit for labor, and children are arguably the largest vulnerable population in the world. The lack of parental presence makes these children targets for slavers looking to provide laborers for tanneries that process leather, rug looms, metal fabrication shops, brick kilns, cocoa farms, or any of a wide array of industries that utilize manual labor. In India, more than 50% of children work outside the home because of the high poverty rate (Population Reference Bureau, 2002). In the United States, the Child Labor Coalition estimates that there are 5.5 million children between the ages of 12 and 17 engaged in labor. Such a large group represents significant chances for exploitation (U.S. Department of Health and Human Services, 2007).

Child Soldiers

The use of child soldiers by various military and rebel factions around the world is a practice that dates back to pre-Roman era tribes. In those societies, child soldiers were utilized as a coming-of-age event for the transformation from child to man, from tribe member to warrior. In the last century, however, the use of child soldiers has largely spawned from a lack of eligible male/female adult combatants in developing nations. Children are forced or coerced into serving a military unit in a variety of roles: soldier, cook, porter, medic, or sexual consort (usually for the benefit of adult officers) (U.S. Department of State, 2011).

In many cases, children are coerced or defrauded into joining military units. Hip-hop artist and former child soldier Emmanuel Jal was lured to a military training camp after the death of his mother (Jal, 2012). Many recruiters target young children like Jal, who was just 8 years old at the time he was inducted, because of the ability to psychologically manipulate the children. Jal remained a soldier in Sudan for 4 more years before his unit faced a major defeat by the northern Sudanese troops. He and several other child soldiers fled into the jungle where they faced starvation, disease, predatory animals, and the prospect of cannibalism for survival. While many of his friends died, Jal was eventually able to make it to a refugee camp (the same camp where many of Sudan's "Lost Boy" refugees resided). He met a British aid worker, Emma McCune, who adopted Jal and helped him leave the camps and enabled him to start on a path that would involve getting an education and discovering a talent for musical expression. He has since used his music to tell the story of his enslavement as a child soldier, his escape, and the challenges he faced leading up to his rescue. He has now become a staunch advocate against child slavery and for global peace (Jal, 2012).

Profile: Lord's Resistance Army

In 2012, U.S. President Barack Obama made good on a pledge to provide military backing to a plan to bring a Ugandan national, Joseph Kony, to justice. The President ordered 100 Special Forces troops to aid in the coordination of African military elements to conduct a search and capture campaign for Kony, the leader of an organization called the Lord's Resistance Army (LRA). Started as a resistance movement against the government of Uganda, the LRA experienced a challenge in that the lack of willing men to sign up to fight the militarily superior government inhibited its campaign. Kony resorted to raiding villages in the northern part of Uganda and kidnapping its children—some as young as 7—to be indoctrinated as soldiers in the LRA. These children—typically forced to kill adult members of their village or, in some cases, fellow children—are subject to intense brainwashing and manipulation by Kony and his officers and then used on the front lines. Like forced laborers and sex slaves, child soldiers are not given a choice but are forced into a life of subjugation.

The impetus for President Obama's action was legislation championed by the nonprofit group Invisible Children based in San Diego, California Led by three young filmmakers who had traveled to Africa expecting to document the genocide in Darfur, the group discovered the plight of the child soldiers in Uganda. The organization's rise and mobilization of high school- and college-age students led to a very successful lobbying machine that in large part helped pass the LRA Disarmament and Northern Uganda Recovery Act of 2009, which authorized President Obama to send the military observers to the region. The Act also authorized $10 million in aid to the Democratic Republic of Congo (DRC), Sudan, and Uganda to promote economic recovery in areas where the LRA had conducted raids (Resolve Uganda, 2010).

Just 1 year prior, Congress passed the Child Soldiers Protection Act of 2008 (CSPA). The Act required a list of governments actively using child soldiers to be included in each annual TIP Report, with monitoring by the U.S. government beginning in 2010. The 2011 TIP Report published the first list of six countries: Sudan, DRC, Yemen, Somalia, Chad, and Burma. Uganda did not make this list because at the time of the 2011 Report, the LRA had moved its primary force into the DRC, carrying out raids and reportedly operating a diamond mine utilizing child labor (U.S. Department of State, 2011).

To counter Kony's operations, Invisible Children launched a new campaign in 2011 designed to install radio towers in villages in the DRC with an eye toward duplicating the process in Chad, the Central African Republic, and South Sudan. These towers allow for a rudimentary "early warning system" for the purposes of reporting atrocities discovered, kidnappings, and other criminal and human rights abuses perpetrated by the LRA and similar groups.

To coordinate with the military initiative in Uganda sponsored by the Obama administration, Invisible Children released a wildly popular campaign, #Kony2012, utilizing the social networking site Twitter and linking back to videos and information on the Invisible Children website. The campaign drew criticism, at times intense, from opponents who saw the campaign and Invisible Children's mission as an oversimplification of the complex issues surrounding Uganda's troubled history, instability in the region, and what Kony was truly doing in Africa (Resolve Uganda, 2012). What the journalists failed to admit, however, was that #Kony2012 had sparked a global conversation on the issue of child soldiers and brought the issue front and center to many, especially those in the United States, who had little to no knowledge that such practices existed in the 21st century.

While Kony and the LRA were the focus of Invisible Children's mission, it should be noted that the Ugandan government had also utilized child soldiers during its more than 20 years of war. In fact, child soldiers have been utilized in many African countries, including but not limited to, Sudan, DRC, Sierra Leone, and Nigeria (U.S. Department of State, 2011).

CAUSAL FACTORS OF HUMAN TRAFFICKING AND EMERGING SOLUTIONS

Human trafficking, at its very essence, is an economic crime. Certainly, the fact that it is a predatory act that involves the brutal treatment and often commercial rape of its victims cannot be overlooked. However, the driving factor in human trafficking is, and will always be, an economic exchange. Whether the act is the sale of sex for money or the sale of labor in exchange for goods or services, economic factors are the most significant driving forces behind the trade in human beings. Specifically, profits drive the crime. Whether the issue is profit in business from the use of free labor or profit from the sale of sexual acts, profit is still the commonality. Even in the case of child soldiers, the enslavement can be "profitable" because the rebel group or government does not have to pay for their labor.

To illustrate this point, a large metro law enforcement agency had been investigating a street-level trafficker who was utilizing 20 victims spread out over three U.S. states. Each of these victims was assigned a $1,000 per night quota, or they faced punishment from the trafficker and his associates. Since the victims typically do not get days off, the trafficker was averaging $15,000 to $20,000 in tax-free income per day, resulting in an annual income of close to $6 million. It's an uphill battle on the street when government programs encourage children to stay in school and to strive for college so that they can make $30,000 to $100,000 annually through hard, legal work, while crimes like human trafficking seemingly offer a quick route to financial success (Law Enforcement Training, 2011).

Abject poverty, then, can be seen as a direct causal factor in promoting human trafficking. This discussion is far more complex, however, than just noting that the poor make excellent victims. It is a societal lack of opportunity for economic security, most especially for women, that often creates a "buyer's market" for procurers of victims. Other regional factors can include political or social instability, armed conflicts, lack of cohesive family units, the presence of domestic abuse or societal attitudes toward spousal abuse, or outright lack of access to education.

According to Caritas (2012), universal factors influencing high rates of trafficking may include:

- Ever more limits and obstacles to legal migration channels to countries with stronger economies and/or regions with better prospects;
- The sophisticated organization, resources, and networking capacity of criminal networks;
- A lack of awareness of the dangers of human trafficking;
- A lack of effective antitrafficking legislation, and if such legislation exists, a lack of effective enforcement;
- Global economic policies that foster exclusion of marginalized people;
- Disintegration of social protection networks;
- Widespread corruption in countries of origin, of transit, and of destination among the persons capable or responsible to combat trafficking.

Given that the issue at stake is economic, the solution then presents itself for quite a few of the source countries of human trafficking victims. It appears that when victims—most often women—are unable to achieve economic security that leads to personal prosperity, access to food, shelter, medical care, and most importantly, education, they become a vulnerable population as mentioned previously. To counter this, significant efforts have risen up in recent years to provide economic opportunity. Many of these are especially targeted at women, though the programs that are open to either men or women are numerous.

Looking to the Supply Chains

The Fair Trade movement is one of the proposed deterrents to human trafficking. By ensuring that all parties in the manufacturing, farming, or other labor process are paid a fair wage in exchange for their work, the possibility for labor trafficking is highly reduced. Fair trade goods have often been stigmatized as being overly expensive, but prices for such goods have come down in recent years to the point where many such products can compete directly with products manufactured through traditional means. Between 2004 and 2007, the Fair Trade Federation reported a 102% growth in sales in the United States and Canada (Fair Trade Federation, 2012).

To put this in better perspective, the International Institute for Tropical Agriculture conducted a study in 2002 and discovered that in Ghana, Nigeria,

Cameroon, and the Ivory Coast, more than 284,000 children were working on cocoa farms (Fair Trade Federation, 2012). These children are typically forced to work long hours for little or no pay and are often sold to the farms by a third party (Bales, 1999).

By advocating for fair trade in the cocoa industry where farmers are paid reasonable wages for their work, the need for exploitation is diminished. In fact, one Ghanian cocoa seller and chocolate developer, Divine, has capitalized on this fact: The farmers are the drivers of pricing and salaries in Ghana. Each year, the farmers gather to determine the prices of the cocoa that will be produced. Divine Chocolate, then, purchases the cocoa knowing that no one has been exploited in the agricultural process and creates a host of cocoa-based confections that are sold internationally (Divine Chocolate USA, 2012).

Shopping as a Form of Activism

Fair trade, however, is not the only economic solution to curbing demand. Some products are referred to as having been "ethically sourced," meaning that they come from supply chains wherein no workers were exploited and, in many cases, the goods were made from renewable resources utilizing green manufacturing processes. In addition, there are several international organizations that have set up programs wherein victims of human trafficking are able to be rehabilitated while generating economic security.

Made By Survivors (www.madebysurvivors.com), a company that operates programs in some of the most economically challenged regions of the world, offers a wide array of paper products, jewelry, textiles, handbags, and other goods made by survivors of sex trafficking. Programs like this do not lessen the initial impact of slavery but provide an avenue for the restoration of a victim and enables the individual to become self-sufficient.

Robin Rossmanith, co-owner of the website Shop to Stop Slavery (www.shoptostopslavery.com), describes the mission of her organization.

> As a consumer, you have a lot of power. If you choose to stop buying items that are produced by slaves, the demand drops. If you purchase items that have been made by survivors of human trafficking, you are supporting a new lifestyle for those individuals. If you purchase ethically sourced products, you increase the demand for such items.
>
> —*Rossmanith, 2012*

The issue of human trafficking is complex. It is not a problem that can be solved quickly, nor is there a single "silver bullet" that will prove to be the solution ending modern-day slavery. It is, however, an issue that can be dealt with by the current generation. Part of the challenge of facing slavery today is that unlike the days of the Trans-Atlantic slave operations, human trafficking is not a public occurrence. Thus, it will take a greater concentration of resources to bring about an end to modern-day slavery. It will require more research, more legislation, more enforcement, more victim-centered care, and more global cooperation.

REFERENCES

Ax, R. K., & Fagan, T. J. (2007). *Corrections, mental health and social policy: International Perspectives*. Springfield: Charles C. Thomas.

Bales, K. (1999). *Disposable people*. Los Angeles: University of California Press.

Bales, K. (2007). *Ending slavery*. Berkeley: University of California Press.

Bales, K., & Soodalter, R. (2010). *The slave next door*. Los Angeles: University of California Press.

Bales, K., & Trodd, Z. (2008). *To plead our own cause: Personal stories by today's slaves*. Ithaca, NY: Cornell University Press.

Caritas.org. (2012, January 12). *Root causes of human trafficking*. Retrieved January 12, 2012, from Caritas.org: http://www.caritas.org/activities/women_migration/caritas_migration_trafficking_and_women.html?cnt=431

Coalition of Immokalee Workers. (2012, January). *CIW Anti-Slavery Campaign*. Retrieved January 21, 2012, from Coalition of immokalee workers: http://www.ciw-online.org/slavery.html

Divine Chocolate USA. (2012, January). *Our story*. Retrieved March 15, 2012, from Divine Chocolate USA: http://www.divinechocolateusa.com/about/story.aspx

Europol. (2005). *Legislation on trafficking in human beings and illegal immigrant smuggling*. Europol Public Information.

Fair Trade Federation. (2012). *Facts and figures*. Retrieved March 24, 2012, from Fair Trade Federation: http://www.fairtradefederation.org/ht/d/sp/i/197/pid/197

Hainsworth, J. (2006). Mail-order brides face exploitation in Canada. Retrieved October 1, 2012, from http://www.wunrn.com/news/2006/10_09_06/101006_cnada_mail.htm

Hoerrner, M. (2008). *Georgia human trafficking operations report*. Atlanta, Georgia: Not For Sale Campaign/Not For Sale Georgia.

Hoerrner, M. (2009a). Personal conversation with law enforcement. Atlanta, Georgia.

Hoerrner, M. (2009b). Personal conversation: U.S. Asst. District Attorney Susan Coppedge.

Hoerrner, M. (2011). Personal conversation: Joe Collins. Atlanta, Georgia.

Human Trafficking and Smuggling Center. (2008). Domestic human trafficking: An Internal Issue.

International Labour Organization. (2012, January 14). *Commercial sexual exploitation of children*. Retrieved January 14, 2012, from International Labor Organization: http://www.ilo.org/ipec/areas/CSEC/lang–en/index.htm

Jal, E. (Performer). (2012, March 27). *An evening with Emmanuel Jal*. Kennesaw State Social Sciences Auditorium, Kennesaw, Georgia.

Jeffreys, S. (2009). *The industrial vagina: The political economy of the global sex trade*. New York: Routledge.

Kangaspunta, K. (2006). Trafficking in persons: Global patterns. International Symposium on International Migration and Development. Turn, June, 28–30.

Kara, S. (2009). *Sex trafficking: Inside the business of modern slavery*. New York: Columbia University Press.

King, G. (2004). *Woman, child for sale*. New York: Chamberlain Brothers.

King-Tisdell Cottage Foundation. (n.d.). *Slavery in savannah*. Retrieved January 12, 2012, from King-Tisdell Cottage Foundation: http://www.kingtisdell.org/Slavery.htm

Kouri, J. (2006, June 1). *Woman enslaved by physicians for almost two decades*. Retrieved March 1, 2012, from Renew America: http://www.renewamerica.com/columns/kouri/060601

Law Enforcement Training. (2011). Nashville, Tennessee.

Maiti Nepal. (2012). *Interception points*. Retrieved March 28, 2012, from Maiti Nepal: http://www.maitinepal.org/?page=introduction_latest_picture

Malarek, V. (2003). *The natashas*. New York: Viking Press.

McCullough, K. (2010). Personal communication.

McGill, C. (2003). *Human traffic: Sex, slaves and immigration*. London: Vision Paperbacks.

National Center for Missing and Exploited Children. (2009). *Protecting victims of child prostitution training course*. Retrived from http://www.missingkids.com/missing kids/servlet/PublicHomeServlet?LanguageCountry=en_US. Georgia.

Nazer, M., & Lewis, D. (2003). *Slave: My true story*. New York: Public Affairs.

Polaris Project. (2012, January 14). *State and federal laws*. Retrieved January 14, 2012, from Polaris Project: http://www.polarisproject.org/resources/state-and-federal-laws

Polaris Project. (2012, January 12). *Survivor stories*. Retrieved January 14, 2012, from Polaris Project: http://www.polarisproject.org/what-we-do/client-services/survivor-stories/464-keisha-domestic-minor-sex-trafficking

Population Reference Bureau. (2002, July). *Children's environmental health: Risks and remedies*. Retrieved March 29, 2012, from Population Reference Bureau: http://www.prb.org/Publications/PolicyBriefs/ChildrensEnvironmentalHealthRisksandRemedies.aspx

Resolve Uganda. (2010, May 24). *LRA Disarmament and Northern Uganda Recovery Act of 2009*. Retrieved March 28, 2012, from Resolve Uganda: http://www.theresolve.org/lra-disarmament-and-northern-uganda-recovery-act-of-2009

Resolve Uganda. (2012, March 23). *10 things critics—and everyone—should know about the kony2012 campaign*. Retrieved March 28, 2012, from Resolve Uganda: http://www.theresolve.org/blog/archives/3071032531

Rossmanith, R. (2012, January). *Mission*. Retrieved April 1, 2012, from Shop To Stop Slavery: http://www.shoptostopslavery.com/about

Rubin, J. (Performer). (2003). *Dying to leave. [Television]*. New York: Public Broadcasting System.

Ruffins, E. (2010, April 30). *Rescuing girls from sex slavery*. Retrieved February 14, 2012, from CNN International: http://edition.cnn.com/2010/LIVING/04/29/cnnheroes.koirala.nepal/

Skinner, B. (2008). *A crime so monstrous*. New York: Free Press.

Strauss, E. M. (2008, July 14). *Domestic sex trafficking in the u.s.* Retrieved March 3, 2012, from ABC News: http://abcnews.go.com/Primetime/story?id=5326721&page=1#. T3k39Kv2YsI

Sun, L. (1998, March 8). The search for miss right takes a turn toward russia: "Mail-Order Brides" of the '90S are met via Internet and on "Romance Tours." *The Washington Post.*

Tanaka, Y. (2002). *Japan's comfort women: Sexual slavery and prostitution during World War II and the US occupation.* New York: Rutledge.

Thomas, H. (1997). *The slave trade: The story of the Atlantic slave trade: 1440–1870.* New York: Simon & Schuster.

U.S. Department of Health and Human Services. (2007). *Human trafficking into and within the united states.* Washington, DC: Government Printing Office.

U.S. Department of State. (2010). *Trafficking in persons report 2010.* Retrieved February 2, 2012, from U.S. Department of State: http://www.state.gov/j/tip/rls/tiprpt/2010/142761.htm

U.S. Department of State. (2011). *2011 Trafficking in persons report.* Washington, DC: U.S. Department of State.

UN GIFT. (n.d.). *Human trafficking: The Facts.* Retrieved March 15, 2012, from United Nations Global Initiative to Fight Human Trafficking: http://www.unglobalcom pact.org/docs/issues_doc/labour/Forced_labour/ HUMAN_TRAFFICKING_-_THE_FACTS_-_final.pdf

United Nations High Commissioner for Refugees. (2007). *Trafficking in persons.* Retrieved February 21, 2012, from UN High Commissioner for Refugees: http://www.unhcr.org/pages/4a16aae76.html

United States Congress, Committee on Foreign Relations. (2004, July 13). *Committee hearing: Human trafficking: Mail order bride abuses.* Washington, DC. Retrieved March 1, 2012.

Whitcomb, C. (2001). *Cold zero: Inside the FBI hostage rescue team.* New York: Little Brown and Company.

CHAPTER 3

Community Models and Resources

MARY DE CHESNAY

*N*ow that community leaders are becoming enlightened about sex trafficking prevalence and incidence in their own backyards, they are mobilizing in multidisciplinary teams to arrest and prosecute the traffickers and to help the victims attain a semblance of mental and physical health. Survivor success stories abound and many survivors have become leaders in the effort to help others escape. This chapter focuses on a variety of initiatives around the United States and internationally that nurses can access to help these most vulnerable women and children.

There are many successful organizations that are designed to help survivors, and it is impossible to discuss all of them. The agencies discussed in this chapter have established a successful track record and a high proportion of their fund-raising goes directly to victim services. Particular attention is given to the shelters that are designed specifically for victims of sex trafficking. These places offer a multi-method approach to survivors: food, shelter, social services, medical and mental health treatment, skills training, and vocational planning.

In the United States, many organizations with an abolitionist mission have dedicated their resources to end slavery. These organizations can be found in both the public and private sectors. Some are faith-based and others have no religious affiliation. Similarly, several international organizations might serve the people of their own countries, but have established international credibility.

This chapter highlights agencies located in the United States, but a few international agencies are included because they exemplify best practices that are culturally based and would be excellent resources for American nurses who find themselves working with victims from other countries. The special circumstances of immigrants, whether documented or not, implies the need for services in English language and acculturation. In many of the origin countries, poverty and lack of education are so prevalent that victims who are trafficked to the United States do not speak English and fear the police, making them all the more dependent on the traffickers who terrify them with threats of arrest, torture, and deportation. They need someone who can counter the traffickers' false assertions about American ways of doing things.

BEST PRACTICES TARGETING DEMAND

Publicizing Demand

Shared Hope International's initiative is to stop demand, for without demand there would be no sex trafficking business. This campaign focuses on the customers ("johns") to call attention to their place in the system and to hold them accountable for their behavior (Shared Hope International, 2012). Previously, efforts have focused on the victims who have been treated as criminals since they are the most vulnerable and easy to arrest. There has also been some focus on pimps but it is difficult to prosecute them due to the victims' unwillingness or inability to testify against them.

There are several reasons for the difficulty. First, many pimps are "romeos" who alternate kindness with violence and who obtain their victims by seducing them into believing they care for them and will be their protectors. These pimps are seen by the girls as boyfriends. They insist upon being called "Daddy" and the other girls in their stables become the victim's new family, engendering loyalty and hope for a future of "happily ever after."

The *Demand* initiative by Shared Hope International and a similar campaign, *Reduce the Demand,* by Free the Captives (Free the Captives, 2012) focuses on the customers, for without the "johns" there would be no prostitution. The national billboard campaign shows a man with a wedding ring and his belt partly undone with the caption: "This man wants to rent your daughter." Other billboards have been placed on major roads to call attention to human trafficking and they often show the national hotline number of 888-3737-888, which anyone can call to report suspected human trafficking. (N.B. the phone number is printed deliberately in this way to capture attention.)

Legislation

In 1999, Sweden became the first country to make the buying of sex rather than the selling of sex a crime and they report a drop in the rate of sex trafficking (Ekberg, 2004). Finland followed but outlawed sex in public places, making both the selling and buying of sex illegal and requiring the johns to know the victims have been trafficked (Viuhko & Jokinen, 2009). Macedonia and Croatia also have legislation targeting demand, but their laws also require the purchaser to know the woman is trafficked (Hughes, 2004). Nevertheless, these countries are making a concerted effort to hold customers accountable.

In the United States, Shared Hope International initiated the Protected Innocence Initiative to promote zero tolerance for child sex trafficking. Their team of researchers conducted a major study in which they examined the antitrafficking legislation in all 50 states to determine the relative effectiveness of the states along six criteria. In December 2011, they published "report cards" for each state and Washington, DC, ranked on effectiveness along several criteria related to criminal penalties for sex trafficking, demand, facilitation, and enforcement. Each state was assigned a letter grade from "A" to "F" with no state earning an "A" and only Illinois, Missouri, Texas, and the state of Washington earning "B" (Protected Innocence Initiative, 2011). Many other states have major activities in progress but do not quite reach all of the goals specified by the Shared Hope team.

Johns' Schools

In an effort to reduce demand, the justice system has an alternative option to jail: sending offenders to Johns' schools. Similar to "driving under the influence" (DUI) schools, Johns schools can be found in many large cities in the Americas, among them Atlanta, Chicago, Toronto, Ottawa, Vancouver, Las Vegas, Portland, Philadelphia, and St. Paul. First set up in San Francisco, Johns schools are typically weekend programs that allow first offenders to attend a day-long workshop where they learn about sexually transmitted infections (STIs), morality, health, laws, community effects of prostitution, and the degradation experienced by women who are prostituted (usually presented by a survivor.) Johns schools allow men to avoid the lengthy court process by attending school and paying a fine, sometimes with a few hours of community service, while the women they have victimized experience the full range of criminal prosecution (Monroe, 2005).

Whether these programs reduce recidivism is uncertain. Kennedy et al. (2004) studied 341 men who attended Johns school and found evidence of attitude changes that suggests that these programs might be effective at reducing recidivism by reversing the notion that prostitution is a victimless crime. According to a study by Monto and Garcia (2001) recidivism rates are low both for men who attend such programs and men who do not attend. They speculate that perhaps it is the arrest itself that deters men from offending a second time. However, it is also possible that first offenders learn from their mistake of getting caught and find more secretive ways of engaging in prostitution.

Automobile Confiscation

California, Michigan, and Florida have passed laws that were upheld upon challenges, some by the American Civil Liberties Union (Hazle, 2004). When a customer is arrested, his car is confiscated and he is held until bail or a fine is posted. In Florida, he attends mandatory Johns school and is evaluated for STIs. If no other offenses occur, he is adjudicated with time served.

BEST PRACTICES FOR SURVIVORS

Comprehensive Care

A holistic approach is critical to success of agencies that are designed to help sex trafficking victims. Comprehensive services should include safety, medical care, social services, legal services, and skill development. The Comprehensive Continuous Integrated System of Care (CCISC) approach has been useful as a best practice for co-occurring mental disorders and substance abuse (Minkoff & Cline, 2004). Designed by Minkoff (1991), the CCISC model has four major components: system level of change, efficient use of resources, incorporation of best practices, and integrated treatment philosophy. Adapting this model for trafficking victims seems to show the best promise for addressing the numerous and complex problems of human trafficking, but whatever model is used should be a collaboration among all the resources available.

Although many agencies that serve victims of sex trafficking provide comprehensive services, the state of Georgia was the first to implement a state-wide response to the problem of commercial sex exploitation of children (CSEC) in the form of a System of Care. At this writing, Georgia remains the only state with a state-wide response, though many large cities have well-developed services in place and efforts in some states, notably Texas, are moving toward a state-wide response. In Georgia, the system of care involves partnerships with law enforcement, prosecutors, health care professionals, social service providers, and educators to provide a full range of services so that survivors have options for the future (state of Georgia, 2012).

Georgia Care Connection Office (GCCO)

The GCCO was created by the Governor's Office for Children and Families in 2009. In order to expand its statewide approach, in 2011 GCCO was administratively attached to the Children's Advocacy Centers of Georgia. The mission of the GCCO is to serve as a single point of contact for the victims of domestic minor sex trafficking, providing continuity of care by assessing the children, linking them with family-centered and youth services, and providing follow-up. The system of care model in place in Georgia provides for ease of communication among many social service providers, law enforcement, prosecutors and medical professionals, and others (www.georgiacareconnection.com/about_gcco).

Streetlight—Phoenix

The mission of Streetlight is to eradicate child sex slavery through a three-pronged strategy of awareness, prevention, and aftercare. Streetlight developed a collaborative network in Phoenix of law enforcement, prosecutors, other nonprofits, the National Center for Missing and Exploited Children, the FBI, Arizona State University, over 70 churches and numerous individuals committed to the mission. To promote awareness, Streetlight produced *Branded*, a documentary that has reached thousands of citizens. Prevention is addressed by working with state legislators to protect children from sex exploitation. Aftercare is provided by Streetlight at its residential facility, which houses under-age victims of sexual exploitation. The residence provides a supportive, healing atmosphere with a mentor mother and family-type environment. Health care, counseling, life skills, and vocational training are provided to help the girls make the transition from the street to a new career (Michael Klinckner, personal communication, 2012).

Natalie's House

Natalie's House in Arizona is a small residential facility for girls who have been exploited. Not limited to trafficked victims, these girls might be runaways or throwaway children who engaged in survival sex. It is the only facility I found that is designed and operated by a nurse. The founder, Janet Olson, is a master's-prepared nurse with extensive experience in treating survivors and a holistic approach. Her program offers a range of trauma-focused therapy, group therapy, social support, life skills development, equine therapy, and fun activities such as sports and crafts in a home environment, staffed 24/7. The rooms are furnished comfortably in a secure building. A keystone of her intervention is to teach the girls how to garden and care for animals. Each girl will have a small plot of land to grow her own vegetables and a chicken to care for. Much more than a group home, the philosophy of Natalie's House is to provide a family setting with supportive adults who can guide and teach the girls (Janet Olson, personal communication, 2012).

Girls Education and Mentoring Services (GEMS): New York City

Founded by a survivor, GEMS's mission is to empower girls and young women from 12 to 24 years old to exit the commercial sex industry and to develop their full potential. Not limited to working individually with survivors, GEMS works actively to change public impressions and to revolutionize the policies and systems that enable the sex trade with the ultimate goals of eliminating commercial sexual exploitation. Rachel Lloyd, a survivor who had been commercially exploited as a teenager in Europe, immigrated to New York City and founded GEMS in 1998. Recognizing the need for specialized services to this population, she started GEMS from her kitchen table and it has grown to a staffed organization with comprehensive services, a highly visible web site, and a track record of influencing legislation (GEMS, 2012; Lloyd, 2011).

Somaly Mam Foundation

A Cambodian child of extreme poverty who was sold in marriage to a soldier at age 9 and was later sold to a brothel where she suffered daily rape and torture,

Somaly Mam managed to escape and forge a new life for herself in France with a new husband (Mam, 2009). Returning to Cambodia, she created a foundation in 2007 to help other girls escape the sex trade. She promotes Action, Advocacy, and Awareness. With partners in Southeast Asia, the Somaly Mam Foundation rescues children and provides rehabilitation services, education, and reintegration to thousands of girls in the region. A special program, *Voices for Change*, enables survivors to participate in awareness and advocacy programs to educate the general public and to mentor other survivors.

New Hope Moldova

An extremely poor country in Eastern Europe, Moldova is known for numerous orphanages where children are discharged at the age of 13 with about $150 to start a new life. This means the children are easy targets for the human traffickers of Europe. Boys are taken into the forced labor and drug businesses while girls are trafficked for sex, and both genders are trafficked for organ harvesting, a trafficking phenomenon that has not received much attention in the scientific literature (Kevin Ellington, personal communication, 2012).

New Hope Moldova, founded by Oleg Reutki, is a Christian organization whose mission is to provide hope for the orphans of Moldova by settling them within families in transition homes where they can be educated into a trade, taught English, and learn the social skills of healthy family life. Children who have been rescued from the traffickers also receive medical and psychological care. Many children who come from the orphanages do not have documents and Mr. Reutki helps them obtain documents so that they can go to school and learn a trade. As a faith-based organization, New Hope Moldova is affiliated with churches such as the Catalyst Church of Woodstock, GA, in the United States and this collaboration facilitates services and fund raising for the activities.

Maiti Nepal

Maiti Nepal, loosely translated as "Mother's House" is an organization founded in 1993 by Anuradha Koirala, a survivor of domestic violence who founded the organization to serve the survivors of violence and trafficking. As a primary country of origin for girls to be trafficked from Nepal into India and Pakistan, Nepal is hampered by low rates of education and employment opportunities, particularly for girls and women, making them vulnerable to the traffickers. Maiti Nepal provides transition homes, teaching programs for HIV/AIDS and life skills, educational opportunities, prevention, advocacy, rehabilitation, and legal consultation. A particularly effective aspect of the program is border patrol in which suspicious vehicles are detained and girls rescued prior to leaving Nepal. Since its beginning, Maiti Nepal has rescued over 12,000 girls from traffickers (Anuradha Koirala, personal communication, 2012; Maiti Nepal, 2011).

Free the Captives

As a theocentric Christian organization, Free the Captives in Houston, TX, approaches the problem of human trafficking from three perspectives: advocacy, liberation, and education. Advocacy involves providing legal services for victims and influencing legislation. Liberation includes victims services; follow up; basic necessities of food, clothing, safe shelter; and skill development. Education is accomplished through a system of public awareness campaigns, the Reducing the Demand program, and an annual conference on human trafficking that reviews the best knowledge to date (www.freethecaptives Houston.com).

Shared Hope International

Headquartered in Vancouver, WA, Shared Hope International was founded by former U.S. congresswoman, Linda Smith to provide services to victims, influence legislation, and educate the public about human trafficking. Their Demand campaign, which focuses attention on the criminal behavior of the johns rather than the victims, is a major aspect of their advocacy. Even though the U.S. State Department (United States State Department, 2012) ranked the United States in Tier 1 of their listing of what countries are doing to fight human trafficking, we have a long way to go. Shared Hope's ultimate goal is to promote a zero-tolerance policy for child sex exploitation.

Other International Resources

The U.S. State Department publishes an annual Trafficking in Persons (TIP) Report that ranks countries in three tiers of effectiveness at addressing human trafficking within their borders. This report is a key resource for understanding the issues in the countries it measures. Amnesty International in its annual report for 2012 cites a continuing lack of global leadership that is effective in combatting human rights violations. The report by country can be read online (Amnesty International, 2012).

SUMMARY

So many organizations designed to help trafficking survivors have been founded around the world that it is impossible to do justice to all of them. The ones highlighted here were chosen because their track records are established or the administrators are expert at treating the population, but this chapter by no means is meant to be inclusive. Table 3.1 is a list of websites of some services familiar to the author that might be good resources for nurses working in those cities.

TABLE 3.1   Resources for Trafficking Victims in United States

Name/City	Mission	Web Site
Nashville, Tennessee	To prevent teens from getting sucked into the underground world of human trafficking.	www.newschannel5.com/ story/16149242/ nashville-sex-trafficking-victim-speaks-out.
Salt Lake City, Utah	To help create awareness and support for those in this state who may be involved in human trafficking.	www.deseretnews.com/ article/865554035/ Survivors-of-sex-trafficking-speak-out-at-Salt-Lake-symposium.html?pg=2
Washington, DC	Prevent Human Trafficking (PHT) promotes sustainable solutions to sex trafficking.	http://preventhuman trafficking. org/core-programs/
Center for the Human Rights of Children/Chicago, Illinois	Recognizing that children require special protections, the Center for the Human Rights of Children pursues an agenda of interdisciplinary research, education, and service to address critical and complex issues affecting children and youth, both locally and globally.	www.luc.edu/chrc/pdfs/ Building_Child_Welfare_ Response_to_Child_ Trafficking.pdf
Campaign Against Sexual Exploitation (CASE)/Alexandria, Virginia	Campaign Against Sexual Exploitation (CASE) provides the tools and resources to better educate local communities about the many issues surrounding child sexual exploitation and how and where to report these crimes.	www.ndaa.org/ncpca_ case_campaign.html
San Francisco Airport Human Trafficking Prevention/ San Francisco, CA	An innovative new program at San Francisco International Airport will train airport personnel to identify and stop human trafficking on commercial airlines.	www.huffingtonpost.com/ 2012/03/13/sfo-human-trafficking-prevention_n_ 1342179.html
International Organization for Adolescents (IOFA)/ New York City, New York	IOFA currently has two main initiatives—the Youth Trafficking Prevention Initiative and the Youth Leadership Initiative.	www.humantrafficking. org/organizations/354
Coalition Against Trafficking in	Coalition Against Trafficking in Women-Asia Pacific (CATW-AP)	www.catw-ap.org/

(continued)

TABLE 3.1 Resources for Trafficking Victims in United States (*continued*)

Name/City	Mission	Web Site
Women—Asia Pacific/Bangladesh, Fiji, India, Papua New Guinea, Philippines, Taiwan, and Thailand	plans to expand its project on educating young men on gender issues, sexuality, and the consequences of prostitution as methods to reduce the demand that fuels sex trafficking, as well as addressing young women's vulnerability to sexual exploitation.	
Catholic Relief Services/Cameroon	Catholic Relief Services and its partners also plan to identify and refer victims of trafficking to shelters and strengthen partner capacity to address victims' basic needs.	www.crs.org/
Department of Justice/Office of Overseas Prosecutorial Development/ Djibouti	This project aims to expand and strengthen the enforcement of Djibouti's antitrafficking laws.	www.usdoj.gov/criminal/ opdat/
World Hope International/ Liberia	World Hope International (WHI) proposes to reduce the incidence of TIP by training communities and stakeholders on trafficking issues. WHI will also identify and respond to survivors of trafficking by providing immediate services such as emergency survival kits, short-term shelter, and domestic repatriation when possible.	www.worldhope.org/
Save the Children Federation/Burma	Save the Children's overarching objective is to establish effective child protection systems in communities and townships. Project activities include awareness-raising and conducting training in communities; collaborating	www.savethechildren.org/

(*continued*)

TABLE 3.1   Resources for Trafficking Victims in United States (*continued*)

Name/City	Mission	Web Site
	within communities to establish child protection systems; and facilitating local and national policy discussions to improve policies and procedures on human trafficking, migration, and child protection.	
International Organization for Migration/ Indonesia	This project's overall goal is to contribute to Indonesia's efforts to fight human trafficking by supporting an ongoing, sustainable mechanism for comprehensive victim recovery, assistance, and protection.	www.iom.int/
Coalition to Abolish Slavery and Trafficking/Mexico	Coalition to Abolish Slavery and Trafficking (CAST) will build the capacity of five local non-governmental organizations (NGO) to lead anti-trafficking efforts in their respective regions through training and technical assistance, development of victim-centered service standards, provision of task-force building efforts, and public awareness campaigns.	www.castla.org/
International Organization for Migration/Haiti	International Organization for Migration (IOM) proposes to combat trafficking of women and children in Haiti through preventive and protective measures.	www.iomhaiti.org/
Free the Captives	A faith-based NGO that provides legal services, medical care, social services, and skill development to survivors of human trafficking. An annual conference increases public awareness.	www.freethecaptives houston.com/ houston-anti-human-trafficking-conference.php
Shared Hope International	Founded by former congresswoman Linda Smith,	www.sharedhope.org/

(*continued*)

TABLE 3.1   Resources for Trafficking Victims in United States *(continued)*

Name/City	Mission	Web Site
	Shared Hope International is one of the foremost organizations combatting human trafficking at a global level. Through research and training sessions, SHI educates, raises awareness, and documents progress.	
Polaris Project	Founded to promote abolition, the Polaris Project has made a major impact on providing services to survivors, through their comprehensive approach, national hotline number at 888-3737-888, public policy advocacy and international advocacy.	www.polarisproject.org/about-us/10-years-of-impact
Somaly Mam Foundation/Cambodia	The Somaly Mam Foundation provides shelter and alternatives for Cambodian girls.	www.somaly.org
GEMS/NYC	Girls' Education and Mentoring Services was founded to provide safety and follow-up to girls on the street.	www.gems-girls.org/
Maiti Nepal/Nepal	Maiti Nepal (Mother's House) is active as a shelter and education resource for Nepali girls as well as political action.	www.Maitinepal.org

REFERENCES

Amnesty International. (2012). *Annual report—Human trafficking.* Retrieved July 1, 2012 from http://www.amnesty.org/en/campaigns/stop-violence-against-women/issues/implementation-existing-laws/trafficking

Ekberg, G. (2004). The Swedish law that prohibits the purchase of sexual services. *Violence Against Women, 10*(10), 1187–1218.

Free the Captives-Houston. (2012). Retrieved December 4, 2011 from http://www.freethe captivesHouston.com

GEMS. (2012). Retrieved March 23, 2012 from http://www.gems-girls.org

Georgia Care Connection. (n.d.). Retrieved July 2, 2012, from http://www.georgiacarecon nection.com/about_gcco

Hazle, B. (2004, January 29). El Cajon beings seizing vehicles for solicitation of prostitution. *SanDiego.com*.

Hughes, D. (2004). Best practices to address the demand side of sex trafficking. Report for the U.S. Department of State under Cooperative Agreement S-INLEC-04-CA-0003. Retrieved June 9, 2012, from: http://www.uri.edu/artsci/wms/hughes/demand_sex_trafficking.pdf

Kennedy, M. A., Klein, C., Gorzalka, B., & Yuille, J. (2004). Attitude change following a diversion program for men who solicit sex. *Journal of Offender Rehabilitation, 40*(1/2), 41–60.

Lloyd, R. (2011). *Girls like us*. New York, NY: Harper Collins Publishers.

Maiti Nepal. (2011). Retrieved November 22, 2011 from http://maitinepal.org

Mam, S. (2009). *The road of lost innocence*. New York, NY: Spiegel & Grau.

Minkoff, P. (1991). Program components of a comprehensive integrated care system for serious mentally ill patients with substance disorders. *New Directions for Mental Health Services, Summer*(50), 13–27.

Minkoff, P., & Cline, C. (2004). Changing the world: The design and implementation of comprehensive continuous integrated systems of care for individuals with co-occurring disorders. *Psychiatric Clinics of North America, 27*(4), 727–743.

Monroe, J. (2005). Women in street prostitution: The result of poverty and the brunt of inequity. *Journal of Poverty, 9*(3), 69–88.

Monto, M. A., & Garcia, S. (2001). Recidivism among the customers of female street prostitutes: Do intervention programs help? *Western Criminology Review, 3*(2), Retrieved June 1, 2012, from http://wcr.sonoma.edu/v3n2/monto.html

Protected Innocence Initiative. (2011). *Shared Hope International*, Retrieved January 4, 2012 http://www.sharedhope.org/WhatWeDo/BringJustice/PolicyRecommendations/ProtectedInnocenceInitiative.aspx

Reduce the Demand for Sex Trafficking. (2012). *Free the captives, Houston, TX*. Retrieved from http://www.freethecaptiveshouston.com/reducing-the-demand-campaign.php

Shared Hope International. (2011). Retrieved January 3, 2012 from http://www.sharedhope.org.

United States State Department. (2012). Trafficking in Person (TIP) Report—2012. Retrieved June 1, 2012, from http://www.state.gov/j/tip/rls/tiprpt/2012/

Viuhko, M., & Jokinen, A. (2009). *Human trafficking and organized crime: Trafficking for sexual exploitation and organised procuring in Finland*. Helsinki, Finland: European Institute for Crime Prevention and Control. Retrieved June 3, from http://www.heuni.fi/Satellite?blobtable=MungoBlobs&blobcol=urldata&SSURIapptype=BlobServer&SSURIcontainer=Default&SSURIsession=false&blobkey=id&blobheadervalue1=inline;%20filename=dod9o.pdf&SSURIsscontext=Satellite%20Server&blobwhere=1266335656633&blobheadername1=Content-Disposition&ssbinary=true&blobheader=application/pdf

CHAPTER 4

Working With Law Enforcement

MARK HOERRNER

*H*uman trafficking is not a crime that stands alone. Rarely is there a case prosecuted by law enforcement that does not involve other elements: assault, battery, rape, torture, visa fraud, exploitation of minors, child pornography, mail fraud, wage and hour violations, harboring of illegal aliens, false imprisonment, peonage, female genital mutilation, obstruction of justice, involuntary servitude, incest, perjury, and even murder. Thus, the potential for multiple psychological, sexual, and physical traumas is extremely high in trafficking victims. It also blurs the lines of jurisdiction for many agencies that investigate these numerous crimes.

For the health care provider, the work with law enforcement must be a highly developed partnership. Law enforcement will endeavor to protect life and property and arrest offenders. Those in the health care field are bound to provide medical care for those in need—including the traffickers. To ensure the safety of health care facility staff and to properly advance the cause of justice, no partnership could be more important.

ENFORCEMENT AGENCIES TASKED WITH HUMAN TRAFFICKING DUTIES

Human trafficking is investigated by a wide array of law enforcement agencies operating at the federal, state, and county/municipal levels. While any policing agency can enforce laws to protect the public at any time and many agencies reach across jurisdictional lines to create active task forces, most law enforcement agencies have a strictly defined function.

Federal Agencies

The U.S. government supports a number of agencies that actively investigate the crime of human trafficking. Two agencies, the Federal Bureau of Investigation (FBI) and Immigration and Customs Enforcement (ICE), are in the forefront of human trafficking investigations. These law enforcement arms typically function independently of one another and are governed by separate command structures, but the enforcement roles of each often overlap. This is positive for the public because it means shared resources and personnel on large-scale investigations, and it means multi-jurisdictional collaborations on large-scale enforcement actions such as multi-county or multi-state arrest sweeps.

Prosecutorial

The primary prosecutorial enforcement arm is the U.S. Department of Justice (DOJ), specifically the divisions of Child Exploitation and Obscenity (CEOS) and Civil Rights, Human Trafficking. CEOS tends to focus on cases of domestic commercial sexual exploitation of children (CSEC) or pornography within the United States (U.S. Department of Justice, n.d.).

Enforcement

Federal Bureau of Investigation

The Federal Bureau of Investigation (FBI) handles human trafficking cases through its Civil Rights division. Nearly 14,000 special agents comprise the FBI's primary investigative pool, with surveillance and investigative support analysts, administrative support, and victim services specialists bringing the total number of employees to 35,664 worldwide (FBI, 2012).

The FBI typically engages in what are known as "enterprise-level" investigations that seek to dismantle the primary and extended networks related to a criminal offense. Because of this, human trafficking investigations can be as short as 6 months to as long as approximately 6 years, according to active agents. The goal of such operations is not to simply put away a trafficker and rescue his/her victims, but to arrest the trafficker and all related individuals involved in the procurement of a victim for sale (Hoerrner, 2009). Forced labor cases are sometimes investigated by the FBI, but documented cases illustrate that more often than not, human trafficking cases are focused on sexual enslavement of adults and children.

One of the more unique collaborations of the last decade has been the FBI's *Innocence Lost* program. Innocence Lost is a partnership with the National Center for Missing and Exploited Children (NCMEC) and the DOJ's, CEOS, which is a division of the FBI (FBI, 2011). Targeted at curbing the commercial sexual exploitation of domestic minors, Innocence Lost was designed to create an ongoing dialogue about domestic minor sex trafficking between the FBI and state/local law enforcement. There have been five multi-state, multi-agency prostituted children sweeps, dubbed "Operation Cross Country" followed by a numerical designation. The 2011 sweep was Operation Cross Country V. The program has spawned 44 task forces and working groups nationwide, and the results have been strong—more than 1,800 children have been recovered from the hands of controllers and kidnappers; more than $3 million in assets have been seized; and more than 800 traffickers have been convicted (FBI, 2011).

Immigration and Customs Enforcement
The agents of ICE are a special division of the Department of Homeland Security (DHS). Within ICE is the Homeland Security Investigations (HSI) directorate. It is this arm of ICE that is tasked with investigating human trafficking for labor, sex, or CSEC. In addition, HSI special agents investigate a host of other crimes including gang activity, drug smuggling, arms trafficking, artifact theft, counterfeit goods operations, workplace immigration issues, cybercrime, cash smuggling, and more (ICE, n.d.). The HSI division alone includes more than 6,700 special agents and a total of more than 10,000 employees assigned nationally and in 47 countries outside the United States (ICE, n.d.).

Other Federal Agencies

Many federal agencies that do not typically see human trafficking as part of their directives may still be involved in slavery investigations. As noted in Chapter 2 and above, human trafficking is an amalgamation of crimes rather than just a single offense. As such, other federal agencies such as the Railway Police, U.S. Postal Inspection Service, U.S. Marshal Service, U.S. Secret Service, Drug Enforcement Agency, Central Intelligence Agency, Defense Intelligence Agency, Federal Protective Service, Diplomatic Security Service, Defense Criminal Investigative Service, and the Bureau of Alcohol, Tobacco and Firearms (DOJ) may coordinate with ICE or the FBI in investigating human trafficking. Additionally, each branch of the U.S. military maintains a criminal investigation division tasked with investigating any claims in which U.S. military personnel may be involved in human trafficking.

State, County, and Local Law Enforcement

State
Most states have either a state police agency or a state investigative agency (such as the Tennessee Bureau of Investigation) that will focus on human trafficking investigations. While investigations involving forced labor are not out of reach for these police agencies, the primary human trafficking investigations are CSEC offenses.

County/Municipality
Local law enforcement can be involved in human trafficking operations if—and this is one of the national shortfalls at the moment—the agency has personnel

trained in human trafficking investigations AND if the department has a criminal investigations division large enough to handle such investigations. It is more common for CSEC investigations to be initiated at this level than any other trafficking cases.

WHO ARE THE TRAFFICKERS

Those who participate in the selling of human beings are opportunists. They may be calculated opportunists but opportunists all the same. They can operate with fox-like intelligence or may influence those they exploit through sheer brutality. They seek the weak and the vulnerable. They look for those who would not be missed by a larger section of society and for those who have already been left behind because of tragic circumstances. But traffickers do not come from or operate in a single geographic region, ethnicity, religious group, or society. Operations can be large or small, comprised of many controllers or just a single manipulative individual.

Anna Rodriguez, originally a victim advocate with the Collier County Sheriff's Department in Florida, is now the executive director of the Florida Coalition Against Human Trafficking (FCAHT). In her work as an investigator, she tripped over human trafficking during the interviewing of two individuals in a domestic violence case. A pair of nonnative U.S. citizens had brought in a young girl from their home country as a domestic servant, and there were allegations that the husband was having sex with the young girl. The young woman turned out to be a victim of involuntary domestic servitude (Trafficking.org, n.d.). From that point, Rodriguez has gone on to uncover dozens of cases of human trafficking, has participated in multiple operations involving trafficking during the Superbowl, and has served annually on a delegation to the Organization of American States in order to train law enforcement and governments on human trafficking trends. Based on her experiences, she developed a list of characteristics of those who traffic in human beings. They:

- are often members of the victim's own ethnic or national community
- are in the United States with legal status and maintain close contact with their country of origin
- may be fluent in English as well as a native language
- may have greater social or political status in their home country than their victims
- may be diplomats or consular figures
- can represent international organized criminal syndicates. (Rodriguez, 2009)

The challenge with traffickers, however, is that they do not fit a single profile; traffickers can come from all walks of life. Most of these bullet points reference the concept of "international" traffickers, which can include people known and unknown to the victims, and are often from the same ethnic group as the victim. While this may enable traffickers to approach the victim in the early stages of the controller–victim relationship, it also often allows traffickers to conceal the victim within the ethnic group by utilizing controllers who know the victim's family or by playing to cultural and language barriers (Rodriguez, 2009).

In the United States, most citizens feel safe because the country promotes the concept of the rule of law. For natives, while some police corruption is expected, it is usually not a concern for those who seek aid from a law enforcement officer. This is not the case in many countries abroad, especially in developing nations where law enforcement is still part of a highly impoverished group.

In Peru, while visiting with a group of street youth, many of whom were victims of prostitution, the children told stories of being arrested for being homeless and taken to local justice centers. The holding cells for children at these justice centers are typically stocked with just a few beds, but several dozen children may be relegated to the cell at any given time. The children told stories of frequent beatings and harassment by police officers. One child, now an adult, related his experience of being buried up to his neck at a police station and beaten or kicked regularly. A young teen girl showed off wounds where she claimed the police had set her on fire. On the day the children were to meet with aid workers and American visitors at a local park, National Police officers fired randomly into the queue as the children waited for a local bus. Luckily, only one child received minor wounds from a grazing (Hoerrner, 2008).

Such experiences create a fear of law enforcement. That fear is not limited to children, and modern-day slavers will capitalize on those experiences to instill a fear of law enforcement in victims. Especially in the United States, it is imperative that health care personnel reassure victims that law enforcement will help victims gain freedom and protection—and not that the victim is being handed to yet another form of trafficker.

Rodriguez has also seen her share of slavers in the United States who are natural-born citizens. Individual controllers may be pimps and panderers with commercial sexual motives or predators with noncommercial sexual motives (Rodriguez, 2009). Domestic minors have been prostituted by relatives, casual acquaintances, close friends, friends of friends, and by kidnappers. In many of the cases, the trafficker has some connection—no matter how tenuous—that gives victims trust in their controller (Rodriguez, 2009). It is upon that trust that the trafficker begins a process of psychological manipulation of the victim, angling the victim toward an enslavement that comes without physical chains but is just as binding.

Rodriguez also believes that traffickers often have other unique traits:

- Many have "diversified trafficking portfolios"—people who traffic humans often smuggle drugs and guns because many routes for all of these are often the same.
- "Mom-and-pop" family operations will often involve extended family members. International traffickers may have family members operating on both sides of a national border

- May be female although arrest records indicate the majority of traffickers are male
- May have independently owned businesses: agents that provide laborers for agricultural work, construction work, restaurants, and janitorial services are examples

For those who have seen the popular human trafficking film "Taken," there are likely two mischaracterizations that arise. The first is that human trafficking happens in foreign venues exclusively. While it does take place abroad, the reality of trafficking young women from Moldova who do not typically have a significant education or support system in their home country versus kidnapping U.S. citizens whose families are likely to raise the alarm with national and international law enforcement cannot be overlooked; as a trafficker, significant consideration will be given to which scenario is least likely to bring unwanted attention from police agencies. Second, the movie gives the impression that most traffickers are part of extensive networks or syndicates. While some of those do exist, as Rodriguez notes, traffickers are more likely to be from either very loose networks or operating independently (Rodriguez, 2009).

RECOGNIZING SIGNS OF HUMAN TRAFFICKING

In the health care profession, frontline emergency services providers will be the most likely individuals to encounter human trafficking victims. Nurses and other practitioners in psychological, maternity, and specialized medicine areas may also encounter victims, and it is important to be on the lookout for signs that might indicate that a person is under the control of another.

While this book is highly detailed in what health care providers might encounter, it bears repeating a few medical conditions that are often found in conjunction with victims of human trafficking if only to suggest that if these afflictions coincide with suspicious actions or answers to the questions below, strong concern should be given to contacting law enforcement and treating the patient as a victim of human trafficking.

Common conditions include: vaginal and rectal damage; pregnancy, especially in minors; chronic diseases such as tuberculosis; sexually transmitted diseases; urinary tract infections; bite or burn marks; malnutrition or dehydration; cuts, bruises, or broken bones, especially if they are indicators of some form of physical torture; bald spots, especially in women; drug abuse; wounds derived from baseball bats or coat hangers; blunt trauma; black eyes; branding or tattoos that may indicate ownership; botched medical procedures by nonprofessionals; missing teeth or dental damage; and repetitive stress injuries or injuries related to heavy lifting or overwork (Belles, 2012).

In cases where a patient/victim is accompanied, it should be noted that if the individual present with the victim is of the same gender, that individual may be a controller. More and more often, primary controllers are female. In the worlds of CSEC and sex trafficking, a controller's primary victim is often referred to as a "bottom" or "bottom bitch." This is actually a rank within sex trafficking operations, and bottoms often act as controllers when the primary controller is absent. Some of the common signs that a patient may be a trafficking victim (Belles, 2012):

- The patient has no identification, especially if the patient appears to be foreign.
- The patient seems to be unable to relate where he/she is geographically.
- The patient seems to have no money or is not in control of his/her money.
- The patient appears to be unable to answer basic questions without checking with an associate or appears to be afraid to talk.
- The patient appears fearful or especially submissive.
- The patient appears unable to describe how he/she arrived at the location or is unable to relate where he/she lives or works.
- The patient lives with his/her employer.
- The person who accompanied the patient does not want to be separated under reasonable circumstances from the patient.
- The patient or the patient's associate appear to be shy or fearful around uniformed security or law enforcement officers.

If any of these above scenarios raises suspicion with health care staff, a standard operating procedure related to suspected human trafficking should be followed. In the event that a location does not have such a policy in place, law enforcement should be notified immediately. This becomes of greater importance if the patient is a minor.

It will be up to the health care professional to determine whether or not to ask questions to determine if a patient is a human trafficking victim in the presence of someone who might be the victim's controller. In most cases, such questions are best asked after separating the victim from an associate. This may require that the health care worker separate the individuals under a pretext, and for the safety of all present staff, security or law enforcement (if employed by the health care facility) should be on the floor.

The *Campaign to Rescue and Restore Victims of Human Trafficking*, a program of the U.S. Department of Health and Human Services (DHHS), recommends the following as suggested interview questions for determining a patient's status as a suspected victim of human trafficking (DHHS, 2008):

- Can you leave your job or situation if you want?
- Can you come and go as you please?
- Have you been threatened if you try to leave?
- Have you been physically harmed in any way?
- What are your working or living conditions like?
- Where do you sleep and eat?
- Do you sleep in a bed, on a cot, or on the floor?
- Have you ever been deprived of food, water, sleep, or medical care?

- Do you have to ask permission to eat, sleep, or go to the bathroom?
- Are there locks on your doors and windows so you cannot get out?
- Has anyone threatened your family?
- Has your identification or documentation been taken from you?
- Is anyone forcing you to do anything that you do not want to do?

Additional questions that may help in a victim determination (Belles, 2012):

- What kind of work do you do?
- How much are you paid for the work you do?
- Are you free to contact family or friends?
- Are you required to check in with someone on a regular basis?

STRATEGIES FOR COORDINATING A LAW ENFORCEMENT RESPONSE

It is becoming more common for health care facilities to have a strategy in place to deal with human trafficking victims. Most facilities have a plan for dealing with victims of crime, and coordination with law enforcement is a standard part of that plan. If such a protocol is not present for victims of human trafficking, it should be developed as soon as possible.

Identifying the Best Law Enforcement Contacts

Many law enforcement agencies receive little training on human trafficking beyond a short seminar during basic academy instruction. Thus, the need to make contacts in the law enforcement world with the knowledge, skills, and training to respond appropriately to referrals from health care workers is high. Given the breadth of experience at the federal level in prosecuting human trafficking, contacting a victim services advocate at ICE or the FBI is an excellent starting point. Often, these individuals have a background in coordinating with multiple service providers and are aware of key personnel who can assist health care professionals in developing response protocols that include both federal and local law enforcement.

Task Forces and Working Groups

One of the best ways to create a strong relationship with law enforcement is to network through local human trafficking working groups or task forces. Simply put, a working group is an informal gathering of professionals exchanging information about human trafficking and offering guidance on how to implement various programs in a geographic area. Task forces tend to be formal gatherings of law enforcement, aid workers, and advocates designed to address specific concerns about human trafficking in the community (DOJ, Office of Victims of Crime, 2010).

Both give the health care worker a positive chance to network with law enforcement professionals. By doing so, law enforcement becomes more comfortable with known contacts from a health care facility; aid workers gain knowledge of the health care worker in order to refer victims not found through law enforcement channels for care; and the health care professional gains knowledge of exactly who to contact within law enforcement with the specialized knowledge and training to properly respond to calls from the health care provider.

Priorities for Health Care Facilities

In preparing for a law enforcement referral program at a facility, one of the first goals is to be educated on the issue. Bringing in an expert to give both general and health care–specific training on human trafficking is imperative. Follow-up information delivered regularly in a newsletter or other forms of regular communication will help reinforce such training and keep the issue present in the minds of health care workers.

To reinforce this information, the DHHS, through the Administration of Children and Families, produces a great deal of printed material for health care providers for dissemination at work. Free posters, information cards, brochures, and more may be ordered online (www.acf.hhs.gov/trafficking/campaign_kits/index.html#health).

Once training has been completed and law enforcement contacts have been put in place, additional training on using the protocol along with roleplaying sessions should take place so that all facility personnel are aware of how to effectively implement procedures. Law enforcement should be included in this training in order to give both parties familiarization with personnel, facility layouts, and ingress/egress procedures. While issues like parking for law enforcement, access to floors and wards, and security office coordination may seem like minor points, these may become large issues in practice. The faster and easier it is for law enforcement to reach the referring health care worker, the safer the situation will become for provider and patient.

PERSONAL SAFETY CONCERNS FOR HEALTH CARE WORKERS

A word of caution: Human traffickers are, by definition, violent criminals. These are predatory individuals with a significant financial (and, often, personal) investment in their victims. After all, victims represent an economic commodity whether it is a prostituted person or a forced laborer.

A perusal of recent cases of human trafficking shows high levels of violence. In the Cortes-Meza case in Atlanta, GA, lead trafficker Amador Cortes-Meza beat one victim with a closet clothes rack before causing a grievous laceration on her scalp by throwing a clothes iron at her head. In addition, he beat the victim in the face and midsection with his fists and broke fingers on one hand. After this battery, the victim was not allowed to seek medical attention (DOJ, 2011). A young girl from Mexico brought to Texas under the pretense of serving as a domestic worker was beaten and sodomized by her trafficker with a broom. When not working, the traffickers chained her to a pole in the back yard of the residence where she was held. Rescue personnel who responded to the scene were hesitant to remove her chains as they had become embedded in her skin (Bales & Soodalter, 2010).

When traffickers are willing to engage in such wanton abuse, it should be assumed that health care professionals who may be stepping between a trafficker and a victim may face the possibility of physical harm from the trafficker. Thus, when a patient is a suspected victim, facility security or law enforcement should be called to the scene in order to protect all parties involved. No health care provider should approach a victim, especially an accompanied victim, alone; two or more individuals should be present.

REFERENCES

Bales, K., & Soodalter, R. (2010). *The slave next door*. Los Angeles: University of California Press.

Belles, N. (2012). Helping human trafficking victims in our backyard. *Journal of Christian Nursing, 29*(1), 30–35.

Federal Bureau of Investigation. (2011, April). *Innocence lost*. Retrieved November 14, 2011, from Federal Bureau of Investigation: http://www.fbi.gov/about-us/investigate/vc_majorthefts/cac/innocencelost

Federal Bureau of Investigation. (2012, Feb). *Quick facts*. Retrieved March 3, 2012, from Federal Bureau of Investigation: http://www.fbi.gov/about-us/quick-facts

Hoerrner, M. (2008). Personal conversation: Lima Street Children. Lima, Peru.

Hoerrner, M. (2009). Personal conversation: Special Agent Kerri McInturf. San Francisco, California.

Immigration and Customs Enforcement. (n.d.). *Homeland security investigations*. Retrieved January 4, 2012, from Immigration and Customs Enforcement: http://www.ice.gov/about/offices/homeland-security-investigations/

Rodriguez, A. (2009). *Labor trafficking*. Florida: Bonita Springs.

Trafficking.org. (n.d.). *Heroes: Anna Rodriguez*. Retrieved December 5, 2011, from Trafficking.org: http://trafficking.org/heroes/anna-rodriguez.aspx

U.S. Department of Health and Human Services. (2008, December 12). *Screening tool for victims of human trafficking*. Retrieved November 8, 2011, from Campaign to Rescue and Restore Victims of Human Trafficking: http://www.acf.hhs.gov/trafficking/campaign_kits/tool_kit_health/screen_questions.html

U.S. Department of Justice. (2011, August 1). *Building bridges: Uniting to combat human trafficking in Georgia*. Atlanta, Georgia.

U.S. Department of Justice. (n.d.). *Civil rights division*. Retrieved October 19, 2011, from U.S. Department of Justice: http://www.justice.gov/crt/index.php

U.S. Department of Justice. (n.d.). *U.S. Dept. of justice agencies*. Retrieved January 7, 2012, from U.S. Department of Justice: http://www.justice.gov/agencies/index-list.html

U.S. Department of Justice, Office of Victims of Crime. (2010). *Anti-human trafficking task force strategy and operations e-guide*. Washington, DC: U.S. Department of Justice, Bureau of Justice Assistance.

CHAPTER 5

Legislation Efforts: The Foundation in the Fight Against Sex Trafficking

JENNIFER McMAHON-HOWARD AND TARA TRIPP

Sex trafficking legislation first emerged in the late 1800s and early 1900s in response to concerns about European women being trafficked across international borders for the purpose of prostitution (Beckman, 1984; Demleitner, 1994; Nelson, 2001). Although the original focus of international treaties and domestic legislation was on the *international* "white slavery" of women and children, these policies were amended over time to address both domestic and international sex trafficking of male and female individuals. In 2000, the United Nations passed the Protocol to Prevent, Suppress, and Punish Trafficking in Persons, Especially Women and Children (UN Protocol, 2000), which is the most comprehensive international policy to address sex trafficking as a severe form of human trafficking. Following the UN Protocol (2000), a similar policy was adopted in the United States—the Trafficking Victims Protection Act of 2000 (TVPA, 2000).

In this chapter, we provide an overview of the development of international sex trafficking treaties as well as federal and state sex trafficking legislation in the United States. First, we discuss the international efforts to combat sex trafficking, which have contributed to the creation of sex trafficking legislation in the United States. Then, we provide a detailed discussion of current federal and state sex trafficking legislation in the United States.

INTERNATIONAL EFFORTS TO COMBAT SEX TRAFFICKING

Since the initial concern about sex trafficking arose from reports of European women being taken from one country and sold for prostitution in another country (Beckman, 1984; Demleitner, 1994; Nelson, 2001), the original focus of sex trafficking treaties and legislation was on the international sex trafficking of women. Thus, it was recognized from the outset that any effort to combat sex trafficking would require collaboration and cooperation between the countries of origin and destination. As a result, 12 European states came together to ratify the 1904 International Agreement for the Suppression of White Slave Traffic, which was acceded to by an additional nine countries.[1] Since not much was known about sex trafficking at the time, these countries agreed to monitor potential trafficking routes (i.e., railways, ports, etc.), coordinate and share information, report suspected trafficking cases to the authorities in the countries of origin and destination, and provide shelter for trafficking victims until they can be sent back to their country of origin (Nelson, 2001). With a growing awareness of the nature and extent of sex trafficking, however, the need to criminalize sex trafficking became apparent. Thus, the 1910 International Convention for the Suppression of the White Slave Traffic required signatories to criminalize the international "procurement of women for prostitution" (Nelson, 2001, p. 558).

While several other international treaties were passed between 1910 and 1949,[2] which extended the provisions to include the prostitution of male and female individuals as well as Whites and non-Whites, the most significant international policy to address sex trafficking is the UN Protocol to Prevent, Suppress, and Punish Trafficking in Persons, Especially Women and Children (UN Protocol, 2000). As stated in the Preamble of the UN Protocol (2000), any successful effort to prevent and combat human trafficking must include "measures to prevent such trafficking, to punish the traffickers and to protect the victims of such trafficking, including by protecting their internationally recognized human rights" (p. 41). Thus, the UN Protocol stressed the importance of the "3 Ps"—protection, prosecution, and prevention.

As a major improvement over the previous international agreements, the UN Protocol addresses multiple forms of trafficking and exploitation, and provides very clear definitions of "trafficking in persons" and "exploitation." According to the UN Protocol (2000), "trafficking in persons" is defined as:

> the recruitment, transportation, transfer, harbouring or receipt of persons, by means of the threat or use of force or other forms of coercion, of abduction, of fraud, of deception, of the abuse of power or of a position of vulnerability or of the giving or receiving of payments or benefits to achieve the consent of a person having control over another person, for the purpose of exploitation ... [Trafficking in persons also includes] the recruitment, transportation, transfer, harbouring or receipt of a child [under the age of 18] for the purpose of exploitation ... even if this does not involve any of the means set forth [above]. (pp. 42–43)

Also, "exploitation" includes "the prostitution of others or other forms of sexual exploitation, forced labour or services, slavery or practices similar to slavery, servitude, or the removal of organs" (UN Protocol, 2000, pp. 42–43). Thus, the UN Protocol (2000) incorporates several *types* of trafficking—sex trafficking, labor trafficking, and organ trafficking. It also recognizes the different *stages* of trafficking (i.e., recruitment, transportation, etc.) and the multiple *means* of trafficking (i.e., by force, fraud, coercion, abuse of power, or vulnerability, etc.). Also, if any of these means of trafficking are present, the UN Protocol specifies that the consent of the victim is irrelevant. Therefore, by addressing the multiple types, stages, and means of trafficking, the UN Protocol takes a comprehensive approach to combating the multifaceted processes involved in human trafficking.

As another major improvement over previous international agreements, which failed to incorporate adequate protections for victims of trafficking, the UN Protocol (2000) made the protection of trafficking victims and their basic human rights a key focus. Indeed, the UN Protocol (2000) contains several articles addressing the need to protect and assist trafficking victims. These articles include provisions for ensuring the physical safety of the victim and protecting the victim's privacy and identity. There are also a number of victim's rights included, such as the right to be informed (i.e., providing the victim with information about criminal proceedings) and the right to be heard (i.e., allowing the victim an opportunity to express his/her views or concerns at appropriate stages of the court process). Also, the UN Protocol (2000) calls for states to provide assistance to victims to help in their recovery (i.e., housing, employment opportunities, counseling, medical assistance, etc.) and to ensure that there are legal avenues for victims to receive victim's compensation for "damage suffered." Furthermore, while previous international treaties failed to address safety concerns when returning a victim back to their country of origin, the UN Protocol (2000) encourages countries to consider "humanitarian and compassionate factors" in developing legislation that grants either temporary or permanent legal status to foreign victims, which will allow the victims to remain in that territory. If the country returns the victim to his or her country of origin, however, then the UN Protocol (2000) dictates that the state and the home country should work together, "with due regard for the safety of that person," to facilitate the victim's return (p. 45).

Finally, the UN Protocol (2000) is the first international treaty to take a proactive approach to human trafficking by addressing the efforts needed to prevent human trafficking. In addition to raising awareness through research and media campaigns, the UN Protocol requires states to cooperate with nongovernment organizations to develop prevention policies and programs. Also, countries should work to address the factors that make victims vulnerable to trafficking (i.e., poverty) and create legislation or make other efforts to decrease the conditions that facilitate human trafficking.

SEX TRAFFICKING LEGISLATION IN THE UNITED STATES

The origin and development of sex trafficking laws in the United States mirror the development of the international treaties. Specifically, the laws on sex trafficking in the United States can be traced back to the Alien Prostitution Importation Act of

1875 and the White Slave Traffic Act of 1910. The Alien Prostitution Importation Act (1875, p. 477) made "the importation into the United States of women for the purposes of prostitution" a felony offense punishable by up to 5 years in prison and a $5,000 fine. This Act was amended in 1903 to include the importation of girls for the purposes of prostitution (Beckman, 1984). Thus, whether the women and girls were brought voluntarily or by force, it was a crime to transport foreign women and girls to the United States for the purpose of prostitution. Furthermore, the White Slave Traffic Act of 1910, which is also referred to as the Mann Act (Chacon, 2006), made it a felony offense to transport or assist with the transportation of a woman or girl "in interstate or foreign commerce . . . for the purpose of prostitution or debauchery or for any other immoral purpose" (White Slave Traffic Act, 1910, p. 825). Until the United States passed the Trafficking Victims Protection Act of 2000, sex trafficking cases could be prosecuted under the Alien Prostitution Importation Act (1875) and/or the Mann Act (White Slave Traffic Act, 1910).

Although the stated purpose of the Mann Act was to prohibit the international and interstate transportation of women and girls who were being forced or coerced to engage in prostitution,[3] it was primarily applied to cases that did not involve forced or coerced commercial sexual activity (Beckman, 1984; Chacon, 2006). That is, a man who took his mistress across state lines and engaged in sex could be penalized for interstate travel involving an "immoral practice" under the Mann Act. Thus, while the original focus of the Act was international and interstate criminal activity, the Mann Act was primarily used to regulate interstate immorality (Beckman, 1984). Additionally, in the cases that *did* involve interstate commercial vice, it is important to note that the women being transported were often charged with conspiracy to violate the Mann Act. For example, in one case, a Mexican woman who was forced to engage in prostitution and turn her earnings over to her pimp was convicted under the Mann Act and subsequently deported (Beckman, 1984). In other cases, however, if the women cooperated with the investigation and testified against the traffickers, then they were not prosecuted for the conspiracy charge (Beckman, 1984).

To address a number of limitations, the Mann Act was amended several times during the 1970s and 1980s. Specifically, the Act was amended in 1978 to include minor boys as potential victims (Beckman, 1984), and then again in 1986 to extend possible victim status to all male individuals (Young, 1998). Congress also attempted to curb the regulation of immorality in 1986 by replacing the phrases "debauchery" and "any other immoral purpose" with "sexual activity for which any person can be charged with a criminal offense" (Conant, 1996, p. 99). The Amendments resolved the problem of gender bias and eliminated the possibility of prosecutions based solely on immoral actions, but they did not rectify all of the Mann Act's limitations for prosecuting sex traffickers.

Victim protection neither appears in the original act nor any of its amendments. Under the Mann Act, victims of forced prostitution were not provided with any alternate housing, psychological treatment, or protection from their traffickers and/or pimps. In fact, in the early years of the Mann Act, victims were barely treated with respect as law enforcement officers frequently arrested the women as leverage to induce testifying against traffickers or pimps (Beckman, 1984). The Mann Act also does not provide any protection for immigrant victims who face possible and probable deportation. Protection needs to be offered so that victims have more confidence in law enforcement which, in turn, may promote the disclosure of more Mann Act violations. Victim protection may also aid the prevention of retaliation by the defendants or co-conspirators.

The Mann Act also suffers from several other significant limitations. While the Mann Act was often used to prosecute men who solicited sex across state lines[4] and cases involving voluntary prostitution across state lines,[5] it was rarely used by itself to prosecute sex trafficking. Also, even though the Mann Act explicitly relates to both "interstate and foreign commerce," it was seldom used in international sex trafficking cases (Young, 1998). Furthermore, the Mann Act does not address intrastate cases of commercial sexual exploitation. Due to these shortcomings, prosecutions under the Mann Act have not focused on sex trafficking.

Trafficking Victims Protection Act of 2000

Even though federal prosecution of interstate and foreign sex trafficking was technically possible under the Mann Act, the United States needed more thorough and direct legislation related to the heinous crime. Therefore, as a part of the Victims of Trafficking and Violence Protection Act of 2000 (VTVPA), the United States passed the Trafficking Victims Protection Act (TVPA). The TVPA (2000) was the first legislation specifically designed to combat human trafficking and directly criminalize labor and sex trafficking. Prosecution, prevention, and protection, or the 3 Ps, outline the relatively new strategy employed by the federal government in the fight against human trafficking.

In order to enhance prosecutorial abilities, the TVPA (2000) established sex trafficking as a crime with the creation of 18 U.S.C. 1591 (sex trafficking of children or by force, fraud, or coercion). Sex trafficking is defined under the TVPA as "the recruitment, harboring, transportation, provision, or obtaining of a person for the purpose of a commercial sex act" (TVPA, 2000, p. 1470). Also, the crime becomes a severe form of trafficking when the "commercial sex act is induced by force, fraud, or coercion, or in which the person induced to perform such act has not attained 18 years of age" (TVPA, 2000, p. 1470).

Additionally, since the focus of the original TVPA (2000) was on *international* sex trafficking, it addressed other illegal conduct that contributes to international sex trafficking. Specifically, the TVPA (2000) created a separate offense, 18 U.S.C 1591 (Unlawful conduct with respect to documents in furtherance of trafficking, peonage, slavery, involuntary servitude, or forced labor), to create additional punishments for those who confiscate, remove, conceal, or destroy another person's immigration documents or create false documents in an effort to traffic that person. Punishment for unlawful conduct in relation to documents that promote trafficking constitutes a fine and/or imprisonment for no more than 5 years.

While the creation of new federal offenses that can be used to prosecute sex traffickers was an important step, the original punishments for sex trafficking were quite lenient, as they did not include a minimum punishment. Specifically, under the original TVPA (2000), the punishments for sex trafficking by force, fraud, or coercion and sex trafficking involving a minor under the age of 14 include a fine and/or imprisonment for any number of years, including life.[6] For sex trafficking of a 14- to 17-year-old minor without the use of force, fraud, or coercion, the punishments include a fine and/or imprisonment for no more than 20 years.[7] Also, according to the TVPA (2000), the court must order the offender to forfeit any assets used in the commission of the trafficking or gained as a result of the trafficking, and the court must order the offender to pay restitution to the victim.

In addition to creating new federal offenses, the TVPA (2000) included provisions to provide protection for victims of severe forms of trafficking. Since successful prosecutions and subsequent punishments depend heavily on the cooperation of sex trafficking victims, such protections are essential (Coonan, 2010). Specifically, due to the unique circumstances that the majority of international sex trafficking victims face as a result of being in the United States illegally, the TVPA (2000) extends certain immigration benefits to victims of severe forms of trafficking who cooperate with law enforcement to prosecute the traffickers.

According to the TVPA (2000), federal law enforcement officials can grant "continued presence" in the United States to victims of severe forms of trafficking who may serve as witnesses during the investigation and prosecution of the traffickers. Granting "continued presence" provides victims with a temporary immigration status. When federal law enforcement officials grant "continued presence" to a victim, the officials who are investigating and prosecuting the traffickers are expected to ensure the safety of the trafficking victims and protect the victims and their families from intimidation and reprisals from traffickers.

The TVPA (2000) also amended the Immigration and Nationality Act (8 U.S.C. 1184) to create a new nonimmigrant visa classification—the T Visa, which extends the eligibility for nonimmigrant status to victims of severe forms of trafficking. In order to be eligible for T nonimmigrant status, an immigrant must meet four qualifications: The individual is a victim of a severe form of trafficking, the victim is physically present in the United States due to trafficking, the victim has demonstrated compliance with law enforcement requests or has not attained 15 years of age, and the victim would experience extreme hardship if removed from the United States (TVPA, 2000).

Another immigration option for sex trafficking victims, the U nonimmigrant visa, was created by the Violence Against Women Act of 2000, which is embedded in the VTVPA 2000. The U nonimmigrant status visa allows immigrant victims of serious crimes, such as rape, kidnapping, torture, involuntary servitude, and forced prostitution, to apply for temporary legal immigration status

(VAWA, 2000). Similar to the T Visa, an immigrant must meet four qualifications in order to be eligible for the U Visa: The immigrant has suffered "substantial physical or mental abuse" due to serious criminal activity, the immigrant has information pertaining to the criminal act, the individual is helpful in the investigation and prosecution of the aforementioned criminal activity, and the crime occurred in the United States or its territories (VAWA, 2000, p. 72). The creation of the U Visa hinged upon a desire for stronger prosecutorial and investigatory abilities while attempting to maintain the "humanitarian interests of the United States" (VAWA, 2000, p. 72). Similar to the T Visa, the U Visa relies on the cooperation or assistance of victims in prosecutorial efforts; however, the U Visa does not require proof of hardship upon removal from the country (Sangalis, 2011).

The TVPA (2000) also extends benefits and services offered by certain federal and state programs to victims of severe forms of trafficking, regardless of their immigration status. Specifically, the TVPA (2000) makes victims of severe forms of trafficking eligible for the benefits offered to refugees, such as food stamps, Medicaid, and medical assistance (Adelson, 2008). The TVPA (2000) specifies that grant funds should be provided to victim service agencies so that they can provide services for victims of trafficking. Also, if victims of severe forms of trafficking are in the custody of the federal government, then the victims must be housed in an appropriate facility and be provided with medical care and assistance. Furthermore, if the victim is in custody, the federal government must protect the victim and the victim's family from harm, intimidation, and/or retaliation from traffickers and ensure that identifying information about the victim and the victim's family is not released to the public. For trafficking victims in other countries, the federal government must assist with programs that will ensure the "safe integration, reintegration, or resettlement" of the victim (TVPA, 2000, pp. 1474–1475).

Finally, in addition to enhancing prosecutorial abilities and providing protections for victims, the TVPA (2000) includes provisions for the prevention of human trafficking. Specifically, the legislation established an Interagency Task Force to Monitor and Combat Trafficking (TVPA, 2000). Agency involvement in the task force ranged from the Secretary of State to the Health and Human Services Department and many other diverse entities (TVPA, 2000). Responsibilities of the task force consist of evaluating the United States' progress in all areas of human trafficking, organizing data, enhancing cooperation between countries, and facilitating interaction with nongovernmental organizations (TVPA, 2000). Greater public awareness and dissemination of information is also acknowledged as a necessity to prevent human trafficking.

TVPA Reauthorizations

Prosecutorial and prevention tools to combat human trafficking increased greatly with the creation of the TVPA in 2000, but victim protection still proved considerably lacking in strength. By 2003, only 289 T Visas were authorized despite the possible 5,000 T Visas that could have been issued and the 672 individuals that applied (Seelke & Siskin, 2008). Reauthorizations of the TVPA in 2003, 2005, and 2008 attempted to address various shortcomings in victim protection, as well as strengthen the ability to prosecute traffickers.

Revising victim protection began with an amendment to the T Visa, which was included in the Trafficking Victims Protection Reauthorization Act (TVPRA) of 2003. Under the TVPA (2000), all victims who were 15 years old or older were required to cooperate with law enforcement in the investigation and prosecution of the trafficker(s) in order to receive a T Visa; the 2003 TVPRA amended this requirement so that any juvenile sex trafficking victim, under 18 years of age, would be eligible for the T Visa regardless of their cooperation with law enforcement officials (TVPRA, 2003). The 2003 TVPRA also furnished T Visa benefits to the siblings of victims and added a civil suit method for victims to litigate against traffickers (Payne, 2009). In 2008, the William Wilberforce Trafficking Victims Protection Reauthorization Act took a step toward the elimination of the cooperation condition for issuance of a T Visa. If the Attorney General deems a victim "unable to cooperate ... due to physical or psychological trauma," then the victim is no longer ineligible for a T Visa (William Wilberforce TVPRA, 2008, p. 5052). Furthermore, the 2008 TVPRA details procedures for locating appropriate places for unaccompanied immigrant minors. The Secretary of Health and Human Services plays a significant role in placing immigrant juveniles in safe and secure facilities and determining if the location will be in the best interest of the child's mental and physical needs (William Wilberforce TVPRA, 2008).

While additional protections for international sex trafficking victims were added by the TVPA reauthorizations, it is important to note that the 2005 TVPRA addressed domestic sex trafficking for the first time and devoted an entire section to combating human trafficking that occurs entirely within United States territory. Including domestic sex trafficking as a "severe form of trafficking," the 2005 TVPRA included provisions to improve grants, assistance, and prosecution efforts toward domestic sex trafficking. The Department of Health and Human Services provides services to juvenile victims of human trafficking (under 18 years of age), such as shelter and psychological counseling (TVPRA, 2005). Additionally, the 2005 TVPRA instructs the Federal Bureau of Investigation to investigate domestic human trafficking.

Other amendments to the TVPA have been made to adapt to challenges that sex trafficking poses in regard to prosecution. Originally, to gain a sex trafficking conviction, the prosecution was required to prove that the offender "knowingly" engaged in efforts that contributed to sex trafficking (TVPA, 2000). The "knowingly" standard proved unwieldy when trying to convict members of a sex trafficking ring whose duties were limited to tasks such as transportation of female victims or financial management (Payne, 2009). To charge an offender with sex trafficking of minors, the offender had to possess the knowledge that a victim was under 18 years of age (Payne, 2009). The high culpability standard limited prosecutorial capabilities as sex traffickers claimed they unwittingly employed juveniles. Therefore, the Wilberforce Trafficking Victims Protection

Reauthorization Act of 2008 changed the "knowingly" standard to one which required only a reckless disregard for the truth to convict sex traffickers (William Wilberforce TVPRA, 2008). Any individual involved in sex trafficking who had a "reasonable opportunity to observe" that the victim was under 18 years of age can be charged with sex trafficking of minors (William Wilberforce TVPRA, 2008). These revisions aid in the strength of prosecution charges.

Additional Federal Legislation Related to Sex Trafficking

Although the TVPA and its subsequent revisions are the strongest method to prosecute traffickers and provide assistance to trafficking victims, they are not the only applicable legislation. Recently, attorneys have used the Racketeer Influence and Corrupt Organizations (2011a, b) (RICO) statute to prosecute traffickers due to the highly organized operations of sex traffickers (Overbaugh, 2009). Under the RICO (2011a) statutes, deception and coercion of trafficking victims outside and within the United States' borders can be viewed as racketeering activity because "racketeering" is defined as "any act or threat involving murder, kidnapping, gambling, arson, robbery, bribery, [or] extortion" (18 U.S.C. 1961). RICO (2011b) further prohibits the receipt of "any income derived, directly or indirectly, from a pattern of racketeering activity or through collection of an unlawful debt" and the maintenance or control of any activities that disrupt or affect interstate commerce (18 U.S.C 1962). Due to the common practice of traffickers demanding fees after arranging illegal transportation into the United States (Young, 1998), RICO can be used to prosecute traffickers who use these deceptive tactics.

The practice of transporting individuals for commercial sex acts also can be prosecuted under the Prosecutorial Remedies and Other Tools to end the Exploitation of Children Today (PROTECT) Act of 2003 (Overbaugh, 2009). The PROTECT Act of 2003 took a stance to prevent sexual tourism and increased maximum sentences for both the coercion or enticement of minors and the transportation of minors to engage in illicit sexual activities. An individual charged with knowingly persuading, enticing, coercing, or inducing a minor (under age 18) to engage in prostitution can be imprisoned for up to 20 years (18 U.S.C. 2422). An individual who transports minors with the intent to have the minor engage in illegal sexual activity should serve no less than 10 years and could serve life imprisonment (18 U.S.C 2423). The PROTECT Act increased penalties for promoting and engaging in sexual tourism and does not have a statute of limitations for sex crimes or child abductions (Overbaugh, 2009). Due to the intricacies of sex trafficking rings and frequent transportation, the PROTECT Act can be employed to prevent and prosecute sex trafficking. The Act can only be used to prosecute sex trafficking of minors, but since juveniles are the most vulnerable category of victims, it is useful to have another prosecutorial tool to ensure penalties for the perpetrators of such grave crimes.

In regard to juvenile victims, there is another possible protection offered under the Homeland Security Act of 2002. Specifically, under the Homeland

Security Act of 2002, an unaccompanied illegal immigrant minor is eligible for a special immigration status. To be deemed a Special Immigrant Juvenile, a minor must demonstrate that "(a) he or she has been declared dependent on a juvenile court located in the United States, (b) he or she has been deemed eligible by that court for long-term foster care, and (c) it has been determined that it would not be in his or her best interest to return to his or her country of nationality" (Pollock & Hollier, 2010, p. 136). Obtaining this status, however, may be very cumbersome for a victim of sex trafficking due to the fact that the minor must be dependent on a juvenile court (Pollock & Hollier, 2010). Thus, Special Immigrant Juvenile Status does not provide a perfect alternative to T Visas for juveniles, but it is a step toward providing victims with more protections.

Overall, the federal legislation passed during the 21st century has made great strides in acknowledging and combating sex trafficking. The TVPA and its reauthorizations created the first laws directly criminalizing sex trafficking and provided awareness for the often secretive world of human trafficking. Also, the TVPA is the first legislation to include protection for sex trafficking victims and to establish interagency forces to assist in discovery and prosecution of the crime. As scholars, legislators, and governmental agencies gather more knowledge about sex trafficking, legislation can be tailored to meet the needs of victims and prosecutors.

State Sex Trafficking Legislation

While federal laws were put in place to combat sex trafficking in the United States, it is widely recognized that state antitrafficking legislation is needed as well (Mariconda, 2009; Smith & Vardaman, 2010). Prior to 2003, there were no state antitrafficking laws; however, between 2003 and 2011, 45 states passed antihuman trafficking laws that criminalized sex trafficking.[8] While almost all states currently have antitrafficking laws, there is significant state-to-state variation in the severity of punishments, the protections for victims, the inclusion of civil penalties, and other state mandates (i.e., law enforcement training, antihuman trafficking taskforces, prevention efforts, etc.) (Bouche & Wittmer, 2009; Mariconda, 2009; Smith & Vardaman, 2010). In fact, there are nonprofit organizations, such as the Center for Women Policy Studies, the Polaris Project, and Shared Hope International, that regularly monitor and rate state antitrafficking laws.[9] Notably, the antitrafficking laws in Florida, Georgia, Illinois, Minnesota, Missouri, New York, Texas, and Washington have received highest scores by all three organizations.

Indeed, Georgia's antihuman trafficking law (O.C.G.A. § 16-5-46), which was enacted in 2006 (Georgia Security and Immigration Compliance Act, 2006) and amended in 2011 (Ga. HB 200, 2011), has been referred to as "one of the toughest state anti-trafficking laws in the nation" (Bluestein, 2011). According to the Official Code of Georgia (2011), the crime of sex trafficking is committed when "a person knowingly subjects or maintains another in sexual servitude or knowingly recruits, entices, harbors, transports, provides, or obtains by any means another person for the purpose of sexual servitude" (O.C.G.A. §

16-5-46). Sexual servitude is defined as engaging in sexual conduct or performing sexually explicit conduct in exchange for anything of value when the conduct is "induced or obtained by coercion or deception or which conduct is induced or obtained from a person under the age of 18 years" (O.C.G.A. § 16-5-46).

Georgia's antitrafficking law provides broad definitions of deception and coercion (O.C.G.A. § 16-5-46). Deception includes providing another person with false information, falsely promising services or benefits that the person will not actually receive, or providing false information to a person in regard to the status of their debt repayment. Coercion includes threating or using physical harm/restraint/confinement, threatening or actually exposing damaging information about a person (i.e., criminal behavior, illegal immigration status, etc.), taking away or destroying another person's passport, immigration, or other government identification documents, or providing a controlled substance. Also, when the law was amended in 2011 (Ga. HB 200, 2011), using financial control and threatening or actually causing financial harm to another person were added to the definition of coercion.

While the original penalty for sex trafficking was imprisonment for 1 to 20 years, with enhanced penalties of 10 to 20 years in prison if the victim was under the age of 18, the 2011 amendment (Ga. HB 200, 2011) increased the penalty for all sex trafficking offenses to 10 to 20 years in prison with a possible fine of up to $100,000. Enhanced penalties of 25 to 50 years in prison were added if deception or coercion was used to traffic a person under the age of 18. Also, the amended law allows for the forfeiture of all property used during the commission of the offense. HB 200 (Ga. HB 200, 2011) also increased the penalties for pimping, pandering, or keeping a house of prostitution when the offense involves a minor under the age of 16.

In addition to increasing the penalties, HB 200 (Ga. HB 200, 2011) also included a number of provisions to assist victims. Specifically, in an effort to help victims recover from their victimization, it added sex trafficking victims to the list of victims who are eligible for the state victim compensation program. It also added an affirmative defense for prostitution when coercion or deception is used to induce a person to engage in prostitution. This protects sex trafficking victims from being charged and convicted for engaging in prostitution. Georgia is only one of a few states who provide such an affirmative defense to prostitution.[10]

HB 200 (Ga. HB 200, 2011) also includes provisions designed to improve law enforcement's response to and treatment of trafficking victims. Specifically, it mandates the development and implementation of guidelines and procedures for identifying sex trafficking victims, reporting incidents, providing specialized training and information for assisting sex trafficking victims (i.e., referrals to victim service and other social service agencies), and providing appropriate detention facilities or a suitable alternative (i.e., shelter or treatment center). While the increased penalties indicate that Georgia is serious about punishing and deterring traffickers, it is the inclusion of the provisions for protecting victims and the mandatory training for law enforcement that shows that Georgia is stepping up the efforts to combat sex trafficking.

CONCLUSION

Overall, since the passage of the UN Protocol (2000) and the TVPA (2000), there have been significant improvements in international sex trafficking treaties as well as in federal and state sex trafficking legislation in the United States. These improvements include the creation of new sex trafficking offenses and increased punishments, protections for sex trafficking victims, and efforts to prevent sex trafficking both internationally and domestically. The creation of such comprehensive sex trafficking legislation should increase the number of sex trafficking prosecutions and convictions, which, in turn, should prevent future trafficking and protect victims.

NOTES

1. Countries that ratified include Belgium, Denmark, France, Germany, Italy, Netherlands, Portugal, Russia, Spain, Sweden and Norway, Switzerland, and the United Kingdom. Those that acceded include Austria-Hungary, Brazil, Bulgaria, Colombia, Czechoslovakia, Lebanon, Luxembourg, Poland, and the United States.
2. These include the Convention for the Suppression of the Traffic in Women and Children (1921), the International Convention for the Suppression of the Traffic of Women of Full Age (1933), and the United Nations Convention for the Suppression of the Traffic in Persons and of the Exploitation of the Prostitution of Others (1949).
3. Congressman James Robert Mann, the author of the Act, stated that the purpose of the Act was "to put a stop to villainous interstate and international traffic in women and girls. . . [it] does not attempt to regulate the practice of voluntary prostitution, but aims solely to prevent panderers and procurers from compelling thousands of women and girls against their will and desire to enter and continue in a life of prostitution" (H.R. REP. NO. 47, 61st Cong., 2d Sess. (1909), as cited by Beckman (1984, p. 1117)).
4. *U.S. v. Vang*, 128 F.3d 1065 (1998); *Bell v. U.S.* 349 U.S. 81 (1955); *U.S. v. Anderson*, 664 F.3d 758 (2012).
5. *U.S. v. Barrington*, 806 F.2d 529 (1986).
6. The Adam Walsh Act (2006) increased this punishment to include a fine and imprisonment for a minimum of 15 years to life.
7. The Adam Walsh Act (2006) increased this punishment to include a fine and imprisonment for a minimum of 10 years to life.
8. For current information on state antitrafficking legislation, go to www.polar isproject.org/what-we-do/policy-advocacy/state-policy/current-laws
9. www.centerwomenpolicy.org/documents/ReportCardonStateActiontoCom batInternationalTrafficking.pdf, www.sharedhope.org/WhatWeDo/Bring Justice/PolicyRecommendations.aspx
10. California, Connecticut, New York, and Washington have passed laws that prevent victims from being prosecuted for prostitution.

REFERENCES

Adam Walsh Child Protection and Safety Act of 2006, Public Law 109-288, §208. (2006).

Adelson, W. (2008). Child prostitute or victim of trafficking? *University of St. Thomas Law Journal, 6*(1), 96–128.

Alien Prostitution Importation Act of 1875, ch. 141, 18 Stat. 477 (1875).

Beckman, M. D. (1984). The White Slave Traffic Act: The historical impact of a criminal law policy on women. *72 Georgetown Law Journal*, 1111.

Bluestein, G. (2011, July 11). Georgia sex trafficking law goes into effect. *Huffington Post.* Retrieved from http://www.huffingtonpost.com/2011/07/11/georgia-sex-trafficking-law_n_894505.html.

Bouche, V., & Wittmer, D. (2009). Human trafficking legislation across the states: The determinants of comprehensiveness. *First Annual Interdisciplinary Conference on Human Trafficking, 2009.* Available at http://digitalcommons.unl.edu/humtraff conf/6.

Chacon, J. M. (2006). Misery and myopia: Understanding the failures of U.S. efforts to stop human trafficking. *74 Fordham Law Review*, 2977.

Conant, M. (1996). Federalism, the Mann Act, and the Imperative to Decriminalize Prostitution. *5 Cornell Journal of Law & Public Policy*, 99.

Coonan, T. (2010). Anatomy of a sex trafficking case. *5 Intercultural Human Rights Law Review*, 313.

Demleitner, N. V. (1994). Forced prostitution: Naming an international offense. *18 Fordham International Law Journal,* 163.

Georgia House Bill 200, 2011 Georgia Laws 54. 3 May 2011.

Georgia Security and Immigration Compliance Act. 2006 Georgia Law 105, § 3/SB 529. 17 April 2006.

Homeland Security Act of 2002, 6 U.S.C. §279. (2010).

Immigration and Nationality Act of 1965, 8 U.S.C. § 1184. (2000).

International Agreement for the Suppression of the White Slave Traffic of 1904, art. 1, 11 L.N.T.S. 83, 85–86.

International Convention for the Suppression of the White Slave Traffic of 1910, 211 Consol. T.S. 45, 1912 GR. Brit. T.S. No. 20.

International Convention for the Suppression of the Traffic in Women and Children of 1921, arts. 2, 5, 53 U.N.T.S. 39, 42.

International Convention for the Suppression of the Traffic in Women of Full Age, Oct. 11, 1933, 150 L.N.T.S., *entered into force* Aug. 24, 1934.

Mariconda, S. L. (2009). Breaking the chains: Combating human trafficking at the state level. *29 Boston College Third World Law Journal*, 151.

Nelson, K. E. (2001–2002). Sex trafficking and forced prostitution: Comprehensive new legal approaches. *24 Houston Journal of International Law*, 551.

Official Code of Georgia. § 16-5-46. Trafficking of persons for labor or sexual servitude. (2011).

Overbaugh, E. (2009). Human trafficking: The need for federal prosecution of accused traffickers. *39 Seton Hall Law Review*, 635–664.

Payne, V. S. (2009). On the road to victory in America's war on human trafficking: Landmarks, landmines, and the need for centralized strategy. *21 Regent University Law Review*, 435–468.

Pollock, J. M., & Hollier, V. (2010). T visas: Prosecution tool or humanitarian response? *Women & Criminal Justice, 20*(1–2), 127–146.

Prosecutorial Remedies and Other Tools to end the Exploitation of Children Today Act of 2003 (PROTECT), 18 U.S.C §2421-2423. (2011).

Racketeer Influence and Corrupt Organizations Act of 1970, 18 U.S.C §1961. (2011a).

Racketeer Influence and Corrupt Organizations Act of 1970, 18 U.S.C §1962. (2011b).

Sangalis, T. R. (2011). Elusive empowerment: compensating the sex trafficked person under the Trafficking Victims Protection Act. *Fordham Law Review, 80*(1), 403–439.

Seelke, C. R., & Siskin, A. (2008). Trafficking in persons: U.S. policy and issues for congress. *Federal Publications*. Available at http://digitalcommons.ilr.cornell.edu/key_workplace/479.

Smith, L., & Vardaman, S. H. (2010). Domestic human trafficking series: A legislative framework for combating domestic minor sex trafficking. *23 Regent University Law Review*, 265.

Trafficking Victims Protection Act of 2000 (TVPA), Public Law No. 106-386, 114 Stat. 1466 (2000).

Trafficking Victims Protection Reauthorization Act (TVPRA) of 2003, Pub. L. No. 108-193, 117 Stat. 2875.

Trafficking Victims Protection Reauthorization Act (TVPRA) of 2005, Public Law No. 109-164, 119 Stat. 3558 (2005).

United Nations Convention for the Suppression of the Traffic in Persons and of the Exploitation of the Prostitution of Others of 1949, resolution 317 (IV) of 2 December 1949, Entry into force: 25 July 1951, in accordance with article 24.

United Nations Trafficking Protocol. (2000). *United Nations Protocol to Prevent, Suppress and Punish Trafficking in Persons, Especially Women and Children, Supplementing the United Nations Convention Against Transnational Organized Crime*, G.A. Res. 55/25, Annex II, at 31, UN GAOR, 55th Sess., UN Doc. A/RES/55/25 (Januray 8, 2001), reprinted in 40 I.L.M. 335, 384–385.

Victims of Trafficking and Violence Protection Act (VTVPA) of 2000, Pub. L. No. 106-386, 114 Stat. 1464–1548.

Violence against Women Act of 2000 (VAWA), 114 Stat § 1464, 1491. (2000).

White Slave Traffic Act of 1910, ch. 395, 36 Stat. 825. (1910).

White Slave Traffic Act - Codified as amended at 18 U.S.C. 2421-2424 (2000). 61st Congress (Session II), chapter 395, p. 825. Public, No. 277 (June 25, 1910 H.R. 12315).

William Wilberforce Trafficking Victims Protection Reauthorization Act (TVPRA) of 2008. Public Law No. 110-457, 122 Stat. 5044. (2008).

Young, B. (1998). Trafficking of humans across United States borders: How United States laws can be used to punish traffickers and protect victims. *Georgetown Immigration Law Journal, 13*, 73–104.

CHAPTER 6

Trials and Tribulations: The Prosecution of Sex Traffickers

JENNIFER McMAHON-HOWARD AND TARA TRIPP

Successfully prosecuting traffickers is considered the "linchpin" for combating all forms of human trafficking, including sex trafficking (Overbaugh, 2009). Without successful prosecutions, traffickers operate with impunity. Therefore, the goal of developing comprehensive antitrafficking legislation, such as the Trafficking Victims Protection Act (TVPA, 2000) and its subsequent reauthorizations (2003, 2005, and 2008), is to increase trafficking prosecutions. Indeed, while the TVPA includes protections for victims, one of the main goals of this comprehensive antitrafficking law is to prosecute and punish traffickers as a means to deter future sex trafficking.

In this chapter, we examine issues related to the prosecution of sex trafficking cases in the United States. First, we discuss the importance of sex trafficking prosecutions. Then, we review the data and literature on federal sex trafficking prosecutions in the United States. Finally, we provide examples of sex trafficking cases that were prosecuted in the United States.

THE IMPORTANCE OF PROSECUTION

Increasing sex trafficking prosecutions should protect victims and deter future sex trafficking (Overbaugh, 2009). In order to prosecute sex traffickers, prosecutors first need the cooperation of the victim(s). By including protections for sex trafficking victims, the TVPA provides an incentive for victims to come forward and testify against the traffickers. In turn, the cooperation of the victim increases the likelihood that traffickers will be caught, convicted, and sentenced. Since the TVPA includes harsh punishments, traffickers are more likely to receive long prison sentences, which should create a strong enough deterrent so that potential traffickers perceive the costs of sex trafficking (i.e., the increased likelihood of being caught, convicted, and sentenced severely) as outweighing the benefits (i.e., financial profit) (Overbaugh, 2009). Indeed, the inclusion of asset forfeiture and mandatory restitution to victims as part of the punishments plays a large role in removing the perceived financial gain for potential future traffickers. Furthermore, incapacitating offenders provides immediate protections for current victims and prevents offenders from continuing their trafficking enterprise (Overbaugh, 2009).

Federal Prosecution of Sex Traffickers

While the majority of states have enacted laws that enable them to prosecute sex trafficking cases, the majority of sex trafficking cases are prosecuted at the federal level (Clawson, Dutch, Lopez, & Tiapula, 2008). With access to more resources, the federal government is in the best position to prosecute human trafficking cases (Overbaugh, 2009). Also, the federal government is able to prosecute traffickers for crimes committed in various states and across international borders, and there are more federal statutes that can be used to prosecute traffickers. In fact, federal prosecutors often rely on these other federal statutes for traffickers who are willing to plead guilty to a lesser charge in exchange for a reduced punishment (Overbaugh, 2009).

Specifically, in addition to prosecuting sex traffickers under TVPA statutes, which include 18 U.S.C. 1589 (forced labor), 18 U.S.C. 1590 (trafficking with respect to peonage, slavery, involuntary servitude, or forced labor), 18 U.S.C. 1591 (sex trafficking of children or by force, fraud, or coercion), 18 U.S.C. 1592 (unlawful conduct with respect to documents in furtherance of trafficking, peonage, slavery, involuntary servitude, or forced labor), and 18 U.S.C. 1594 (general provisions, including conspiracy), federal prosecutors also can pursue charges under 18 U.S.C. 1581 (peonage), 18 U.S.C. 1583 (enticement into slavery), and 18 U.S.C. 1584 (sale into involuntary servitude). Federal prosecutors also can pursue charges under chapter 117 (transportation for illegal sexual activity and related crimes), which includes 18 U.S.C. 2422 (coercion and enticement) and 18 U.S.C. 2423 (transportation of minors). In international sex trafficking cases, federal prosecutors can charge offenders under immigration laws, such as 18 U.S.C. 1546 (fraud and misuse of visas, permits, and other documents), 18 U.S.C. 1324 (bringing in and harboring certain aliens), 18 U.S.C. 1327 (aiding or assisting certain aliens to enter), and 18 U.S.C. 1328 (importation of aliens for immoral purpose). With such a vast array of statutes at the federal government's disposal, prosecutors are able to prosecute each member of the trafficking ring. That is, the person who created false documents for trafficking purposes, the individuals who transport the victims, and the leaders of sex trafficking rings can all be prosecuted.

Furthermore, prosecuting a sex trafficking case at the federal level is best for cases involving undocumented victims; with the federal government having control over the immigration status of victims, federal law enforcement officers, and prosecutors are in the best position to help the victim establish a legal and temporary immigration status (Overbaugh, 2009). Also, since international sex trafficking cases may require the cooperation of other countries, the involvement of the federal government is needed to facilitate these efforts.

Number of Sex Trafficking Prosecutions

Since the passage of the TVPA (2000), the number of federal sex trafficking prosecutions and convictions has increased significantly. At the federal level, child sex trafficking cases are prosecuted by the Department of Justice's Child Exploitation and Obscenity Section (CEOS) and the United States Attorney's Office. Looking at these federal child sex trafficking cases, research indicates that from 2001 to 2006, the number of suspects prosecuted under federal child sex transportation statutes[1] increased from approximately 100 to 500 (Motivans & Kyckelhahn, 2007). Thus, it is clear that there has been a significant increase in the number of federal child sex trafficking prosecutions.

The available data also suggest that U.S. Attorneys are successful in securing convictions in child sex trafficking cases. Based upon a review of all federal prosecutions of child sexual exploitation offenders in 2006, a report from the Bureau of Justice Statistics indicates that 567 child sex transportation suspects had their cases closed by U.S. Attorneys in 2006 (Motivans & Kyckelhahn, 2007). Approximately 64% of these suspects were prosecuted and 36% had their cases dropped. For the 365 who were prosecuted, 86% pled guilty, 5.8% were convicted at trial, 8.2% had their cases dismissed, and 0.2% were found not guilty at trial. Of the 335 who were convicted, 97.6% received a prison sentence, 2.1% were sentenced to probation only, and 0.3% received only a fine. Thus, once federal prosecutors decide to move a child sex transportation case forward, they are quite successful in securing a conviction and a prison sentence.

Similar to the increase in the federal prosecutions and convictions for child sex trafficking cases, there has also been an increase in prosecutions and convictions for other federal sex trafficking cases. The majority of these other sex trafficking prosecutions (not involving a child) are handled by the Department of Justice's Civil Rights Division (CRD) and the United States Attorney's Offices (U.S. Department of Justice [DOJ], 2010). According to the Attorney General's Annual Report on Trafficking in Persons (DOJ, 2010), there is clear evidence that the volume of these federal sex trafficking prosecutions has grown substantially from 2001 to 2009 (see Figures 6.1–6.3).[2] During the first 3 years (2001–2003) after the passage of the TVPA (2000), there were 19 cases filed, 74 defendants charged, and 54 convictions in federal sex trafficking cases involving force, fraud, or coercion. During the next 3 years (2004–2006), there were 71 cases filed, 200 defendants charged, and 116 convictions. Then, during the following 3 years (2007–2009), there were 69 cases filed, 166 defendants charged, and 163 convictions.

Since the convictions secured in a given year may involve cases that were filed in previous years, we cannot determine a conviction rate for federal sex trafficking cases based upon the data from the Attorney General's report (DOJ,

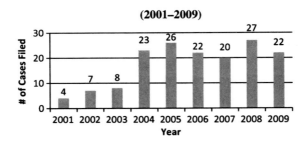

FIGURE 6.1 Sex trafficking cases filed.
Source: DOJ, p. 62.

2010). Other sources of data on human trafficking prosecutions, however, suggest that there is a high conviction rate in federal human trafficking cases. In a review of 298 human trafficking cases prosecuted under the TVPA between 2001 and 2007, Clawson et al. (2008) found that 77% resulted in a conviction—47% of the cases involved plea negotiations and 30% resulted in a conviction at trial. Thus, once the decision is made to prosecute a human trafficking case, U.S. Attorneys are likely to secure a guilty verdict in the majority of the cases. In these cases, punishments ranged from probation to 50 years in prison, with an average sentence of $6\frac{1}{2}$ years (Clawson et al., 2008).

Data from the Attorney General's reports (DOJ, 2007, 2010) suggest that sentence lengths may be increasing. Of the 62 offenders who were convicted of a federal human trafficking offense in 2007, 53 were sentenced to prison. These prison sentences ranged from 1 to 480 months (40 years), with an average prison sentence of 9.4 years (DOJ, 2007). In 2010, there were 112 offenders convicted of a federal human trafficking offense and 104 were sentenced to prison. These prison sentences ranged from 3 to 644 months (53.67 years), with an average sentence of 11.8 years (DOJ, 2010). Thus, both the range and the average length of sentence were higher in 2010 compared to 2006.

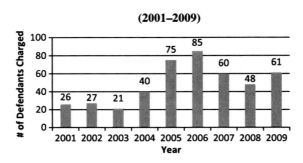

FIGURE 6.2 Sex trafficking defendants charged.
Source: DOJ, 2010, p. 62.

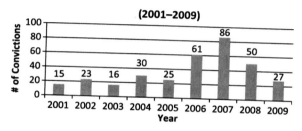

FIGURE 6.3 Sex trafficking convictions.
Source: DOJ, 2010, p. 62.

CHALLENGES AND BARRIERS TO SEX TRAFFICKING PROSECUTIONS

While federal prosecutors are successful in securing convictions in human trafficking cases, not all human trafficking cases are prosecuted. According to a Bureau of Justice Statistics report on federal prosecutions of human trafficking,[3] U.S. Attorneys closed 377 human trafficking cases between 2001 and 2005 (Motivans & Kyckelhahn, 2006). While 39% of these cases were prosecuted, 59% were closed because the U.S. Attorneys declined to prosecute the case. The reasons for not prosecuting the case include: "lack of evidence of criminal intent (29%), weak or insufficient admissible evidence (28%), prosecution by other authorities or facing other charges in federal court (14%), no federal offense evident (9%), and other (20%) reasons" (Motivans & Kyckelhahn, 2006, pp. 1–2).

Federal prosecutors face a number of challenges or barriers to prosecuting sex trafficking cases. Since sex trafficking investigations and prosecutions rely heavily on the testimony of the victim(s), there are a number of issues related to sex trafficking victims that can create barriers to prosecution. One of the greatest challenges for law enforcement officers and prosecutors is gaining the trust and cooperation of the victim(s). Owing to fear of being deported and/or arrested for prostitution, sex trafficking victims may fear and/or distrust law enforcement (Coonan, 2010). Also, since traffickers may threaten to harm the victim and/or the victim's family in an attempt to keep victims from going to the authorities, the victims may be too afraid to identify and testify against their trafficker(s) (Clawson et al., 2008; Coonan, 2010). If the safety of the victim and the victim's family cannot be ensured, then victims are likely to be uncooperative and/or reluctant to testify (Clawson et al., 2008). Furthermore, if victims do not have financial support and a safe place to stay, they may recant and return to their trafficker(s) (Clawson et al., 2008). Without the testimony of the victim, prosecutors are not likely to secure a conviction. As a result, prosecutors may have to decline to prosecute a case.

Another barrier to prosecution in sex trafficking cases is the high burden of proof needed to establish that the trafficker(s) used force, fraud, or coercion to get the victim(s) to engage in a commercial sex act (unless the victim is under the age of 18). In doing so, the prosecutor must prove that the victim did not consent to the commercial sex act(s) (Coonan, 2010). It may appear relatively simple to prove that an individual did not want to engage in commercial sex acts, but the issue becomes particularly complicated when victims initially consent to be smuggled into the country and/or consent to work (in a nonsexual manner) for a trafficker. In some cases, victims who face poverty, homelessness, and/or desperation are lured into prostitution by traffickers who promise them a better life (Coonan, 2010). Many victims, domestic or international, desire new opportunities and willingly follow the trafficker whose end goal is not apparent to the victims. While this aspect of trafficking is recognized under the UN protocol, which includes "the abuse of power or of a position of vulnerability" as one of the means of trafficking, the TVPA only recognizes trafficking committed by "force, fraud, or coercion." Also, when the specified means of trafficking are present, the UN protocol explicitly states that the consent of the victim is irrelevant (UN Protocol, 2000), however, the TVPA is silent on the issue of consent (Kandathil, 2005). Therefore, in the United States, some defendants may use the consent of the victim(s) as a defense.

While some sex trafficking victims initially agree to engage in sex work, they may end up working under inhumane and coercive conditions (Coonan, 2010; Kandathil, 2005). If physical force or restraint was not used, it is extremely difficult for prosecutors to secure a conviction for sex trafficking (Kandathil, 2005). Even when victims have been beaten, abused, and/or psychologically manipulated by their traffickers, however, prosecutors may still have a difficult time convincing the court that these are "real" victims (Coonan, 2010; Kandathil, 2005). Also, international sex trafficking poses a unique challenge because immigration issues fill the political and social arena; juries may place undue emphasis on the fact that victims arrived in the United States illegally (Overbaugh, 2009).

Since a jury may not grasp the complexities of a sex trafficking situation, they may not understand why the victim(s) initially consented to engage in sex work and/or why the victim(s) did not escape their captors. Jurors also may be unsympathetic to those who knowingly violated immigration laws (Overbaugh, 2009). Therefore, in such cases, prosecutors may decide to prosecute the offender for other federal offenses, such as violations of immigration law, conspiracy, and Mann Act offenses, where the consent of the victim is irrelevant (Coonan, 2010; Kandathil, 2005). The problem with not prosecuting the offender for a "severe form of trafficking" under the TVPA, however, is that the victims may not be provided with the same protections (Kandathil, 2005).

Other barriers to prosecuting sex trafficking cases arise as a result of a lack of funding and resources (Clawson et al., 2008). Owing to the length of time that it takes to investigate and prosecute federal sex trafficking cases, which can take twice as long as other federal cases, there is a significant amount of funding and personnel resources needed to prepare a case. At the same time, funding and resources are needed to provide the sex trafficking victims with necessary services (Clawson et al., 2008). As a result, U.S. Attorneys are not able to pursue all sex trafficking cases that come to their attention.

STRATEGIES FOR SUCCESSFUL SEX TRAFFICKING PROSECUTIONS

There are a number of factors, however, that can help lead to a successful prosecution. Since successfully prosecuting a sex trafficking case often hinges on the cooperation and testimony of the victim(s), investigations and prosecutions must be "victim-centered" (Coonan, 2010). That is, the well-being of the victim must be considered as a priority. Law enforcement officials and prosecutors must be patient with the victim(s), develop rapport with each victim, demonstrate concern for the victim's well-being, and gain the victim's trust (Clawson et al., 2008; Coonan, 2010). Therefore, both law enforcement officers and prosecutors need to receive training to understand the complex issues involved in sex trafficking cases and to learn how to work with victims (Clawson et al., 2008). This training should include "sensitivity training in working with traumatized persons and persons of different cultures" (Clawson et al., 2008, p. 21). Also, since victims often have legitimate safety and financial concerns, these cases require coordination and cooperation between local and federal law enforcement officers, prosecutors, and victim service organizations (Coonan, 2010).

Even though sex trafficking prosecutions depend heavily upon victim testimony, testimonies are not the only evidence admitted during a trial. Sex traffickers control every aspect of a victim's life, and this information can be proven and used against traffickers in court. The most convincing physical evidence that is utilized by prosecutors is often found at the locations where victims live or engage in forced sexual acts (Moossy, 2009). Prosecutors frequently use photographs of the traffickers and victims together that have been taken by law enforcement agents or the victims themselves (Hughes, 2005). Law enforcement agents during search and seizures should take pictures of the living conditions of victims and any locks or restraints throughout the location because these photographs can be used to illustrate manipulation and complete control over the victims (Moossy, 2009). Lists of contacts, email messages, and advertisements for sexual services provide evidence against the traffickers (Hughes, 2005). Debt and income ledgers demonstrate the financial side of the sex trafficking business (Moossy, 2009). Following the money is beneficial due to the substantial amount of money generated by sex trafficking (Moossy, 2009). Diaries given to the victims by the traffickers can be very useful in court. Victims may detail their experiences and emotions while living and working for the traffickers against their will (Hughes, 2005). Through a combination of victim testimony and physical evidence, compelling cases and successful prosecutions emerge.

Examples of Successful Sex Trafficking Prosecutions

By examining several sex trafficking prosecutions, we can see how prosecutors are able to secure convictions in sex trafficking cases. First, we discuss the prosecution of an international sex trafficking case (*U.S. v. Cortes-Meza,* 2011), which involved a sex trafficking ring who brought 10 women and girls from Mexico to the United States and forced them to work as prostitutes. Next, we discuss the prosecution of an interstate sex trafficking case, which involved a sex trafficking ring responsible for the prostitution of juveniles within the United States (*U.S. v. Pipkins*, 2004). Finally, we discuss the prosecution of a sex trafficking case in which a mother prostituted her daughter (*U.S. v. O'Connor*, 2011). While the contexts of these sex trafficking cases differ, the strategies used by prosecutors to secure convictions in each of the cases are similar. Specifically, each of these cases demonstrates the importance of victim testimony, using a wide range of federal charges, and plea bargains in securing convictions in sex trafficking cases.

U.S. v. Cortes-Meza *(2011)*
Beginning in 2006, Immigration and Customs Enforcement (ICE) investigated a sex trafficking ring in metro-Atlanta and discovered that Juan, Francisco, and Amador Cortes-Meza along with three other men were the perpetrators (*U.S. v. Cortes-Meza*, 2011). The men had lured approximately 10 Mexican women, including four juveniles, to the United States with the promise of a better life (ICE, 2011). Upon arrival in the United States, the traffickers informed the women that they would be working as prostitutes to payoff a smuggling debt. The traffickers forced the women to work in prostitution by using a combination of physical assault, verbal abuse, psychological manipulation, romantic gestures, and false promises (*U.S. v. Cortes-Meza*, 2011). In 2008, a grand jury indicted Juan, Francisco, Amador, and the three accomplices on a total of 34 charges (*U.S. v. Cortes-Meza*, 2011). Francisco Cortes-Meza pled guilty to "commercial sex trafficking by force, fraud, or coercion" in violation of the TVPA (*U.S. v. Cortes-Meza*, 2011, p. 2). Juan Cortes-Meza pled guilty to "sex trafficking of a child by force, fraud, or coercion, in violation of 18 U.S.C. § 1591(a) and one count of importation of an alien for immoral purposes" (*U.S. v. Cortes-Meza*, 2011, p. 2). Francisco received a total of 20 years imprisonment, and Juan received a sentence of 16 years and 8 months imprisonment.

On the other hand, Amador Cortes-Meza, the leader of the sex trafficking ring, proceeded to trial in the fall of 2010. Prosecutors relied heavily on victim testimony to corroborate claims of physical abuse, fear of the traffickers, and the overall trafficking scheme. Nine of the 10 victims testified against Amador (ICE, 2011). The victims identified the houses in which they were confined, recounted horrendous memories of brutal beatings, and revealed their fear of the traffickers (ICE, 2011). One victim testified that she met Amador at 14 years of age, and Amador had convinced her that he loved her (ICE, 2011). She was then smuggled into the United States, forced into prostitution for 3 years, and, at one point, had a knife pulled on her by Amador (ICE, 2011). These victim recollections assisted in Amador's final conviction. The jury found Amador guilty of sex trafficking minors, "sex trafficking by force, fraud and coercion, transporting minors for the purpose of prostitution, smuggling aliens into the United States for purposes of prostitution, and conspiracy to do the same" (ICE, 2011). Amador's sentence was 40 years imprisonment with an additional

5 years of supervised release and mandatory restitution, ranging from $6,000 to $80,000, for eight of the victims (ICE, 2011).

U.S. v. Pipkins *(2004)*

In one infamous case in Atlanta, Georgia, *U.S. v. Pipkins* (2004), it is clear that U.S. Attorneys were able to overcome some of the barriers and challenges to prosecuting a sex trafficking case. In this case, federal prosecutors indicted 15 pimps involved in juvenile sex trafficking from 1997 to 2001 (*U.S. v. Pipkins*, 2004). Specifically, the pimps recruited young women from various states, such as Tennessee, prostituted the girls in Georgia, and occasionally in other states, and used Internet sites to locate clients (*U.S. v. Pipkins*, 2004). Thirteen of the 15 predominantly male pimps listed in the grand jury indictment pled guilty to trafficking-related charges, but two defendants, Charles Floyd Pipkins (also known as "Sir Charles") and Andrew Moore (also known as "Batman") proceeded to trial (*U.S. v. Pipkins*, 2004).

The trial, and its subsequent appeals, revealed the high degree of organization and intricacies within the sex trafficking ring. The criminal ring had organized hierarchies for both pimps and the women. The hierarchy for women included a "bottom girl" at the top of the chain of command and a "wife-in-law" for supervisory responsibilities (*U.S. v. Pipkins*, 2004). A pimp hierarchy contained "popcorn pimps," "hustlers," or "wannabes" at the bottom of the ladder, and "players" occupied the highest respected level of pimps (*U.S. v. Pipkins*, 2004). Sir Charles had allegedly reached "player" status. Moore received the label "guerrilla pimp" because he used intimidation and violence to influence the behavior of the women under his control (*U.S. v. Pipkins*, 2004). The women were obligated to engage in sex in exchange for money, surrender all earnings, obey all orders, and engage in sexual intercourse with the traffickers when the men desired (*U.S. v. Pipkins*, 2004). Multiple pimps aided each other in securing more women, bailing the girls out of jail, geographically dividing the areas for prostitution, "mentoring" new girls, and traveling across state lines (*U.S. v. Pipkins*, 2004). Demonstrating this extreme level of cooperation and organization helps a prosecution to obtain Racketeering Influenced and Corrupt Organizations Act (RICO) enterprise convictions. Therefore, prosecutors secured testimony from both pimps and victims of the enterprise. Four of the pimps from the original indictment and 14 of the girls testified on behalf of the government, which proved especially vital for acquiring RICO enterprise charges against both Pipkins and Moore (*U.S. v. Pipkins*, 2004).

Ultimately, Pipkins and Moore were found guilty of "conspiring to participate in a juvenile prostitution enterprise affecting interstate commerce through a pattern of racketeering activity," which constitutes a RICO violation (*U.S. v. Pipkins*, 2004). The jury also found Pipkins guilty of "enticing juveniles to engage in prostitution" in violation of the Mann Act, "using interstate facilities to carry on prostitution" (18 U.S.C. § 1952), extortion (18 U.S.C. § 1951), involuntary servitude (18 U.S.C. § 1584), "transfer of false identification documents" (18

U.S.C. § 1028), and "distribution of marijuana and cocaine to minors" (21 U.S.C. § 859) (*U.S. v. Pipkins*, 2004, p. 1287). The jury convicted Moore on additional charges of "enticing juveniles to engage in prostitution," "using interstate facilities to carry on prostitution," four counts of extortion, six counts of involuntary servitude, and "distribution of marijuana and cocaine to minors" (*U.S. v. Pipkins*, 2004, p. 1287).

The defendants challenged the RICO conspiracy violations and whether the sentencing guidelines were properly administered (*U.S. v. Pipkins*, 2004). Pipkins appealed on the grounds that his acts did not constitute extortion and that there was not enough evidence to convict him of involuntary servitude and the transfer of falsified documents (*U.S. v. Pipkins*, 2004). The Eleventh Circuit Court of Appeals analyzed the prosecution's evidence of organized and cooperative interactions between the defendants and other pimps (*U.S. v. Pipkins*, 2004). Testimony from one of the victims demonstrated that Pipkins had enticed girls to work for him and obligated that the girls received identical tattoos (*U.S. v. Pipkins*, 2004). Both Pipkins and Moore worked alongside other pimps in southwest Atlanta and shared resources. All of these facts and others led the Court to confirm the RICO conspiracy charges.

Additionally, Pipkins challenged the extortion conviction by claiming that the girls voluntarily gave their earnings to him because of a prearranged contract (*U.S. v. Pipkins*, 2004). Through the testimony of several of the women, the prosecutor was able to establish that the girls turned over their money due to fear of retaliation from their pimps (*U.S. v. Pipkins*, 2004). Therefore, the extortion convictions were upheld (*U.S. v. Pipkins*, 2004). In regard to Pipkins's claim that the girls were free to leave at any time, the Court rejected the argument (*U.S. v. Pipkins*, 2004). The Court cites victim testimony that proved intimidation tactics were used against the juveniles (*U.S. v. Pipkins*, 2004). Pipkins was also unsuccessful in his attempt to overturn the transfer of false documents conviction. Sentence guidelines were found to be applied correctly, and the original sentences were affirmed—30 years of imprisonment for Pipkins and 40 years of imprisonment for Moore.

In this case, prosecutors relied significantly on RICO and Mann Act charges in order to ensure lengthy sentences for the two leaders of the sex trafficking ring. This case illustrates how federal prosecutors often seek charges other than TVPA violations in order to ensure convictions against sex traffickers. The prosecutors were able to secure convictions for individual criminal acts such as distribution of drugs as well as the overall forced prostitution of juveniles.

U.S. v. O'Connor *(2011)*

The case of *U.S. v. O'Connor* (2011) demonstrates that the TVPA and related charges can be applied to a broad range of cases. While both *U.S. v. Cortes-Meza* (2011) and *U.S. v. Pipkins* (2004) involved large-scale sex trafficking rings, *U.S. v. O'Connor* (2011) shows that the existence of such a sex trafficking ring is not necessary to yield a federal trafficking charge. In this case, charges were only filed against two individuals—Linda O'Connor and Dean Sacco.

Linda O'Connor sexually abused, condoned sexual abuse, and profited from the sexual exploitation of her juvenile daughter, referred to as S.O. (*U.S. v. O'Connor*, 2011). O'Connor was unable to make rent payments and provided her daughter to the landlord, Dean Sacco, to compensate for the lack of rent (*U.S. v. O'Connor*, 2011). Sacco arrived from out of state to take sexually explicit pictures and engage in sexual intercourse with S.O. when she was approximately 12 years old (*U.S. v. O'Connor*, 2011). At times, O'Connor would actually participate in the illicit activity. Social services became involved when S.O. attempted suicide and was hospitalized. S.O. tried to reveal the abuse by men, but O'Connor maintained custody of her and the sexual abuse continued (*U.S. v. O'Connor*, 2011). On several occasions, O'Connor and S.O. traveled from Deposit, New York, to Binghamton, New York, where S.O. was forced to prostitute herself as her mother sat in the same room watching television (*U.S. v. O'Connor*, 2011).

Federal charges were brought against both Sacco and O'Connor. Evidence against Sacco included a used condom with S.O.'s DNA, a previous victim who testified to sexual abuse by Sacco, and published writings by Sacco that detailed his pedophiliac interests (*U.S. v. O'Connor*, 2011). Testimony from S.O., social workers, law enforcement officials, and friends of S.O. helped to secure convictions of both Sacco and O'Connor (*U.S. v. O'Connor*, 2011). Sacco and O'Connor were convicted of sex trafficking of a child in violation of the TVPA. Sacco was also convicted of "buying a child for the purpose of producing child pornography" and "coercing a child to engage in sexually explicit conduct for the production of child pornography," in violation of 18 U.S.C. § 2251. He was also convicted of "travel in interstate commerce with intent to engage in illicit sexual conduct with a minor, in violation of 18 U.S.C. § 2423(b) [Mann Act], and possession of child pornography, in violation of § 2252A(a)(5)(B)" (*U.S. v. O'Connor*, 2011, pp. 2–3). Sacco was sentenced to life imprisonment. A jury found O'Connor guilty of the additional charges of "selling a child for the purpose of producing child pornography," and "permitting her child to be used for the production of child pornography" (*U.S. v. O'Connor*, 2011, p. 3). She was sentenced to 30 years imprisonment and a lifetime of supervised release (*U.S. v. O'Connor*, 2011).

As it has been noted, sex trafficking presents itself in a variety of forms. Federal laws are in place to prosecute large-scale international and domestic sex trafficking cases as well as isolated incidents. The TVPA, RICO, child pornography laws, falsifications of documents, and other related offenses can be used to effectively prosecute sex traffickers.

NOTES

1. The "child sex transportation" offenses include sex trafficking of children (18 U.S.C. 1591) and transportation for illegal sexual activity involving coercion and enticement (18 U.S.C. 2422) and the transportation of minors (18 U.S.C. 2423).

2. Since there may be several months between the time that a defendant is charged and the time that he/she is convicted, a defendant who is charged in one year may not be convicted until the following year. Therefore, the number of defendants charged in a given year may not be directly related to the number of convictions in that same year.
3. This includes cases prosecuted under any of the statutes contained in 18 U.S.C. 1581 to 1594.

REFERENCES

Clawson, H. J., Dutch, N., Lopez, S., & Tiapula, S. (2008, September). Prosecuting human trafficking cases: Lessons learned and promising practices. Retrieved on March 1, 2012, from https://www.ncjrs.gov/pdffiles1/nij/grants/223972.pdf

Coonan, T. (2010). Anatomy of a sex trafficking case. *Intercultural Human Rights Law Review, 5*, 313.

Hughes, D. (2005). The demand for victims of sex trafficking. *Women's Studies Program: University of Rhode Island, Cooperative Agreement Number S-INLEC-04-CA-0015*, Kingston, RI: University of Rhode Island.

Immigration and Customs Enforcement (ICE). (2011). Head of sex trafficking ring sentenced to 40 years in prison: Amador Cortes-Meza smuggled young victims from Mexico and forced them into prostitution [News Release]. Retrieved from http://m.ice.gov/news/releases/1103/110324atlanta.htm?f=m

Kandathil, R. (2005). Global sex trafficking and the Trafficking Victims Protection Act of 2000: Legislative responses to the problem of modern slavery. *Michigan Journal of Gender & Law, 12*, 87.

Moossy, R. (2009). Sex trafficking: Identifying cases and victims. *National Institute of Justice Journal 262*, Washington, DC: U.S. Department of Justice.

Motivans, M., & Kyckelhahn, T. (2006). Federal prosecution of human trafficking, 2001–2005 (Rep. No. NCJ215248). Washington, DC: Bureau of Justice Statistics.

Motivans, M., & Kyckelhahn, T. (2007). Federal prosecution of child sex exploitation offenders, 2006 (Rep. No. NCJ219412). Washington, DC: Bureau of Justice Statistics.

Overbaugh, E. (2009). Human trafficking: The need for federal prosecution of accused traffickers. *Seton Hall Law Review, 39*, 635–664.

Trafficking Victims Protection Act of 2000 (TVPA), 18 U.S.C. §1590–1594, 22 U.S.C. §7101–7110 (2000).

Trafficking Victims Protection Reauthorization Act of 2003, 18 U.S.C. §1590–1595, 22 U.S.C. §7101–7110 (2003).

Trafficking Victims Protection Reauthorization Act of 2005 (TVPRA 2005), 18 U.S.C. §1590–1595, 22 U.S.C. §7101–7110 (2006).

United Nations Trafficking Protocol. (2000). *United Nations Protocol to Prevent, Suppress and Punish Trafficking in Persons, Especially Women and Children, Supplementing the United Nations Convention Against Transnational Organized Crime*. G.A. Res. 55/25, Annex II, at 31, UN GAOR, 55th Sess., UN Doc. A/RES/55/25 (January 8, 2001), reprinted in 40 I.L.M. 335, 384–385.

United States Department of Justice. (2007). Attorney general's annual report to congress and assessment of U.S. government activities to combat trafficking in persons, fiscal year 2007. Retrieved March 1, 2012 from http://www.justice.gov/archive/ag/annualreports/tr2007/agreporthumantrafficing2007.pdf

United States Department of Justice. (2010). Attorney general's annual report to congress and assessment of U.S. government activities to combat trafficking in persons, fiscal year 2010. Retrieved March 1, 2012 from http://www.justice.gov/ag/annualreports/tr2010/agreporthumantrafficking2010.pdf

U.S. v. Cortes-Meza, 411 Fed. Appx. 284 (2011).

U.S. v. O'Connor, 650 F.3d 839 (2011).

U.S. v. Pipkins, 378 F.3d 1281 (2004).

William Wilberforce Trafficking Victims Protection Reauthorization Act of 2008, 22 U.S.C. §7101–7110 (2011).

CHAPTER 7

Sexual Trafficking: Designing Experiential Learning for Health Professional Students

BARBARA A. ANDERSON

ENCOUNTERING SEXUAL TRAFFICKING

Sexual trafficking is a global and national problem grounded in crime and poverty. A victim of sexual trafficking is highly vulnerable to the power of the trafficker, including abuse, extortion, sexual slavery, overwhelming debt to the enslaver, and assaults upon physical and mental health (Bennett, 1999). These issues are well described elsewhere in this book. This chapter focuses on educating the health professional student about the realities of this global public health problem within the context of vulnerability and resiliency. It draws upon the experience of the author, a nursing and public health educator, in leading students to an understanding of the dynamics of sexual trafficking, the consequences from an individual and aggregate perspective, and strategies to build resilience and cope with this tragedy.

Many health professional students have never had a professional encounter with a person who has been trafficked or who is currently in a sexual trafficking situation. They may have observed prostitutes on the streets at night or been exposed to stories through the media. Rarely, however, have they had a face-to-face human encounter or one in which they were expected to be a therapeutic agent. They often hold strong opinions about the moral character of persons engaged in trafficking, as do their mentors: practicing professionals and educators. While teaching a public health field-based class in Thailand, an American professional colleague expressed that he was flattered that the "girls here seem to like me and to be enjoying their work." Speechless at first, I attempted to explain the roots of sexual exploitation and extortion. To his credit, he listened, shocked as he learned the facts about sexual trafficking in Thailand. Most professionals who encounter the vulnerability and tragedy of sexual trafficking experience this moment of awareness.

I recall my first encounter with a prostitute, an adolescent on the streets of Manaus, an Amazon River city in Brazil. While strolling through Manaus, I locked eyes with a young woman of the streets. I read a duality of messages. She seemed callous, yet vulnerable; brazen, yet fearful; raucous yet innocently young and hurt. She seemed hungry and alone. I slipped a coin into her palm, realizing that her hand felt like any other hand I had ever touched. Kiely (2005) describes such encounters as crossing contextual borders, the beginning of transformational learning.

Such learning experiences are highly valuable for students, promoting tolerance of differences, raising awareness of biases, and increasing sensitivity to human needs (Ryan, Twibell, & Brigham, 2000; Ryan & Twibell, 2002). Such experiences also reveal ethical dilemmas. In discussing these dilemmas, educators often use Rawls' framework of social justice for ethical decision making. This framework puts the individual and the dilemma in question behind a *veil of ignorance*, a moral blinding that assumes the essential human right to justice regardless of the situation or individual culpability (Rawls, 1971). Rawls's *veil of ignorance*, described under the section titled Preparation for Learning, is a penetrating framework to facilitate discussion of ethical dilemmas, cross-cultural perspectives, and cultural biases.

Sexual trafficking is a phenomenon that occurs in a cultural context different from the lived experience of most health professional students. Examining the ethical and social justice ramifications of this issue may be very uncomfortable, especially if the discussion uses Rawls's framework of putting the prostitute or the trafficker behind the veil of ignorance. This framework invites the learner to cross a contextual border, examining biases and awareness of social messages about the culpability of prostitutes. Unfortunately, the topic of sexual trafficking, fraught with such questions, is rarely addressed in cross-cultural learning experiences. Yet it is a critical dimension of learning for health professionals if they are to develop compassionate and skillful care for these most vulnerable of persons.

EDUCATIONAL APPROACHES

Problem-Based Learning

The prevailing curricular approach to any discussion of sexual trafficking is problem based. It assumes the health professional student will learn to assess the problem and the issues surrounding the problem, identify active interventions toward solution, and lead the afflicted toward health. The problem with this problem-based approach is that it orients the student to look for problems before examining the phenomenon. Sexual trafficking is not a recent event. It has occurred throughout history, fueled by lucrative and powerful economic interests that prey upon the vulnerable and the poor. It creates economic incentives and social stratification for the benefit of power structures. To this end, it has been wrapped in salient social messages justifying the creation of social outcasts, such as prostitutes and traffickers (Anderson, 2005; Friedman, 2005; Sen, 2006).

Starting with a problem-based approach precludes exploration of individual or aggregate resiliency, the dynamics of the community in which the phenomenon occurs, the impact of sexual trafficking upon the community, and the community's response.

Resiliency-Based Learning

Newman (2003) defines resiliency as ". . . the process of adapting well in the face of adversity, trauma, tragedy, or even significant sources of stress" (p. 42). de Chesnay (2005) describes the qualities of resiliency as hope, positive action, and movement toward wholeness. Health professional students learning about sexual trafficking are rarely led through a process of examination from a resiliency perspective. They do not know how to look for indicators of resiliency among a vulnerable population, such as victims of trafficking. They have difficulty identifying and processing the community's responses to the issue. These responses can include criminalization, accusation, ignoring, acquiescence, pity, or actions offering alternatives to the victims of trafficking. These community responses and actions are the hallmarks of the interface between community and vulnerability. Failure to study this interface within the context of the community where it occurs leads to a narrowed thinking process, trading the shadow for the substance.

Resiliency-based learning assumes that the community, vulnerable populations within the community, and health professional students learn from and teach each other. Curricular methods include participant observation in the community and deep reflection (Scott, Harrison, Baker, & Wills, 2005; Tanner, 2006) supporting the learning of emotional intelligence (Leonard & Swap, 2004).

EDUCATIONAL DESIGN

There are five key components necessary to facilitate experiential learning about sexual trafficking for health professional students:

- Interdisciplinary education
- Faculty participation
- Preparation for learning
- Face-to-face encounter
- Transformational learning

Interdisciplinary Education

Health professional students are frequently taught in discipline-specific silos. This approach to the education of health care professionals creates tunnel vision about the issue at hand and the perspectives of other health care disciplines. It also limits breadth in studying phenomena occurring in the community and limits the acquisition of active listening skills to one's colleagues, the community, and the vulnerable. The landmark report, *The Future of Nursing: Leading Change, Advancing Health*, emphasizes the critical need for health professional students to be engaged in interdisciplinary education and in full partnership with colleagues from all walks of health care, as well as the community and those they serve (Institute of Medicine and the Robert Wood Johnson Foundation, 2010). Interdisciplinary learning in the context of exploration of a phenomenon within a community and using a resiliency perspective can increase individual learning exponentially.

In an interdisciplinary graduate level public health course, I told the Master's of Public Health (MPH) students the following true story from my field experience. My purpose in using this story was to discuss the dynamics behind sexual trafficking. Perhaps it achieved that purpose, but the serendipity and the real learning in this classroom experience was the interaction and disciplinary perspectives of these MPH students from multiple health care disciplines.

CASE STUDY #1
A CLASSROOM LECTURE ON THE DYNAMICS OF SEXUAL TRAFFICKING

A young woman worked the streets of a crowded African city. She came from a rural village seeking to help her impoverished family, certain she could find a job as a waitress or a domestic servant. Those jobs were taken. When every opportunity eluded her, in desperation, she turned to the one sure way to make a living in this harsh urban environment. Her experiences tortured her soul and wreaked havoc on her young body. She felt she could not go home again, yet she continued to send money to her parents until she had no extra money when the two babies came along. Tonight she had to make some money. The children had not eaten for two days. She spied a foreign man walking alone and approached him. He waved her away. She was desperate. She continued to follow him. She offered him anything he wanted, with or without a condom, any kind of sex he desired. He started to push her away again, but something stopped this young public health volunteer worker. In the local language that he had learned in his training program, he asked what she needed that she was so desperate on the streets. No one had ever asked her that question before. Weeping, she explained she had to feed the children tonight.

The classroom was silent. A few students looked around in discomfort. One looked angry and another wiped tears from her eyes. Finally, I

(continued)

broke the silence, asking, "So, what were the dynamics of sexual trafficking in this case?" No one answered that question. The discussion among these MPH students, learning together in the classroom, reflected their discipline-specific approaches but also their willingness to learn from each other:

> "Good thing that guy didn't have sex with her. She's high risk for HIV-AIDS" *MD*

> "Exactly! This is the kind of story that needs to hit the press. It's so about life!" *Journalist*

> "But nobody's going to live very long without some food" *Social worker*

> "I wonder about her children—where are they, alone in this city, hungry, probably sick. Does she know how to take care of the children?" *RN*

> "Does she even know how to take care of herself? I wonder how she was feeling having to offer any kind of sex to this stranger." *Psychology major*

> "Yah, but she's doing the best she can. I keep telling you guys that this is exactly the kind of situation that women face in poor urban environments. *Inner city community development worker*

> "That's right. She is living within the context of a community that defines her role and her value." *Undergraduate anthropology major*

> "She needs our support and our compassion. I wonder what the young man did about this situation?" *Protestant minister*

At that point, the class was over but the discussion had just begun. The conversation was animated, as the students picked up their books and left the classroom. They were listening to different perspectives, reaching out from their discipline-specific silos. The learning had begun.

Faculty Participation

For an educator, it is a limited experience to describe the "dynamics of sexual trafficking" within the protection of the classroom. It is a much deeper experience to lead students, in the classroom or in the field, through a deep experiential learning experience. In particular, field experiences that include participant observation and deep reflection require exquisite sensitivity to the learning environment. "Experiential learning is fraught with uncertainty as field experiences can change rapidly. Yet these serendipitous events often provide the richest learning" (Dyjack, Anderson, & Madrid, 2001, p. 245).

The health professional student is generally a novice in the area of sexual trafficking. Benner (2000) describes the educator's role in moving a student from novice toward expert by providing coaching, monitoring, and effective management of rapidly changing situations. Faced with the tragedy of sexual trafficking in the classroom situation but more so in the field, students can easily become overwhelmed. The faculty role is:

- Coaching students through the experience with reflection and introspection
- Getting out of the way and letting the student experience learning
- Monitoring the field situation for opportunities to learn and for "time out" if the situation becomes emotionally overwhelming or dangerous
- Managing situations as they move quickly from one dynamic to another

Preparation for Learning

Orientation and preencounter preparation are essential for the student to maximize learning and to adapt during the learning encounter (Ryan & Twibell, 2002). This is particularly important when preparing students to cope with the tragedies surrounding trafficking. I have developed a six-step approach to preparing students for field experiences that may include exposure to trafficking.

The Veil of Ignorance

The first learning activity is to discuss Rawls's veil of ignorance as a model in decision making within the context of social justice. The value of discussing this construct is that is unveils biases and helps the learner to consider ramifications of social justice for those who society proclaims least worthy of justice. It places the individual and the dilemma in question behind a veil of ignorance, a moral blinding that assumes the right to social justice (Rawls, 1971). While not always a comfortable approach for students, it is a powerful tool to facilitate discussion about vulnerability, social value, and biases. Benner, Surphen, Leonard, and Day (2010) describe this kind of learning environment as a forum for the development of moral imagination.

Meaning and Metaphor

Signature stories that reveal meaning, world view, culture, and lived experience are powerful ways to draw students into deep reflection about profound social issues (Anderson, 2009, November 3). The case study above exemplifies the many ways in which students may view a situation. Telling stories, especially in an interdisciplinary setting, allows everyone to share in the perceptions of others around a common experience: the story. Examining metaphors as they arise helps students to experience the world of trafficking through symbols.

A metaphor uses a concrete image to project an abstract concept. In the 1800s, a common metaphor to describe a prostitute was *soiled dove,* projecting an image of a gentle bird that had become dirty. The prostitute was not *like* a soiled dove—she *was* a soiled dove. Other examples of metaphors around trafficking, projecting a concept from an image, include "she is a piece of trash" or "he is the dark side." Discussing how language frames the social construct often reveals how differently students, one from another, understand words. "Human understanding is by no means guaranteed because conversants share the same dictionary" (Barnhund, 1994, p. 27). Discussion of metaphor and meanings helps students to use symbols to identify biases, express fears about new experiences, and glimpse cross-cultural differences around highly charged social issues.

Crossing Contextual Borders

Learning can be further enhanced through practice in crossing contextual borders. One way is to visualize the experience of trafficking from different perspectives: the young trafficked child, the drug-addicted youth on the streets of a large city, the middle-man pimp caught in the crosshairs of the trafficking mafia, or the father whose daughter has been kidnapped and abducted into a trafficking ring. This experiential learning starts with a call to imagine how one would feel in these situations. This exercise can be followed by having students create and enact stories from different perspectives. Before taking a group of health professional students into community settings that involved interface with sexual trafficking, this kind of visioning, crafting stories, and enacting events not only develops awareness but moves toward adaptation when faced with the reality. Benner et al. (2010) describe this approach as integrative teaching, preparing the student with knowledge, skills, and moral imagination.

CASE STUDY #2
CROSSING CONTEXTUAL BORDERS:
THE STORY OF A YOUNG LAWYER

William, a young law student, needed to complete a pro bono experience. He came to see me, knowing that I have worked with vulnerable populations. I suggested he consider working with an awarded, highly regarded community organization addressing the needs of refugees, including many youth who had been forced into sexual slavery. One of my graduate students was completing an internship at this site and agreed to serve as his preceptor. The son of physicians, he was a child of privilege. Yet he had experienced the vulnerability of growing up Black in America. He yearned to understand vulnerability and resilience as experienced by others. He got the hardest assignment of all—working with the legal aid needs of trafficked refugee youth. A key part of William's learning was to enter into the contextual worlds of refugees, vulnerable youth, sexually trafficking, and the stresses of a chronically underfunded community organization. Under his preceptor, he explored these issues from a community-based perspective. This orientation and preparation enabled

(continued)

him to enter into this pro bono experience with breadth and awareness. This experience also shaped his life. As a lawyer, he now works to promote social justice through legal aid for the homeless.

Focusing on Resilience

Practicing health care professionals encountering the realities of sexual trafficking may become overwhelmed, judgmental, or withdrawn. None of these responses offers a therapeutic approach to the victim of trafficking. Identifying vulnerability and resilience, as demonstrated by the victim and the community, are ways to help health care professional students develop the skills to work effectively with persons who have been trafficked.

Egyptian-born Shyima Hall, at the age of 8, was sold into slavery by her family. Her enslavers smuggled her to California where she lived under the most oppressive of circumstances. She was denied basic education, affection, and childhood while slaving 16 hours a day for a wealthy family that kept her captive. Five years later, acting on a tip, the U.S. Immigration Services rescued her and her enslavers were prosecuted, imprisoned, and later deported. Shyima survived the foster care system, bonding with caring individuals. Now, as a young adult, she has received American citizenship, has a job, and is enrolled in a community college (Wilson, 2011, December 10). Shyima's resilience is the center of her story. Identifying and discussing the hallmarks of her resilience has been a powerful classroom exercise preparing students who are preparing to encounter trafficking. Educational tools used include:

- Role playing various players in the drama of this trafficking
- Giving examples of how Shyima and the community exhibited resilience
- Crafting a decision tree for survival, as the students think Shyima might have done it
- Writing a journal of observations and feelings before and after this classroom exercise

The Encounter

Encountering sexual trafficking can be a deliberate educational experience or a serendipitous event. After extensive preparation, I have taken students to field sites, both in the United States and in other nations, for the purpose of studying public health issues, including trafficking. Face-to-face encounters in the field are filled with stress, dissonance, intensity, and transformational learning. Pre- and post-experience briefings are essential.

Covenant House is a community-based organization providing shelter, counsel, and rehabilitative services to street children and youth in the United States and across the world. This privately funded organization makes a clear distinction between two categories of vulnerable children and youth on the streets.

"Children *in* the streets" are those many children and youth around the world, including the United States, who have a family of some composition to return to after selling commodities on the streets. "Children *of* the streets" are those children and youth who live entirely on the streets, most often neglected, abused, and sexually exploited. These children and youth are emotionally fragile yet often highly resilient.

Supervising health professional students who interface with this population require vigilance in managing situations as they move quickly from one dynamic to another. Coaching and monitoring are critical functions for the educator but getting out of the way and letting the students experience the stories, the compassion of the staff, the veil of ignorance in action, are just as important. My health professional students who have been privileged to work with street children both at Covenant House and at Casa Alianza, Covenant House in Honduras, Central America, have experienced transformational learning as a result of face-to-face encounters with the children, the staff, and the community caring for these children.

Another kind of encounter, harsher and requiring careful monitoring, preparation, and pre- and post-briefing, is the situation where the community does not reach out to victims of sexual trafficking. The ramifications of the economics of global trafficking are very real in key sites around the world, such as Patpong, the infamous site of sexual tourism in Bangkok, Thailand. This site exists because it is well supported by tourism from around the world. While trafficking of adults and children is illegal in the country, it is widespread and lucrative. Blending into the noise and chaos, students can glimpse the world as experienced by the children and youth for sale, gaining deep learning on vulnerability and resiliency.

CASE STUDY #3
CROSSING CONTEXTUAL BORDERS: YOUNG WOMEN FOR SALE

Angela, a graduate student in community health nursing, elected to study sexual trafficking. As part of a field-based course I taught, she did participant observation in Patpong. Participant observation did not mean she engaged in trafficking or being trafficked, but rather that she became an astute observer of the phenomenon while physically in Patpong, an urban quarter of Bangkok. Prior to the field experience, Angela had done extensive research into the economic roots and public health ramifications of this issue. She had reflected deeply on social justice, the multiple underlying social factors, and her own motivation for studying the needs of young trafficked women. Her journal reflected her observations and her inner experiences as she watched the marketing of the women. She listened to

(continued)

their stories in their limited English. She often sat hand-in-hand with the young women on the street curbs—women from northern Thailand, Cambodia, Vietnam. She was careful not to alienate the pimps or to interfere with business. In exploring her experience, she remarked that nothing in the classroom could have prepared her completely for this reality. Angela chose to have this experience and her faculty coached her, monitored the situation, and allowed her the freedom to have this transformational experience. Today, as a community health nurse, she works with trafficked victims within the United States.

In Mumbai, India, my health professional students have encountered even harsher realities of sexual trafficking: the caging and selling of children. Certainly Shyima experienced this in her captivity in the United States. One nongovernmental organization (NGO) in Mumbai explained their approach to child trafficking by buying the children from the dealers so that kidnapped children could be reunited with their families. In the case of children sold by their families, usually for economic reasons, they did not attempt reunification, expecting that the child would be sold again. Rather, they provided shelter, foster care, and education to those children, often until they were able to obtain a free living situation. This highly controversial approach certainly engendered deep reflection by the students on the economic roots of trafficking, the veil of ignorance, and the role of community response.

Encountering community efforts to address trafficking can be a powerful learning experience for students. I had served as a United States Agency for International Development (USAID) consultant on a number of health-related projects including a project in northern Thailand. This program had three purposes:

- To support local health professionals in their health education efforts with the community on the trafficking risks to children
- To foster awareness and community action for protecting the children from kidnapping by traffickers who prey on children in rural northern villages
- To provide technical assistance to villagers in the development of small businesses to stimulate the local economy and indirectly decreasing the voluntary sale of children due to economic hardship within families

After completing this assignment and with consent from the local community leaders and my Thai field partners, I included a site visit to these villages in a field-based graduate level course for health professional students. These health professional students learned how the people in the community generated solutions for protecting their children. This experience was deep learning about the multiple dimensions of trafficking, the ability of the community to mobilize for action, and the resilience of the community.

Transformational Learning

Benner et al. (2010) describe transformation as "... the development of the senses, aesthetics, perceptual acuities, relational skills, knowledge and dispositions...." (p. 87). Riner (2011) expands on this concept, defining transformational learning as "... a process whereby individuals engage in critical reflection to develop new perspectives, skills and behaviors" (p. 315). This learning is not necessarily a comfortable experience. Deep, transformational learning involves dissonance, recurring reflection, moments of deep awareness (the ah-ha moment), and transformed reality. This reality is often a duality, described by Evanson and Zust (2006) as "bittersweet knowledge."

In a qualitative study of nursing students who had completed an international experience in a very poor area of Guatemala, the authors examined the impact of this experience on the students' later personal and professional lives. They used focus group interviews and individual written narratives. They identified three themes arising from the experience of crossing contextual borders. These themes were *coming to understand,* described as a positive experience; *unsettled feelings,* reflecting discomfort and dissonance; and *advocating for change,* a transformational and ongoing response to the experience (Evanson & Zust, 2006).

Likewise, encountering sexual trafficking is a powerful and lasting experience for the health professional student. Deep learning requires experiential learning about the phenomenon and the vulnerability and resilience of individuals and communities. In order for this experience to be transformational, that is, informing beliefs, attitudes, and skills in future interface with victims of trafficking, the health professional student needs to experience this deep, often uncomfortable, learning.

The educator needs to be very deliberative in designing the learning experience. This requires active faculty participation in preparing and coaching students through the experience with tools of reflection and introspection. It necessitates getting out of the way and letting the student experience the learning. It requires careful monitoring with rapid assessment and intervention to avoid emotional overload or danger, as the situation demands. It requires a bold approach to education and trust in the ability of the health professional students to engage in difficult but transformational learning.

REFERENCES

Anderson, B. (2005). *Reproductive health: Women and men's shared responsibility.* Sudbury, MA: Jones and Bartlett Publishers.

Anderson, B. (2009, November 3). *Meaning and metaphor: Relating to cross-cultural differences and diversity among students of nursing.* Presentation at Kennesaw State University School of Nursing, Kennesaw, GA.

Barnhund, D. (1994). Communication in a global village. In L. Samavar, & R. Porter (Eds.), *Intercultural Communication: A Reader,* p. 27. Belmont, CA: Wadsworth.

Benner, P. (2000). *From novice to expert: Excellence and power in clinical nursing practice*. New Jersey: Prentice-Hall Health.

Benner, P., Surphen, M., Leonard, V., & Day, L. (2010). *Educating nurses: A call for radical transformation*. San Francisco: Jossey-Bass.

Bennett, T. (1999). Preventing trafficking in women and children in Asia: Issues and options. *Impact on HIV, 1*, 9–13.

de Chesnay, M. (Ed.). (2005). *Caring for the vulnerable* (1st ed.). Boston: Jones and Bartlett.

Dyjack, D., Anderson, B., & Madrid, A. (2001). Experiential public health study abroad education: Strategies for integrating theory and practice. *Journal of Studies in International Education, 5*(3), 244–254.

Evanson, T., & Zust, B. (2006). "Bittersweet knowledge:" The long-term effects of an international experience. *Journal of Nursing Education, 45*(10), 412–419.

Friedman, B. (2005). *The moral consequences of economic growth*. New York: Knopf.

Institute of Medicine and the Robert Wood Johnson Foundation. (2010). *The future of nursing: Leading change, advancing health*. Washington, DC: National Academies Press.

Kiely, R. (2005). A transformational learning model for service-learning: A longitudinal case study. *Michigan Journal of Community Service Learning, Fall*, 5–22.

Leonard, D., & Swap, W. (2004). Deep smarts. *Harvard Business Review, 82*(9), 88–97, 137.

Newman, R. (2003). Providing direction on the road to resilience. *Behavioral Health Management, 23*(4), 42–43.

Rawls, J. (1971). *A theory of justice*, Boston: The Belknap Press of Harvard University Press.

Riner, M. (2011). Globally engaged nursing education: An academic program framework. *Nursing Outlook, 59*, 308–317.

Ryan, M., & Twibell, R. (2002) Outcomes of a transcultural nursing immersion experience: Confirmation of a dimensional matrix. *Journal of Transcultural Nursing, 13*, 30–38.

Ryan, M., Twibell, R., & Brigham, C. (2000). Learning to care for clients in their world, not mine. *Journal of Nursing Education, 39*, 401–408.

Scott, S., Harrison, A., Baker, T., & Wills, J. (2005). An interdisciplinary community partnership for health professional students: A service-learning approach. *Journal of Allied Health, 34*(1), 31–35.

Sen, A. (2006). *Identity and violence*. New York: W. W. Norton.

Tanner, C. (2006). The next transformation: Clinical education. *Journal of Nursing Education, 45*(4), 99–100.

Wilson, P. (2011, December 10). Breathing free. *Los Angeles Times*, pp. AA1, AA4.

CHAPTER 8

Trafficking and Women of Color: Hidden in Plain Sight

VANESSA ROBINSON-DOOLEY AND EDWINA KNOX-BETTY

*H*uman trafficking is a major issue for the United States and the world. "Human trafficking includes both sex trafficking and labor trafficking and is the second largest, and fastest growing, criminal industry in the world" (The Advocates for Human Rights, 2009, p. 1). Research, practitioners, and advocacy groups have documented the devastation of this criminal industry. What has not been discussed in great detail is the diversity of experience of the girls and women. The focus of this chapter is to provide the reader with a glimpse into the experiences of women of color (WOC). This chapter will provide a definition of the term "women of color" and an explanation of why it is important to review this issue and its impact on this population. This chapter will also discuss the vulnerabilities and risk factors that are unique to this population and require consideration in any efforts at treatment and rehabilitation. Finally, practice recommendations will be provided that include a focus on the culturally competent interventions and a multidisciplinary approach by social work and nursing.

The authors provide this focus on WOC as a call to all those working in any capacity with victims of human trafficking. We encourage you not to read this chapter as a request for "special attention" to WOC, but more as recognition that certain societal and systemic structures may impact your ability to assist WOC. We hope that readers will be informed and then inspired to use this information in practice.

WOMEN OF COLOR: WHO ARE WE?

The term "women of color" has its roots in the women's movement dating back to the late 1970s. In 1977 the National Women's Conference, provided an opportunity to evaluate and make recommendations on the role of women in the United States through a discussion of specific issues and ideas. Approximately 2,000 delegates from 50 states and six territories participated in the conference, which was authorized by public law and supported with federal funds. They were required to include varied economic, racial, ethnic, religious, and age groups. Although the National Women's Conference was not a lawmaking body and could only propose nonbinding recommendations, it was directed to arrive at a national plan of action to help remove sex barriers and utilize women's contributions better.

Organizers of the conference had developed a three-page "Minority Women's Plank" that many of the minority women in attendance thought was inadequate; it was criticized as not representing the interest of minority women. A group of Black women from Washington, DC, formed a group and created a document called "The Black Women's Agenda" to substitute for the "Minority Women's Plank" that was in the proposed plan of action that they wanted the delegates to vote on.

When the group took the "Black Women's Agenda" to the rest of the attendees, "minority" WOC wanted to be included in the "Black Women's Agenda." The Black women agreed, but could no longer call it the "Black Women's Agenda." It was in those negotiations that the term "women of color" was created. The women did not see it as a biological designation, but a solidarity definition, and a commitment to work in collaboration with other oppressed WOC that have been "minoritized."

The term "women of color" was then, and is now, intended to transcend and embrace shades of color. It is intended to unite women with the following shared global experiences with relationship to varied Western- and European-based cultures:

- Race, class, gender-based oppression, and all intersections
- Militarism, targets of war, and police state
- Displacement
- Loss of autonomy
- Violence as the norm
- Stolen legacy
- Economic disenfranchisement
- Cultural/racial appropriation and genocide

In recent years the term has been questioned by many for valid reasons related to personal identity and definition, and because the word "color" is not the primary issue for many women with shared ethnicity and race (adapted from WOCN website). It is important to remember the history of the term "women of color" and as we work with WOC, we respect their right to self-identify.

STATISTICS ON WOC AND SEX TRAFFICKING

Estimates of the number of trafficked persons vary greatly. The secrecy of the population makes compiling comprehensive data close to impossible. What one finds when examining the statistics is that "women and children" are how trafficking victims are globally defined. Obscured in these million-plus counts are the often-overlooked WOC.

Trafficking is illegal and yet it is extremely difficult to extrapolate the scale of the criminal activity from statistics on arrest and convictions because many victims do not come forward for fear of retribution. Trafficking is a serious health threat and yet it is extremely difficult to extrapolate the scale of the health threat from statistics on medical facilities/emergency department visits and admissions, because many victims do not disclose the nature of their injuries/diseases. In cases involving WOC, there is fear of both law enforcement and the health care systems. Subsequently, if or when victims come to the attention of police officers and medical personnel, they are still very often "hidden in plain sight." WOC are particularly lost in numbers; thus they typically go unidentified and thus underserved.

In searching for numbers on WOC in particular it is not surprising how little is found. A research study about the prostitution and trafficking of 105 Native Women produced by Minnesota Indian Women's Sexual Assault Coalition and Prostitution Research and Education (2011) has found that:

- The women were prostituted and trafficked in multiple locations including indoor (strip clubs, private homes, hotels, bars, escort), and street prostitution.
- About half of the women had been trafficked, almost all engaged in prostitution in order to survive, often under pimp or gang control.
- Extreme and frequent violence was committed against these women over the course of their lives: 79% had been sexually assaulted by an average of four perpetrators; 92% had been raped; 84% had been physically assaulted in prostitution; and 72% had suffered traumatic brain injuries from violence in prostitution.
- Racism was linked to sexism in prostitution and caused the women great emotional distress.
- A majority of the women had symptoms of posttraumatic stress disorder (PTSD) and dissociation as a result of sexual violence.
- 98% of the women were currently or previously homeless; 92% wanted to escape prostitution but did not have other options.
- Many women expressed a need for counseling, health care, domestic violence shelters, rape crisis centers, homeless shelters, and substance abuse treatment centers that incorporated Native cultural traditions into the healing services provided (Minnesota Indian Women's Sexual Assault Coalition and Prostitution Research and Education, 2011).

The authors of the study stress that the women's strengths as well as their vulnerabilities must be seen in the context of a history of colonial harm on Native people, racism, poverty, and a lack of housing, lack of equitable health care, and lack of job/educational opportunities.

The small number of published materials, their geographically limited nature, and the absence of rigorous population-based studies prevent a good estimate of how many Native women and youth experience sex trafficking. Even so, similar findings across these publications suggest that this group is overrepresented among trafficking victims. In a 2006 statewide survey, 14 Minnesota human services providers, nurses, and law enforcement personnel reported working with a total of 345 Native victims of sex trafficking over the previous 3 years (Center on Domestic Violence, 2011).

The same challenges hold true for documenting the experiences of other WOC. Much of what we can surmise comes from the knowledge we have about the regions, countries, and areas of the world women and children are trafficked from. Conservative estimates conclude that over 100,000 women, a number predicted to increase by the end of 2010, are trafficked out of Latin America annually for the purpose of prostitution (Ugarte, Zarate, & Farley, 2003). Richard (2000) estimated that of the individuals trafficked into the United States annually, one-third of them are from Latin America. The danger of sex trafficking between the United States and Mexican border has also been discussed, emphasizing the risk posed due to high unemployment (Ugarte et al., 2003). Reports also indicate that women and children are being trafficked from other countries that include the Caribbean, Dominican Republic, and the Philippines (Pan American Health Organization, 2001).

The Bureau of Justice Statistics (BJS) report *Characteristics of Suspected Human Trafficking Incidents, 2008–2010* (Banks & Kyckelhahn, 2011) describes the characteristics of human trafficking investigations, suspects, and victims in cases opened by federally funded task forces between January 2008 and June 2010. The task forces identified 527 confirmed human trafficking victims. Among the confirmed incidents, sex trafficking victims were overwhelmingly women (94%). On the basis of cases where race was known, sex trafficking victims were more likely to be Black (40%).

VULNERABILITIES AND RISK FACTORS

The purpose of this section is to introduce the reader to the vulnerabilities believed to increase the risk and trauma of sex trafficking for WOC. These vulnerabilities or risk factors include the challenges associated with living in poverty, early abuse, and sexualization of children, and the glamorization by media of the concept of *pimping*. It is surmised that these vulnerabilities have a significant impact on WOC and increase their risk for sexual trafficking. This list is not exhaustive and should be assumed to represent only some of the factors that might contribute to the challenges for WOC. It is hoped that this discussion of these factors will begin the conversation about the challenges for this population of women.

Poverty

Research indicates that trafficked women are typically poor, have few job prospects, limited access to education, and may come from rural areas, depending on the country of origin (Omelaniuk, 2005). Although existing research identifies the role of economics in human trafficking, it has failed to probe the complex relationship among poverty, discrimination, and other sociocultural factors such as minority status (Box, n.d., p. 28).

According to the 2010 U.S Census, the poverty rate for Hispanic and Black women rose even more than the poverty rate for women generally—for Hispanic women to 25.0% in 2010 from 23.8% in 2009, and for Black women to 25.6% in 2010 from 24.6% in 2009 (U.S. Census Bureau, 2011). The economic downturn worsened the experiences of women-headed households, particularly families headed by single Black and Hispanic women. In 2009, four out of 10 Black and Hispanic women-headed households were poor—nearly twice the rate of White women-headed households living below the poverty line (WOC Policy Network, 2010).

One common tactic of sex traffickers is to target and lure poor unsuspecting women with promises of legitimate jobs. Minorities are disproportionately affected by poverty, thus they may be more likely to migrate for better economic opportunities (Omelaniuk, 2005). We can imagine, if not fully understand, how a WOC, trying to escape the snares of poverty, may willingly travel with a "boy-friend" or "employer" because she has been promised paid work upon arrival at the destination. In other cases, the women may receive an advance, often for food, clothes, and makeup, and later they are told they must work for free to repay this debt. This is a common practice known as *debt-bondage*. It does not matter whether the women thought they were making a choice or were "tricked," what they were seeking was economic opportunity.

Early Trauma/Sexualization

Countless studies have confirmed that early childhood abuse increases risk for later victimization. Runaways or homeless girls report that sexual molestation within the family and/or the community is a major problem. O'Connor and Healy (2006) reported that for children under the age of 12, it was a family member who introduced the child to prostitution and sexual exploitation. There is an increased risk for WOC because they often report abuse at an early age. Forty percent of African American women report coercive sexual contact or abuse by the age of 18 (WOC Network, 2006). Ninety-two percent of American Indian girls have reported being forced to have sexual intercourse against their will (NCAIR, 2005), while 6.8% of Asian/Pacific Islanders women report some forced sexual trauma in their lives (USDOJ, OJP, 2006). Hispanic women (11.9%) report being raped at some point in their lifetime (2006). These girls are at increased vulnerability to violence on the streets, in homeless shelters, and within the foster care system. They are also at increased risk of entering the sexual exploitation industry as prostitutes. Hughes (2007) reported that as much as 70% of women involved in prostitution were actually introduced to the industry and hence exploited for sexual pleasure before reaching the age of 18. They are prime targets for being trafficked and prostituted.

Owing to the sensitivity of the subject, child sexual abuse in the African American community is severely underreported. Historically, law enforcement has been used to control African Americans through police brutality and racial profiling. This history of racial discrimination, including the popular stereotype of the Black man as sexual predator, often fosters the victims (and those in the family/community) into silence. It is mostly through retrospective studies that we recognize the impact that this trauma has on Black women as they mature into adulthood. According to an ongoing study conducted by Black Women's Blueprint (2011), 60% of Black girls have experienced sexual abuse before the age of 18.

Media Glamorization

In this era of immediate gratification and reality television, everything is made to seem glamorous and desirable. Our children have become consumers and the focus of aggressive marketing by legitimate industries. It is not a surprise that this same mentality of marketing and glamorization has also become a part of the criminal enterprise of sex trafficking. It has been suggested that in the United States the culture of "pimping and prostitution" has been glamorized (Shared Hope International, n.d., p. 2, b). The precursor to sex trafficking, the acts of pimping and prostitution, are often glamorized in television, movies, and video games. The idea that these activities are somehow normal interactions or interactions that might lead to another life might seem foreign to many, but for those living with trauma or marginalized by poverty and oppression, this is not a significant leap. Individuals living in poverty and despair are often more susceptible to the glamour and media because it is a way of "dreaming" about life on better terms.

The glamorization of pimping and prostitution can often result in normalizing the idea of tolerance for the unspeakable crimes associated with trafficking. This idea of cultural tolerance can be seen in multiple settings that are frequented or utilized by people of color. These include "venues of daily life, including clothing, songs, television, and video games" (Kotrla, 2010, p. 183). One example, oversexualized clothing for children, can be seen by walking through American malls. Stores dedicated to young children (aged 7–11), especially young female children, now sell items such as thongs, bikinis, miniskirts, and form fitting clothing that would be suggestive even for some adult women. There is even a show that glamorizes toddlers for being dressed, in full makeup, looking as much like adult women as possible. Often the sexier the outfit for the toddler, the cuter the child is considered. This new trend has somehow become "cute" and overlooked as something that might be sexualizing our children too early.

Another area of entertainment that contributes to the understanding/perception of WOC is television as an entertainment outlet. Multiple examples of songs can be found where women (or girls) are referred to as "ho's" and are encouraged to perform acts for their male suitor. The songs can often be aggressive and advocate acts of violence against women. A shocking example of the concept of normalization of this culture can be found at the 78th Academy Award in 2005. The song title *"It's Hard Out Here for Pimp"* from the movie *Hustle & Flow*, won the Academy Award for Best Original Song (Kotrla, 2010).

The constant use of the term "pimp" in some cultures continues to glamorize a group of people that serve to degrade women. The act of being a "pimp" is often seen as "cool" or "winning" (Shared Hope International, n.d., a) and these men are also seen as popular culture figures "... admirable rebels, as hip and stylish" (Lagon in Kotrla, 2010). The term can be heard in multiple rap songs, videos, and as roles in video games marketed to children. Kotrla (2010) reports locating an online game, "as a player you get to slap your hoes, pimp the streets, kill the competition, and ally with your friends to the pimp world by storm" (p. 183). This type of play may seem harmless, but it is not. It glamorizes a world of oppression and encourages children to believe that violence and degradation against women is an acceptable form of entertainment. It normalizes violence in impressionable children and contributes to the ongoing tolerance of the sexualization of children.

Access to Health Care

The inability to access adequate health care can also be a contributing factor that continues the victimization of WOC. There are several factors that contribute to the challenges that WOC face in accessing adequate health care. These factors include living in poverty, lower levels of education, and lack of insurance. There are also additional social barriers that could include language, fear, and treatment.

The issue of poverty (mentioned earlier in this chapter) also impacts access to health care by WOC. WOC have higher rates of poverty and lower levels of education when compared to White women (Sharps & Campbell, 2006). These factors impact their access to health care in multiple ways. Poverty could result in lack of access to adequate nutrition to sustain a healthy lifestyle or to manage illness. A life in poverty might involve living in a community with limited health care providers and thus means WOC are unable to obtain regular and consistent care. Lack of transportation, which can often be a result of living in poverty, compounds a WOC's ability to access adequate care. "Given the context of their lives, which often includes lower levels of education, higher rates of poverty, and higher vulnerability to intimate partner violence (IPV), contributes significantly to ... health disparities, including access to care, processes of health care and health outcomes" (Sharps & Campbell, 2006, p. 1). The challenges of poverty are compounded for WOC dealing with the trauma of being trafficked. Their medical concerns could include traumatic injuries and sexually transmitted diseases, all needing ongoing and consistent care for recovery. If the resources are not available and accessible for these women because they live in poverty, they will not get the needed treatment.

Lack of education is another barrier to access to health care for WOC. Lack of education may contribute to a lack of understanding or knowledge about the health care system and how to access the care she might require. Additionally, it is known that limited education is a contributing factor to poverty.

Lack of insurance is another factor that impacts a WOC's access to health care. It is a common misconception that most individuals living at or below poverty levels qualify for publicly funded health insurance. The reality is that low-income women (and other poor adults) do not necessarily qualify for publicly funded insurance. Regulations require that adults have children or a disability to qualify for this insurance. "Medicaid thresholds have been expanded and relatively few states have comparable access expansions to Medicaid for working parents or poor adults without children, leaving many low income women uninsured" (James, Thomas, Ranji, Lillie-Blanton, & Wyn, 2009, p. 101).

PRACTICE RECOMMENDATIONS

In order for any practice techniques to be effective, there must be a multidisciplinary approach to treatment. The foundation of this treatment must be culturally competent and be a combination of efforts by social workers and nurses. This effort must involve a commitment to cultural competence, a focus that is "woman centered," and use of an arsenal of tools that are effective for building a multidisciplinary team approach to treatment. Power and control issues must be "checked at the door" and a commitment to leveling the playing field must be agreed upon by the team. The survivor must be an equal partner in treatment plan development.

Cultural Competency

Cultural competency is one of the main ingredients in closing the disparities gap in health care. It is the way patients and doctors can come together and talk about health concerns without cultural differences hindering the conversation, but enhancing it. Quite simply, health care services that are respectful of and responsive to the health beliefs, practices, and cultural and linguistic needs of diverse patients can help bring about positive health outcomes.

Culture and Language May Influence

- Health, healing, and wellness belief systems
- How illness, disease, and their causes are perceived both by the patient/consumer
- The behaviors of patients/consumers who are seeking health care and their attitudes toward health care providers
- The delivery of services by the provider who looks at the world through his or her own limited set of values, which can compromise access for patients from other cultures

The increasing population growth of racial and ethnic communities and linguistic groups, each with its own cultural traits and health profiles, presents a challenge to the health care delivery service industry in this country. The provider and the patient each bring their individual learned patterns of language and culture to the health care experience, which must be transcended to achieve equal access and quality health care (Office of Minority Health, 2005).

Health care is a cultural construct arising from beliefs about the nature of disease and the human body; cultural issues are central in the delivery of health services treatment, and prevention. By understanding, valuing, and incorporating the cultural differences of America's diverse population and by examining one's own health-related values and beliefs, health care organizations, practitioners, and advocacy groups can support a health care system that responds appropriately to, and directly serves, the unique needs of populations whose cultures may be different from the prevailing culture (Katz, M. personal communication, November 1998).

Being aware of individual self-identification is also an important part of working toward cultural competence. Though it may be obvious to us as service providers that trafficked women are "victims," rarely does a WOC self-identify as such. Working from a culturally competent strength perspective, it is empowering to ask women how they identify and then use that term/label in all future communications.

Woman Centered

A woman-centered approach to health is a human rights–based approach that seeks to ensure that every individual has access to basic health, education, and other social services, including sexual and reproductive health. It provides a framework for prevention, care, and treatment that recognizes the roles women play in their communities, as well as the risks and obstacles each woman faces in accessing her own health care (Center for Health and Gender Equality, Policy Statement, 2010).

A woman-centered approach allows the woman to feel empowered by maintaining control of the process. It is intended to support growth and healing by respecting and accepting all of what the woman brings into the process (Women-Centered Approach Transforms Abortion Care in Europe, 2005). Fundamentally, it is the belief that when women are given unconditional support, they find their own answers.

Multidisciplinary Practice

Social service and medical providers have entered into an era of limited budgets and increased need. Clients are coming to providers with multiple issues that could include medical, mental health, and social needs. Agencies are now tasked with providing several levels of care with limited resources. Reliance on multiple disciplines to provide service has become common. The multidisciplinary approach to practice requires utilizing the skills of professionals to provide the client with efficient and effective service. The professions of social work and nursing are two professions that are trained to deal with the multiple issues that trafficking victims bring to service providers. The vulnerabilities and risks that WOC bring as trafficking victims creates a need for providers to be well trained in handling trauma and its effects.

There are tools and interventions that are well suited for this multidisciplinary approach to serving WOC and other trafficking victims. These tools are techniques that have been used in assessment processes and are believed to be especially helpful in working with WOC dealing with the trauma of human trafficking. The *eco-map, genogram, bio-psychosocial spiritual assessment,* and the *behavioral health referral* are tools and methods that are integral to gathering the necessary information to thoroughly assess the client and provide the foundation for building an effective treatment plan.

The genogram is a family diagram developed from information collected from the client about their family history. Monica McGoldrick and Randy Gerson brought the concept of genograms to the forefront through the publication of their book titled *Genograms in Family Assessment* in 1985. Initially the genogram was a tool used by clinicians, but it has become increasingly applicable to other human service settings. Building a useful genogram requires the collection of a detailed history and nature of relationships from the individual. The client is asked to share the names and background of family members, the nature of the relationship to that family member (divorce, marriage, etc.), and the emotional context of the relationship (tense, close relationship, abusive, stressful, etc.). Shapes, lines, and demographic data are displayed in the shapes. Patterns emerge about the function of family for the client. Practitioners use differing styles in how they design the genogram, but the general model can be expanded to include most historical content. Human service professionals understand the importance of collecting these details from the client. The detailing of the familial relationships in their lives provides a "picture" of how the client interacts with multiple systems and how the client functions within the family environment. This information and diagram will often provide a display of family patterns that assist in explaining family functioning. This information is important to begin any treatment planning for a WOC and trafficking victims.

The Eco-map was developed by Ann Hartman, a social worker, as part of her work with child welfare (Hartman, 1995). This tool is another graphic display, but this one is focused on the client's perception of the important people, agencies, and social networks in his/her life. This information is collected in the assessment process with the client. People and social networks are displayed in circles that are filled in by the client. The strength of these relationships is displayed with lines between the circles (strong, detached, fragmented, etc.). Although this process may sound very similar to the genogram[,] they are different tools. Eco-map development can assist with determining the social interactions and social functioning of the client. "Ecomaps provide an aerial view of the external influences at play on people involved in a genogram, hence they are a tool useful for depicting relationships of families and groups" (Kennedy, 2010, pp. 1–12). The Eco-map provides an opportunity for the client to discuss and describe those multiple external influences that affect their daily lives. The external influences then give the practitioner and the client an opportunity to process the nature of their influence. Most importantly, this tool is done from the client's perspective and often this pictorial view of the external influences can bring some realizations to the client that they were not able to talk about in the past.

The bio-psychosocial assessment is a model of assessment first proposed by the psychiatrist George L. Engel (Engel, 1977). Engel (1977) proposed a theory that would look differently at the medical model in treating disease with patients. The bio-psychosocial assessment is an intensive interview that gathers information about the client's medical needs (bio), mental health concerns (psycho), and social networks and social supports (social). Recently, social workers have advocated for collecting data on clients' faith or spiritual beliefs. An understanding of these areas are important to understanding your client as a holistic being. The collection of the data for this assessment can be a long undertaking because it should include interviews with the client and review of medical records and other secondary documentation that may be provided by the client. What should result is a detailed report that assists with developing a treatment plan with a multidisciplinary team.

Finally, it is recommended that a *behavioral health referral* be a standard of practice, especially for practitioners who might be working in isolation and serving WOC. This referral would involve sending the client to an agency or practitioner for a mental health assessment to determine the client's psychological needs. We must not let the "stigma" of mental health prevent us from providing the assessment and treatment we anticipate women who have been trafficked will need.

The above discussion is a brief overview of each suggested tool, but the readers are encouraged to increase their knowledge about these tools, and put them into practice.

CASE STUDY: DESTINY

Destiny is a 26-year-old Latina woman. She was brought to the emergency department in handcuffs by a policeman who reports upon arresting her when he noticed she had a bloody nose, was battered, and badly bruised. Destiny's blouse was torn partly exposing her breast. The policeman tells the nurse he was patrolling the "track" known for street prostitution. Destiny is cradling her left arm as she rocks back and forth mumbling to "mentir... mentir." Destiny becomes increasingly upset and starts to cry as the police officer continues talking with the nurse. The nurse tells her to "calm down, sugar," to this Destiny responses with an angry outburst,

(continued)

shouting in Spanish what sounds like profanities at the policeman. The nurse looks to the police officer and says, "if she is going to continue to be violent I will not be able to help her." The officer removes the handcuffs and responds "I don't care what ya'll do with the crack-ho" and he leaves.

The nurse motions for Destiny to follow her into a small examining area; she closes the curtain and begins her line of questioning. In broken English, Destiny manages to communicate to the nurse that she recently relocated to the area and is currently living in a local extended stay hotel. She does not have an emergency contact. She reports that she has been on her own since she was 16. The nurse asks Destiny for a urine sample and shows her to the restroom. The nurse goes to the nursing station and recounts the details of her encounter with Destiny. When she returns Destiny is no longer there, a woman in the adjoining area reports Destiny left with a "tall good-looking man."

Analysis

Destiny left home at 16 after years of sexual abuse by her brother and being raped twice by men in the community. Before meeting her pimp, Destiny lived on the streets for years supporting herself by committing petty crimes—stealing food and clothes and tips left on tables at 24-hour diners. Destiny was trafficked from Miami to Las Vegas and then to Atlanta by her pimp. Destiny's 6-month-old baby was taken from her at birth when she tested positive for cocaine, which she has been using for years after she realized it helped to "calm" her. The police officer was one of Destiny's regular unpaying "johns" who was a friend of her pimp. The pimp had inflicted the injuries after Destiny failed to make her nightly quota. Both men were certain Destiny would never report either of them, as they often told her "who would believe a cracked-out ho" and "I can arrest you at any time."

Take a moment in determining what could have been done to provide Destiny quality and culturally competent care? Since this is a hospital setting, how could a social worker have been involved in the service provided to this patient?

Here are a few practice points from the authors, but there are many other areas that could be addressed for this case.

1. Her rights to privacy and confidentiality had been respected.
   Culturally competent woman-centered practice: Create a safe environment so that the woman can share her history and her story (allowed her to cover her exposed breast, not assuming it was okay because she was "a prostitute").
2. She had been asked if it was safe for her to return to her home.
   Culturally competent woman-centered practice: Assess safety immediately. (Remember her room at the hotel is her "home.")

3. She had been offered the services of an interpreter.
   Culturally competent woman-centered practice: Ask if she would prefer to speak with a Spanish-speaking woman or another woman of color. Do not assume you are the best person for her to speak with.
4. She had her arm examined.
   Culturally competent woman-centered practice: Appropriately attending to her obvious/presenting injuries. (This could have provided opportunity to build rapport/trust.)
5. She had been informed why she was being asked for a urine sample.
   Culturally competent woman-centered practice: Explain what is being done/ asked and the reasons. Do not assume that your client understands tests and requests that may seem standard to you.
6. She had been offered a referral/opportunity to meet with a social worker.
   Culturally competent woman-centered practice: Provide her with resources that she may utilize immediately and/or in the future. Provide them in a form that she can keep safe, secure, and secret if needed.

IMPLICATIONS FOR PRACTICE

The above case provides an example of a client dealing with sex trafficking and presenting at medical facility. The analysis discussion focused on how the practitioners could be culturally competent and "woman-centered" in the provision of care. This case can be analyzed even more by discussing how social work and nursing, working as a multidisciplinary team, could provide effective service and develop a treatment plan for Destiny. How could each discipline use some of the tools discussed to assist this client? This chapter focused on WOC and their vulnerabilities and risks related to the trauma of being exploited and trafficked for sex. WOC may have additional challenges that need to be addressed based upon systemic issues that include poverty, media glamorization, and access to health care. Suggestions for practice were provided that included tools that could benefit WOC and other victims of sex trafficking. This is just the beginning of the conversation; the challenge is to build upon what has been learned here and to increase the effectiveness and efficiency of the treatment provided to victims of sex trafficking.

REFERENCES

Banks, D., & Kyckelhahn, T. (2011). Characteristics of suspected human trafficking incidents, 2008–2010. United States Bureau of Justice Statistics. Retrieved from http://www.bjs.gov/index.cfm?ty=pbdetail&iid=2372.

Black Women's Blueprint. (2011). Retrieved from http://newsone.com/1680915/half-of-black-girls-sexually-assaulted.

Box, H. (n.d.). Human trafficking and minorities: Vulnerability compounded by discrimination. *Human Rights and Human Welfare, 28–37.*

Center for Health and Gender Equity, a Woman-Centered Approach to the U.S. Global Health Initiative Policy Statement. (2010). Retrieved from http://www.gender health.org/files/uploads/change/publications/womancenteredapproach.pdf.

Center on Domestic Violence. Retrieved, 2011 from http://www.vawnet.org.

Engel, G. L. (1977). The need for a new medical model: A challenge for biomedicine. *Science, 196*, 129–136. doi: 10.1126/science.847460.

Hartman, A. (1995). Diagrammatic assessment of family relationships. *Families in Society, 76*(2), 111–122.

Hughes, D. (2007). Enslaved in the USA. Retrieved from http://www.nationalreview.com/articles/221700/enslaved-u-s/donna-m-hughes#.

James, C. V., Thomas, M., Ranji, U., Lillie-Blanton, M., & Wyn, R. (2009). Putting women's health care disparities on the map: Examining racial and ethnic disparities at the state level. The Henry J. Kaiser Family Foundation. Retrieved from http://www.kff.org/minorityhealth/7886.cfm.

Kennedy, V. (2010). Eco-maps. *MAI Review, 3*. Retrieved from http://www.review.mai.ac.nz/index.php/MR/article/viewFile/371/546.

Kotrla, K. (2010). Domestic minor sex trafficking in the United States. *Social Work, 55*(2), 181–187.

McGoldrick, M., & Gerson, R. (1985). *Genograms in family assessment.* NY: Norton.

Minnesota Indian Women's Sexual Assault Coalition and Prostituting Research and Education. (2011). Retrieved from, http://www.prostitutionresearch.com/c-trafficking.html

National Congress of American Indians Resolution (NCAIR)(2005). #TUL-05-101. Retrieved from http://www.ncai.org/ncai/data/resolution/annual2005/TUL-05-101.pdf

O'Connor, M., & Healy, G. (2006). The links between prostitution and sex trafficking: A briefing handbook. Retrieved from http://www.humantrafficking.org/publications/401.

Office of Minority Health. (2005). What is cultural competency? Retrieved from http://minorityhealth.hhs.gov/templates/browse.aspx?lvl=2&lvlID=11.

Omelaniuk, I. (2005). Trafficking in human beings. United Nations Expert Group Meeting on International Migration and Development. Retrieved from http://www.un.org/esa/population/meetings/ittmigdev2005/P15_IOmelaniuk.pdf

Pan American Health Organization. (2001). *Trafficking of women and children for sexual exploitation in the Americas.* Washington, DC: Women, Health and Development Program. Pan American Health Organization; 2001 [cited 2008, November 30]. Retrieved from: http://www.paho.org/English/AD/GE/TraffickingPaper.

Richard, A. O. (2000). International trafficking in women to the United States: A contemporary manifestation of slavery and organized crime. DCI Report, United States Department of State. Retrieved from https://www.cia.gov/csi/monograph/women/trafficking.pdf

Shared Hope International. (n.d., a). Demand: A comparative examination of sex tourism and trafficking in Jamaica, Japan, the Netherlands, and the United States. Retrieved from http://www.sharedhope.org/Resources/DEMAND.aspx.

Shared Hope International. (n.d., b). Demand: Fact sheet. Retrieved http://www.sharedhope.org/Resources/DEMAND_fact.aspx.

Sharps, P. W., & Campbell, J. C. (2006). The contribution of intimate partner violence to health disparities for women of color. *Family Violence: Prevention & Health Practice*. Retrieved from http://futureswithoutviolence.org/health/ejournal/archive/1-4/ipv_health_disparities.php.

The Advocates for Human Rights. (2009). The facts: Sex trafficking.

Ugarte, M. B., Zarate, L., & Farley, M. (2003). Prostitution and trafficking of women and children from Mexico to the United States. *Journal of Trauma Practice*, 2(3/4), 147–165.

USDOJ, OJP. (2006). *Extent, nature, and consequences of intimate partner violence: Findings from the national violence against women survey*. Retrieved from https://www.ncjrs.gov/pdffiles1/nij/210346.pdf

U.S. Census Bureau, Income, Poverty, and Health Insurance Coverage in the United States: 2010—Report and Detailed Tables (2011). Retrieved from http://www.census.gov/hhes/www/poverty/data/incpovhlth/2010/index.html.

Women of Color Network Facts & Statistics Collection. Sexual violence: Communities of color. June 2006, IPAS.

Women of Color Policy Network. (2010). Income and poverty in communities of color. Retrieved from http://wagner.nyu.edu/wocpn/publications/files/IncomeAndPovertyInCommunitiesofColor.pdf.

Women-Centered Approach Transforms Abortion Care in Europe. IPAS, Retrieved May 2, 2005, from http://www.ipas.org/Library/News/News_Items/Woman-centered_approach_transforms_abortion_care_in_Europe.aspx.

II

Clinical Perspectives

First-Person Accounts of Illnesses and Injuries Sustained While Trafficked

MARY DE CHESNAY, CHERYSE CHALK-GAYNOR,
JENNIFER EMMONS, EMILY PEOPLES, AND
CHANDLER WILLIAMS

*T*he purpose of the study was to identify types of injuries sustained by women and children prostituted in the sex trade. If nurses and other medical personnel are to help these women and children recover from their enslavement, they need to understand the complexity of deprivation and violence experienced in the trade. Whether runaways, kidnapped, or sold by family members into the sex trade, these women and children find themselves in living conditions that are beyond the belief of most nurses, even those of us who have specialized in rape, child sexual abuse, or intimate partner violence. In order to understand the complexity of their health issues, we must first gather data that help us understand their experiences. The specific aim of this study was to compile data on the types of injuries and illnesses experienced by women and children in the sex trade. The first author served as the principal investigator and the coauthors were coinvestigators. The design was a qualitative content analysis of public statements by victims. Data from the study as well as previous clinical experience of the principal investigator determined the types of conditions focused on in Part II of this book.

STATEMENT OF THE PROBLEM

Research Question

What types of injuries and illnesses are experienced by women and children enslaved in the sex trade? Obviously, nothing can substitute for the words of the victims themselves. The best type of study would involve interviewing people who have experienced the injuries in order to elicit the richness of detail that accompanies the stories told by the people who experienced them. However, to address such a personal and painful topic during interviews would be placing the participants at risk of recalling traumatic memories without appropriate support and would be unethical by the standards to protect human subjects in research. Therefore, the question was asked in such a way that this preliminary study could be conducted from publicly spoken words of the victims as represented in the media and on the web.

Significance

When trafficking victims seek health care, they tend to have serious injuries or illnesses that might be camouflaged by their false stories about how they obtained the illness or injury. They disguise the real reasons for their injuries to protect themselves from retaliation by the traffickers. They may lie, disguise their living arrangements, exhibit Stockholm syndrome, and resist attempts to help them escape. Whatever the presenting problem, it is highly likely that trafficking victims will have underlying malnutrition, sleep deprivation, poor dental health, and possible poorly healed fractures, history of head trauma, and other forms of abuse. Nurses need to understand that their presenting problem may be only the tip of the iceberg and should be prepared to conduct a thorough assessment. Only when we understand these people holistically can we treat them adequately.

Review of Literature

The literature was not reviewed a priori in order to avoid the bias that comes from prior knowledge of what other scholars have published. After the types of injuries were listed during data analysis, several sources were found that addressed the mental health and physical health issues of prostituted women and children.

Two major projects conducted under the auspices of the U.S. Department of Health and Human Services (DHHS) reviewed the literature on medical and mental health needs of victims of trafficking (Clawson, Dutch, & Williamson, 2008, 2010). The physical health issues include fractures, headaches and memory loss (head trauma from beatings), gastrointestinal disorders, infectious diseases, dental problems, malnutrition, pregnancy, and gynecological disorders. At least a quarter of all victims reported physical assaults and over two-thirds reported sexual assaults (Clawson, Dutch, & Williamson, 2008; Estes & Weiner, 2001; Raymond et al., 2002; Zimmerman et al., 2003, 2006). Psychological issues include mood disorders, anxiety, dissociation, and posttraumatic stress disorder (PTSD) (Clawson, Dutch, & Williamson, 2008; Family Violence Prevention Fund, 1999, 2005; International Organization for Migration, 2006; Raymond et al., 2002; Zimmerman & Watts, 2003; Zimmerman & Borland, 2009; Zimmerman et al., 2003, 2006, 2008).

In an ethnographic study in Great Britain, Sanders (2004) found that while the women she studied did have concerns about health conditions such as HIV/AIDS and other sexually transmitted diseases, they were more concerned about violence, which they experienced on a regular basis. Sanders's participants expressed that they felt they had knowledge and resources to handle health risks (the British system is socialized and many education projects have targeted sex workers). However, violence from clients is more prevalent and less predictable. Even more complex than physical risks from violence are the emotional costs of sex work. It is irrelevant in this sense whether the woman is trafficked. She still feels the emotional pain of engaging in work for which she feels shame.

Taylor (2011) examined substance abuse and emotional factors such as depression, PTSD, and anxiety in a literature review. Taylor proposed several intervention models for clinicians. Owing to the high rate of HIV and substance abuse comorbidity, crisis intervention services are needed to help women transition out of life, and long-term therapy is needed for mental health issues.

Baker et al. (2003) studied a purposive sample of 75 Midwestern inner-city sex workers about their health concerns. Since they would have needed signed consent forms to interact directly with the women, they merely observed as the women interacted with the staff of a mobile clinic and wrote field notes after the interaction. The women expressed many health concerns including respiratory (asthma, colds, tuberculosis), drug-related injuries such as lip burns from hot crack pipes, ulcers, rape, beatings, fractures, and sores on their bodies. All asked for condoms. The mental health issues were prevalent with depression and thoughts of suicide mentioned.

Although human trafficking is usually discussed either as sex trafficking or forced labor, some children who are victims are found when the two forms overlap. In particular, the restavek children of Haiti are at high risk for sexual abuse, though they are usually trafficked as domestic slaves. The term "restavek" refers to the long tradition in Haiti of sending the children from poor communities to the city to live with more affluent families in the hope that they will be educated and have a better life than with their parents. Restaveks are likely to be from poor families, be darker skinned, and subject to mental, physical, and sexual abuse (Janak, 2000).

Another factor that contributes to the physical and mental injuries and illnesses of young women who engage in nonconsensual sexual activity is early marriage. In some cultures, women are devalued except in the sense that they can be bought and sold like cattle by their families to improve the lives of the families. Parents who cannot provide for their children will often give up their daughter to have one less mouth to feed. They have a double benefit, one less mouth to feed and the bride price paid to them for the daughter. Child brides are at risk for early pregnancy and often give birth to stillborns after long and difficult labor (Hampton, 2010). A particularly gruesome outcome of early childbirth is vesico-vaginal fistula, leading to incontinence, and embarrassment, which results in banishment from the husband's home.

METHODOLOGY

Design

This qualitative study used the technique of content analysis to identify types of injuries and illnesses reported by victims of sex trafficking. Public statements by victims in books, news articles, and websites were examined for statements about the injuries sustained by the victims. No attempt was made to count frequencies because we recognize that the data sources may not represent the entire population. The intent is rather to present the array of injuries and illnesses in order that clinicians learn to ask the right questions of these patients.

Sample

Over 300 stories by individuals were reviewed and 178 victim reports of health issues, including multiple issues per victim, were included in the final typology. Stories represented American and foreign women and children who had spoken publicly about their experiences. The Institutional Review Board of Kennesaw State University approved the project.

Instrumentation

Stories were read carefully for material related to the research question on types of injuries and illnesses. A search for the previous 5 years was conducted using keywords linking sex trafficking with injuries, trauma, mental health issues, pregnancy, and specific injuries (fractures or broken bones, burns, abrasions, hematomas, wounds, and gunshots). Sometimes stories led to additional keywords to check, such as "burns" led to "acid burns." We also used "torture" and "beatings" to link with human trafficking and eliminated cases that referred to forced labor rather than sex trafficking. Most victims experienced multiple injuries and we found additional injuries such as "knocking out teeth" and "dragging by hair around room." The keywords were searched in the story and placed into tables that listed mental and physical types of injuries and illnesses.

Limitations

It can be considered a limitation of the study that there is no way to verify the truth of the statements made in the news accounts. However, we do not consider this a serious limitation because the reporters could verify the injuries. While we do not accept that every statement printed in the news media is true, we reviewed so many stories that if even a small percentage of stories would be true, the extent of the problem of injuries to prostituted women and children is great enough and verified clinically with our own experience that nurses should pay attention to the source of any injury presented by a patient.

Procedures

The researchers for this study included a professor of nursing, a nursing student, and four prenursing honors students. The professor was responsible for design, Institutional Review Board (IRB) approval, data collection, data analysis, and writing the final report. The students collected data and assisted in the analysis by submitting their tables and assisting with review of literature.

After IRB approval was secured, the students and principal investigator (PI) read widely in the literature (websites, news media, and books) to elicit stories that contained first-person accounts of injuries. Stories were content analyzed by listing each injury as it appeared in each story. The data were then placed into tables that reflect a typology of physical and mental health injuries and illnesses. Once the data were collected, the literature on health issues and needs of survivors was searched to determine whether the data would verify the theoretical literature.

RESULTS

The stories were coded into two categories of data: physical health issues and psychological issues. Since the data are not known to be representative of the population of women and children forced into the sex trade, quantitative measures were not employed. It was not a concern in this study to quantify the injuries, but rather to describe in some detail what these people experience from the limited information available in the news accounts. Table 9.1 lists the types of physical injuries and illnesses found. Table 9.2 lists the psychological issues.

Physical Injuries and Illnesses

It is clear that prostitution is dangerous work. There are numerous accounts of health issues and many are related to beatings, rape, and torture.

Psychological Issues

The mental health issues suffered by these people are profound and long lasting. Complicated by physical illnesses and injuries that sap energy to heal, the psychological effects are perhaps more damaging.

Personal Accounts

In the next section of results, we present some of the quotes from the first-person accounts. At first, we tried to categorize them under either physical or mental health issues, but found this to be arbitrary and we lost the impact of the words. The stories are presented here as they were printed to convey

TABLE 9.1   Physical Injuries and Illnesses

Injury	Illness
Slapped/rough treatment	STIs: gonorrhea, chlamydia, and HIV/
Rape–genital trauma	AIDS
Rape with foreign object-one victim had	Tuberculosis
pieces left inside her leading to infection	Frequent colds, sore throats
and eventually death	Untreated chronic diseases (asthma,
Cigarette burns	gastro intestinal disorders)
Anal rape or fisting and associated back	Substance abuse-medical issues
pain or head trauma	(detox, withdrawal)
Beatings, bruises/abrasions	Pelvic inflammatory disease
Whipped with belt or pimp stick	Gastrointestinal disorders
Threatened or shot with gun	
Cut with knife/razor	
Had face cut with potato peeler	
Hit with car—ran over her repeatedly	
Dragged by hair; clumps missing	
Unwilling pregnancy—sometimes safe	
abortions and sometimes keep the child	
(pimps allow to keep as method of control)	
Unsafe abortion	
Burns—battery acid and hot iron	
Hitting in face and knocking out teeth	

TABLE 9.2   Psychological Issues

Depression
Dissociative reaction
Suicide attempts/ideation
Anxiety
Panic attacks
Agoraphobia
Poor self-esteem, feelings of worthlessness
Shame and guilt
Fear for family members (threats by traffickers)
Substance abuse as an escape mechanism

holistically some of the experiences of the survivors and their families. Some stories fit in several categories, but there are certain concepts we would like to emphasize.

Family Experiences

"I learned that within hours of being taken, my daughter had been drugged and raped by her pimp," she said. "Within 24 hours of my daughter being gone, she was being repeatedly sold for sex."

www.cbn.com/cbnnews/us/2011/May/Cities-Fight-Back-Against-Sex-Trafficking-/

Living in Fear
Jasmine worked on and off as a prostitute in South Africa, surviving what she described as the horrors that come with that life. She said the men raped her, threatened her with beatings if she tried to escape, controlled her day-to-day movements, and fined her if she left her small apartment without their permission. "My perception of human trafficking was being chained to a bed, or like in a small little box, and being sent to another country, and I didn't think of it internally," she said. "She was told, 'You will be a sex worker, and you will be a prostitute,' but she wasn't told she was going to be a slave."

http://sports.espn.go.com/espn/otl/news/story?id=5251940
www.columbian.com/news/2011/nov/15/child-sex-trafficking-on-rise-crime-upcoming-indus

Entry Into the Life
She ended up with a family friend, a woman who forced her to work as a prostitute, and sell drugs. That is when she met James Jackson, the man she called Jay, who persuaded her to go with him to Portland, Oregon. He promised to show her a better life, but moments after they arrived, Jackson told her she had to "sell her ass," court records show. When she objected, he choked and punched her until she agreed to be a prostitute.

www.washingtontimes.com/news/2011/apr/23/sex-trafficking-us-called-epidemic/print

Elesia Lopez is a survivor of the child sex trafficking system in Portland. At Elesia's 13th birthday party, her mother sold her to a man for $5,000 to feed a drug habit. Elesia was given to the man as his personal sex slave. "He took what he thought he owned and raped me multiple times."

www.washingtontimes.com/news/2010/jul/28/portlands-dark-world-of-child-sex-trafficking/print

Now 32, Jasmine has barely known a life outside prostitution. She said her mother, a former prostitute and drug addict, saw to selling Jasmine's virginity to a Japanese sailor when Jasmine was 12 or 13. "She said she brought me into the world and she always supported me and paid for the bills and everything, and it's now my turn to give back," Jasmine said, recalling her mother's decision to sell her daughter's innocence. "It was just normal. It was just expected of me to do."

http://abcnews.go.com/US/domestic-sex-trafficking-increasing-united-states/ story?id=10557194

For 22 months, Charimaya was regularly beaten, raped, and burnt with cigarette butts in the notorious Kamathipura red-light area. Then in 1996, Charimaya and hundreds of other prisoners were rescued in one of the largest-ever police raids on Mumbai's brothels. Sunita was sold to the same brothel when she was 15 but rescued soon afterwards. "There were nearly 200 girls from Nepal," Danuwar says. "Many of them were 12 or 13." One died of AIDS in the rescue home.

www.ipsnews.net/2011/09/nepal-no-brakes-on-sex-trafficking/

Injuries and Illnesses

Trying to escape only left Jessica full of fear and her body full of scars. "There is a scar on my face because he took a potato peeler and took the skin off my face and ate it … and said, 'you are mine forever'" she said.

www.newschannel5.com/story/16149242/nashville-sex-trafficking-victim-speaks-out

---

Srey Pov's family sold her to a brothel when she was 6 years old. She was unaware of sex but soon found out: A Western pedophile purchased her virginity, she said, and the brothel tied her naked and spread-eagled on a bed so that he could rape her. "I was so scared," she recalled. "I was crying and asking, 'Why are you doing this to me?'" After that, the girl was in huge demand because she was so young. Some 20 customers raped her nightly, she remembers. And the brothel twice stitched her vagina closed so that she could be resold as a virgin. Each time she rebelled she was locked naked in the darkness in a barrel half-full of sewage, replete with vermin and scorpions that stung her regularly.

http://nohumantrafficking.org/?p=1612

Brutality

"They made the first girl stand in the middle of the room. They ordered her to take off her top. She hesitated so they beat her. Then it was my turn. I lifted my top for a second and pulled it right down. Then I noticed the curtains fluttering out the open window …. Time slowed. I heard a ringing in my ears and the room faded. I remember that I said a prayer—'God give me wings.' I ran across the room and jumped over the men on the couch and out the window." When

Marina woke up in the hospital she had shattered one leg and broken the other. She had a concussion and some internal bleeding. It was only then that she discovered that the Russian woman she had paid to take her to Italy had taken her to Istanbul instead and sold her to modern-day slavers.

www.globalpost.com/dispatch/worldview/091203/moldova-sex-trafficking

---

Anna: "I work here as a prostitute, I lost my virginity here, and then I got sick. I want to go home and please help me." The Philippine embassy staged a rescue and helped return Anna home to the Philippines. She is free but not well—I'm afraid I have AIDS.

[After our interview, Anna was diagnosed with human papillomavirus, a sexually transmitted disease that can lead to cervical and other cancers. She will soon undergo a test for HIV/AIDS.]

www.msnbc.msn.com/id/20182993/ns/dateline_nbc/t/sex-trafficked-annas-story/

"They may have physical injuries which can impact, especially for young women, their sexual and reproductive health."

www.npr.org/2011/11/14/142300731/gangs-enter-new-territory-with-sex-trafficking

---

Control

"We're talking sometimes gang rapes, beatings, torture, sleep deprivation, starvation—all kinds of tactics—isolation, moving people from city to city so they no longer know where they are," Rosetti said. Germann said her pimp is also the father of her 5-year-old daughter.

www.notforsalecampaign.org/about/slavery/

She and her husband, who was a drug dealer, threatened to beat me if I tried to leave, and said if I went to the police, I would be deported. They said no one would care what happened to me, and no one would help. Girls who would not cooperate were taken down to the basement of the bar, where they were beaten across their backs, where it would not show but would still be painful, possibly causing damage to their kidneys. I was afraid they would use drugs and alcohol to force me to prostitute myself—I had seen other girls given cocaine and beaten into submission. If we go to police, bad things will happen to our families, and everyone will hear we are prostitutes. I was in Marseille almost 1 year and sold to a man and a woman who took me to Amsterdam. I slept in a small room with no heat and little food, sometimes only what is left over from their meals. Sometimes I did not eat for 1 or 2 days. They are drug addicts and would forget about me—except to bring men. When there were no customers, the man would hit me and burn me with cigarettes and force me to do things sometimes with the woman there also. He said this to make me remember he is the master.

http://jammedtruestories.blogspot.com/

When Pooh was just 12, Datqunn Sawyer, a pimp, befriended her and took her to the apartment where he lived with at least half a dozen other girls, she testified. She saw him throw a girl down a set of stairs, breaking her arm, she said. Pooh was soon put on the streets to prostitute herself and even given a quota: She had to have sex with five to 15 men every day, she testified. Sometimes, when she had a "good day" she said she was rewarded with McDonald's. As the months wore on, there was one day, after Sawyer dropped her off at the so-called "track" along Cicero Avenue that she testified she just could not do it. She took off her high heels, sat down on the concrete and wept, she said. That is when she said Sawyer, 32, appeared from the alley. "You stupid b—-, you're supposed to be making my money," he said as he snapped at her. He grabbed her discarded heel and beat her head with it until she started bleeding, she said. The young women each testified that Sawyer, who did not have a job, used a silver-studded leather belt or a heavy, wooden pimp stick to beat the girls. At 6 months' pregnant, Peaches said Sawyer split her head open with a glass ashtray.

www.suntimes.com/news/metro/8832695-418/witness-in-sex-trafficking-trial-i-was-only-a-child.html

Sawyer [alleged Chicago pimp] also used threats and beatings to enforce a rigid set of rules that left him in control of the victims. To maintain control he had sex with the victims and impregnated three of them, officials said.

http://articles.chicagotribune.com/2011-11-21/news/chi-man-convicted-of-sex-trafficking-minors-20111121_1_trafficking-ring-trafficking-minors-victims

Najeri is afraid to run away. Her pimp, she said, has told her what happens to the bodies of runaways. "The morgue comes by the hospital and incinerates it before anybody can be alerted that an American died," she said. "That struck fear in my heart." She continued, "I don't have the power or the ability to do that," she said.

www.nbclosangeles.com/news/local/Riverside-Girl-Trapped-in-Tijuana-Child-Sex-Trade–133094943.html

"One little girl finally told her captor just to kill her—she couldn't do it anymore. The pimp refused, telling her he makes too much money off her. If she wouldn't do what he told her to, he would kidnap her 8-year-old little sister and pour battery acid over her face while she watched. The little girl complied, living in a dog cage when she wasn't being sold to man after man."

www.traffick911.com/page/what-is-human-trafficking

Women who are not trafficked abroad find themselves obliged to take their chances on the violent streets of Odessa. Those selling sex on Kolontayevskaya street are familiar with the brutality that characterizes the trade. Upsetting the pimps carries a high price. Milla said: "They drive us to the city outskirts and we are raped and beaten. They leave us there. No one does anything because they pay the police." One woman told the *Observer* how she was gang-raped by eight men recently. She took 2 days off to recover before heading back to the street. Another had been forced to have nine abortions by her mama [female trafficker]. Some had been shot.

www.asafeworldforwomen.org/trafficking/europe.html

One girl was trafficked to the Balkans and condemned to an underground dungeon. When rescued, she had been starved of natural light so long her skin was blue. Methods used to export women vary. Oxana, 35, who was transported from Ukraine to a Birmingham brothel, describes how she was forced inside a box placed on a lorry and driven overland through Europe. "It went very quiet for a time. I don't know but I guess I came over by boat." Sofiya, 26, said: "They said my job was sex. A client came in, and I started screaming." She was sold to a trafficker in Izmir, who owned two Moldovan girls, then on to another, joining 38 women kept on the roof of a five-floor hotel. She was repeatedly beaten. After 8 months she was arrested during a police raid, imprisoned in Istanbul for 30 days, and shipped back to Odessa.

www.guardian.co.uk/law/2011/jul/02/odessa-ukraine-sex-trafficking-investigation

---

Sold into prostitution at 12 by her grandfather, Somaly Mam was brutalized and raped—sometimes up to 10 times a day—throughout her teenage years. She feels as though she will never completely overcome the horror she experienced, getting locked in a cellar with snakes, getting raped on a constant basis, and watching her friend get shot and killed. Part of the healing process, Mam shared from her own experience, is being honest and open with the pain she and the survivors have endured. Now divorced, Mam said she is not interested in sex or developing intimate relationships. The smell of sperm and getting close with men is just too painful a reminder of the torture to which she was subjected. Though she is abstaining from relationships, Mam makes sure to remind herself to tend to her needs, to stay strong and healthy to fulfill her work.

www.huffingtonpost.com/2011/11/30/somaly-mam-sex-trafficking-slavery-hiv-aidscambodia_n_1119460.html

---

Fifteen-year-old "Debbie" is the middle child in a close-knit Air Force family from suburban Phoenix, and a straight-A student—the last person most of us would expect to be forced into the seamy world of sex trafficking. One evening Debbie said she got a call from a casual friend, Bianca, who asked to stop by Debbie's house. Debbie went outside to meet Bianca, who drove up in a Cadillac with two older men, Mark and Matthew. After a few minutes of visiting, Bianca said they were going to leave. "So I went and I started to go give her a hug," Debbie told "Primetime." "And that's when she pushed me in the car." While she was putting tape on me, Matthew told me if I screamed or acted stupid, he'd shoot me. So I just stayed quiet." Debbie said she was then drugged by her captors and other men were brought into the room, where she was gang raped. "And then that's when I heard them say there was a middle-aged guy in the living room that wanted to take advantage of a 15-year-old girl," she said. "And then he goes, 'Bend her over. I want to see what I'm working with.' And that's when he started to rape me. And I see more guys, four other guys had come into the room. And they all had a turn. It was really scary." In a rundown, garbage-strewn apartment, her captors were trying to break her down. "They were asking me if I was hungry," she said. I told them no. That's when they put a dog biscuit in my mouth, trying to get me to eat it. I ended up in the dog kennel." Lying on her back in the tiny space, her whole body went numb.

http://abcnews.go.com/Primetime/story?id=1596778&page=1

Asha (6 years old). She started putting makeup on Asha's face. A few minutes later the woman came back with a man. The woman told Asha what to do. Asha did not want to do such things. The woman slapped her. Asha cried. The woman slapped her again. "No! No! I will not do such things." The woman cursed Asha in Nepali and then left. A few minutes later, she returned with another man. His lip curled in a mocking snarl. She had never seen such a look. "So, you don't want to work, eh?" He pulled off his belt and began to beat Asha. He beat her until the pain filled her body. Then he left. Asha curled up on her cot and whimpered softly. Three times that day he beat her. When the time came to eat, they brought nothing to Asha. Still the little girl resisted. The torture lasted for days. Without light, Asha lost track of time. Without food she grew weak. One of the other girls told Asha it was useless to resist. She told Asha of another girl who had been put in a room with a cobra until she changed her mind about doing as she was told. Seven years watching girls become sick with the "Bombay Disease." [Mumbai formerly was named Bombay—refers to HIV/AIDS.]

http://jammedtruestories.blogspot.com/

But the girl's "father" was really a convicted felon, and the girl, who had a record of prostitution in Texas, was an accomplice in the abduction. "Her dad took us to this house and said he'd be right back and he left us there," Newell recounted in a taped interview. "And I asked for some water because I was thirsty. And I drank the water and I blacked out." The water had been laced with a drug. When she woke up, Newell was groggy and couldn't move. "My legs were being held down, and the guy that was raping me was holding my hands back," she said in a quiet voice. "I kept screaming, 'Stop, please don't do this. Leave me alone.' But I was so weak, I couldn't fight them off. Like I was, I was so really out of it. And I blacked out a few times and I kept coming back to. And I was still being raped every time I woke up." After three days of being raped and beaten and drugged, Newell was dirty, bloody, bruised and barely alive. She was airlifted to a hospital and had to be resuscitated twice. In addition to her serious injuries, she had been infected with an STD. Newell said that her captor told her she had been sold on the Internet for $300,000 to a man in Texas. Fortunately, she was rescued before delivery could be made. During Newell's ordeal in Florida, her captor took money from a number of men who raped her. When she screamed, he held a gun to her head and threatened to blow her brains out.

http://jammedtruestories.blogspot.com/

"I didn't know really good how to cook, he threw the food at me and it was hot," she said. She never went to school, and she said she would go days without being fed. The stress of the domestic servitude impacted her psychologically. "I'd pee in the bed almost every day, and (my father) hits me and hits me and hits me. So they decided to put a bed outside and I sleep there," recalled Ana. That "bed" she said was nothing more than a blanket on the ground. "He was high and took a machete from his car, and chased me out of there," she recalled.

http://miami.cbslocal.com/2011/08/17/south-florida-human-trafficking-victims-shares-her-story/

British immigration officials knew that Katya, a vulnerable 18-year-old from Moldova, had been trafficked and forced into prostitution, but ruled that she would face no real danger if she was sent back. Days after her removal from the United Kingdom, her traffickers tracked her down to the Moldovan village where she had grown up. She was gang-raped, strung up by a rope from a tree, and forced to dig her own grave. One of her front teeth was pulled out with a pair of pliers. She discovered that the friend she had been kidnapped with had been murdered by traffickers in Israel who had drugged her and thrown her off a seven-story building.

www.guardian.co.uk/law/2011/apr/19/sex-trafficking-uk-legal-reform

---

Anna's trafficker kept her in submission through physical abuse—beating her, raping her, and slicing her with knives.

www.state.gov/j/tip/rls/tiprpt/2010/142751.htm

Once, Mary's employer threw boiling water on her and continued to beat her after she collapsed in pain. She was denied medical attention. Her clothing stuck to her wounds. Her employer ordered Mary to have sex with another maid on video. When Mary refused, the woman put a hot iron on her neck and threatened her with more beatings. After 2 years, a doctor noted wounds, scars, and blisters all over Mary's body.

www.state.gov/j/tip/rls/tiprpt/2010/142751.htm

In the beginning my naivety[sic] and lack of self-esteem from the abuse I had suffered made it easy for me to believe he was my protector. Later when I began to see what he really was, a predator and pimp, he controlled me with severe beatings and death threats. He beat me with coat hangers, tried to throw me out of his car, and threw me down several flights of stairs. I was married and found out I was infertile because of all the abuse and trauma my young body had been through.

http://communities.washingtontimes.com/neighborhood/world-view/2012/apr/27/breaking-silence-personal-story-sex-traficking/

They invited her to a barbecue. "I said no because I had homework," said Marinela. "When Cornel heard that he just banged my head on the wardrobe and said, 'Put your coat on.' Marius saw my ID card on the table near the TV and took it and my phone. I asked him: 'Why are you taking my passport?' and he just stared at me." There, hours after being abducted, she was raped. "I said, 'I want to go home'—so they beat me up. From that day they kept me prisoner. They wouldn't even let me go outside in case somebody saw me."

www.guardian.co.uk/uk/2011/feb/06/sex-traffick-romania-britain

---

"I was sold to a gentleman from the U.S. by my sister when I was 13 years old. I already had a baby. In the exchange, I was sold under the agreement that he would help me out with my kid because my baby was ill. I ended up being trafficked to Anchorage, Alaska. He basically kidnapped my baby away from me and didn't allow me to see him. At that time, I was forced to have sex with men and women. Our diet was basically rice and beans and nothing else. At the main market, at least in my case, I was 14, about to be 15, I was sold to have sex with other women."

http://homebrewedchristianity.com/2012/05/02/hell-on-earth-a-sex-trafficking-survivors-story/

Witchcraft

Victims of human sex trafficking have told how they were enslaved by witchcraft, torture, and death threats in modern-day Scotland. Nine came from Africa, one from South America. In one of the testimonies to a Glasgow charity, a 21-year-old told how she was branded and forced to take a "witchcraft oath" to prevent her escaping. She said: "I had to take the oath. I was given this mark on my hand. I was told that this mark, if you tell anyone what has transpired, you are going to die." "They gave me a razor blade to eat, they took my armpit hair, they removed my nails from my toes and my fingers. They removed the hair on my body, they tied it up and put it in this shrine, then they tear my body and told me that if I tell anyone,'you will just die.' "It was so painful, they were so rough, they didn't care, they just wanted satisfaction."

www.dailyrecord.co.uk/news/editors-choice/2012/01/27/sex-trafficking-victims-reveal-horror-of-witchcraft-and-torture-being-used-to-enslave-women-in-scotland-86908-23722132/

DISCUSSION

The major conclusion to be drawn from this study is that the lives of women and children who are trafficked are characterized by brutality, destruction of self-esteem, and control by violence and threats of violence to family members. They may enter the life through their families' desperation or greed, their own need to experience adventure, the loneliness that makes them vulnerable to the "romeo" pimps, or by kidnapping.

It is not surprising that multiple rapes and beatings were common in the lives of women and children who had been trafficked. Other forms of torture such as cigarette burns were also common. In extreme cases, battery acid burns and being hit by a car reveal the extent of violence these women experienced on a regular basis. Traffickers maintained control with psychological abuse. Messages of worthlessness damage the self-esteem of even the most confident person. A lifestyle not of their value system but in which they find themselves entrapped produces shame and guilt among survivors. Threats to harm families help the traffickers maintain control by focusing the victim's attention on the fact that while she cannot control what happens to herself, she can control what happens to her family.

Implications for nurses and other medical personnel are to create a safe, nonjudgmental context for the patient to tell her story and to provide holistic treatment that addresses both physical and psychological needs. The complexity of problems, the physical trauma, the sense of shame, and guilt with psychological distress all combine to make prostituted people among the most difficult to treat.

There are four main implications for nursing as a profession to address when working with victims of sex trafficking: developing and funding new treatment and aftercare models in collaboration with other professionals and community leaders, producing awareness campaigns for the general public, promoting education for nurses and other professionals, and political advocacy to promote a zero-tolerance for human trafficking. The American Nurses Association, the

American Academy of Nursing, and other professional groups in health care are working on these issues. As individual nurses, we should examine our own attitudes toward these vulnerable people and educate ourselves to provide safe and respectful treatment. The authors suggest that readers review the websites used for this study and the numerous other sources on human trafficking listed in the chapter of resources in this book.

Further research should be conducted that validates these data with more detailed stories told by survivors themselves in order to obtain a more complete picture of their experiences. Once this is done, outcome studies with interventions designed specifically for the population can provide the evidence basis to specify best practices for each of the conditions for this population. Meanwhile, application of best practices for the injuries and illnesses mentioned should not be denied to these victims on the basis of ignorance.

REFERENCES

Baker, L., Case, P., & Policicchio, D. (2003). General health problems of inner-city sex workers: A pilot study. *Journal of the Medical Library Association, 91*(1), 67–71.

Clawson, H. J., Dutch, N. M., & Williamson, E. (2008). *National symposium on the health needs of human trafficking: Background document.* Washington, DC: Office of the Assistant Secretary for Planning and Evaluation, U.S. Department of Health and Human Services.

Estes, R., & Weiner, N. (2001). *The commercial sexual exploitation of children in the U.S., Canada, and Mexico.* Philadelphia: University of Pennsylvania.

Family Violence Prevention Fund. (1999, October). *Preventing domestic violence: Clinical guidelines on routine screening.* San Francisco, CA: Author.

Family Violence Prevention Fund. (2005). *Turning pain into power: Trafficking survivors' perspectives on early intervention strategies.* San Francisco, CA: Author.

Hampton, T. (2010). Child marriage threatens girls' health. *Journal of the American Medical Association, 304*(5), 509–510.

International Organization for Migration. (2006). *Breaking the cycle of vulnerability: Responding to the health needs of trafficked women in east and southern Africa.* Pretoria, South Africa: Author.

Janak, T. (2000). Haiti's Restavec slave children: Difficult choices, difficult lives. *The International Journal of Children's Rights, 8,* 321–331.

Raymond, J. G., D'Cunha, J., Dzuhayatin, S. R., Hynes, H. P., Rodriguez, Z. R., & Santos, A. (2002). *A comparative study of women trafficked in the migration process: Patterns, profiles, and health consequences of sexual exploitation in five countries (Indonesia, the Philippines, Thailand, Venezuela, and the United States).* Brussels, Belgium: Coalition Against Trafficking Women International.

Sanders, T. (2004). A continuum of risk? The management of health, physical and emotional—Risks by female sex workers. *Sociology of Health and Illness, 26*(5), 557–574.

Taylor, O. (2011). The sexual victimization of women: Substance abuse, HIV, prostitution and intimate partner violence as underlying correlates. *Journal of Human Behavior in the Social Environment, 21*, 834–848.

Williamson, E., Dutch, N. M., & Clawson, H. J. (2010). *Evidence-based mental health treatment for victims of human trafficking.* Prepared for the Office of the Assistant Secretary for Planning and Evaluation (ASPE), U.S. Department of Health and Human Services. Retrieved from http://aspe.hhs.gov/hsp/07/humantrafficking/Mental Health/index.pdf

Zimmerman C., & Borland R. (Eds.) (2009). *Caring for trafficked persons: Guidance for health providers.* Geneva, Switzerland: IOM.2009. Retrieved from http://publications.iom.int/bookstore/free/CT_Handbook.pdf

Zimmerman, C., Hossain, M., Yun, K., Gajdadziev, V., Guzun, N., Tchomarova, M. et al. (2008). The health of trafficked women: A survey of women entering posttrafficking services in Europe. *American Journal of Public Health, 98*(1), 1–5.

Zimmerman, C., Hossain, M., Yun, K., Roche, B., Morison, L., & Watts, C. (2006). *Stolen smiles: A summary report on the physical and psychological health consequences of women and adolescents trafficked in Europe.* London: UK. London School of Hygiene and Tropical Medicine. Retrieved from http://www.humantrafficking.org/uploads/publications/Stolen_Smiles_July_2006.pdf

Zimmerman, C., Yun, K., Shvab, I., Watts, C., Trappolin, L., Treppete, M. et al. (2003). *The health risks and consequences of trafficking in women and adolescents: Findings from a European study.* London: UK. London School of Hygiene & Tropical Medicine. Retrieved from http://www.lshtm.ac.uk/php/ghd/docs/traffickingfinal.pdf

Zimmerman, C., & Watts, C. (2003). *WHO Ethical and Safety Recommendations for Interviewing Trafficked Women.* Geneva, Switzerland: World Health Organization.

APPENDIX A: LINKS TO VICTIMS' STORIES FOUND ON WEBSITES

http://jammedtruestories.blogspot.com/

http://www.polarisproject.org/what-we-do/client-services/survivor-stories

http://abcnews.go.com/Primetime/story?id=1596778&page=1#.T5c4xbNSSrk

http://www.guardian.co.uk/uk/2011/feb/06/sex-traffick-romania-britain

http://www.oregonlive.com/gresham/index.ssf/2010/10/former_sex_trafficking_victim.html

http://www.aagw.org/Education/TrueStories/True9M

http://www.kmbc.com/r/29615870/detail.html

http://www.castla.org/survivor-stories

http://www.dw.de/dw/article/0,,5935051,00.html

http://www.newschannel5.com/story/16149242/nashville-sex-trafficking-victim-speaks-out

http://www.sunjournal.com/city/story/1095292

http://www.state.gov/j/tip/rls/tiprpt/2010/142751.htm

http://www.safehorizon.org/index/what-we-do-2/our-stories-82.html

http://stoptraffickfashion.com/books-resources/the-slave-across-the-street-by-theresa-flores/

http://journals.lww.com/journalofchristiannursing/Fulltext/2012/03000/Helping_Human_Trafficking_Victims_In_Our_Backyard.13.aspx

http://www.wusa9.com/news/local/story.aspx?storyid=119188

http://allafrica.com/stories/201206010872.html

http://www.bangkokpost.com/news/local/256970/sex-workers-reveal-hazards

http://www.cbsnews.com/8301-504083_162-6162491-504083.html

http://www.columbian.com/news/2011/nov/15/child-sex-trafficking-on-rise-crime-upcoming-indus/

http://www.huffingtonpost.com/2011/11/17/chinese-human-trafficking-ring_n_1099736.html

http://www.cbn.com/cbnnews/us/2011/May/Cities-Fight-Back-Against-Sex-Trafficking-/

http://abcnews.go.com/US/domestic-sex-trafficking-increasing-united-states/story?id=10557194

http://www.npr.org/2011/11/14/142300731/gangs-enter-new-territory-with-sex-trafficking

http://eternity.biz/news/how_god_lifted_me_out_of_the_sex-trade_rat_hole/1111060551/

http://articles.chicagotribune.com/2011-11-21/news/chi-man-convicted-of-sex-trafficking-minors-20111121_1_trafficking-ring-trafficking-minors-victims

http://www.ipsnews.net/2011/09/nepal-no-brakes-on-sex-trafficking/

http://www.washingtontimes.com/news/2010/jul/28/portlands-dark-world-of-child-sex-trafficking/

http://www.nytimes.com/2011/11/25/us/raising-awareness-of-sex-trafficking-one-lecture-at-a-time.html

http://www.nbclosangeles.com/news/local/Riverside-Girl-Trapped-in-Tijuana-Child-Sex-Trade-133094943.html

http://articles.timesofindia.indiatimes.com/2011-11-21/goa/30425588_1_crime-branch-trade-victim-protective-home

http://articles.timesofindia.indiatimes.com/2011-11-21/goa/30425588_1_crime-branch-trade-victim-protective-home

http://news.change.org/sex-trafficking

http://www.globalpost.com/dispatch/worldview/091203/moldova-sex-trafficking

http://articles.cnn.com/2009-11-25/opinion/carr.human.trafficking_1_trafficking-victims-protection-act-tvpa-lena?_s=PM:OPINION

http://articles.cnn.com/2009-11-25/opinion/carr.human.trafficking_1_trafficking-victims-protection-act-tvpa-lena?_s=PM:OPINION

http://www.washingtontimes.com/news/2011/apr/23/sex-trafficking-us-called-epidemic/

http://www.smudailycampus.com/news/sex-trafficking-rises-in-dfw-1.1917849

http://www.guardian.co.uk/law/2011/jul/02/odessa-ukraine-sex-trafficking-investigation

http://www.suntimes.com/news/metro/8832695-418/witness-in-sex-trafficking-trial-i-was-only-a-child.html

http://www.huffingtonpost.com/2011/11/30/somaly-mam-sex-trafficking-slavery-hiv-aids-cambodia_n_1119460.html

http://abcnews.go.com/Primetime/story?id=1596778&page=1

http://www.nytimes.com/2011/11/17/opinion/kristof-the-face-of-modern-slavery.html

http://sports.espn.go.com/espn/otl/news/story?id=5251940

http://jammedtruestories.blogspot.com/

http://www.polarisproject.org/what-we-do/client-services/survivor-stories

http://www.castla.org/survivor-stories

http://miami.cbslocal.com/2011/08/17/south-florida-human-trafficking-victims-shares-her-story/

http://www.youtube.com/watch?v=W5u2IUF8JUw

http://www.youtube.com/watch?v=nC1oeF6_b44

http://www.oregonlive.com/gresham/index.ssf/2010/10/former_sex_trafficking_victim.html

http://www.guardian.co.uk/law/2011/apr/19/sex-trafficking-uk-legal-reform

http://www.state.gov/j/tip/rls/tiprpt/2010/142751.htm

http://www.kmbc.com/Sex-Trafficking-Victim-Describes-Break-For-Freedom/-/11664900/12264050/-/item/1/-/6g4kym/-/index.html

http://www.newschannel5.com/story/16149242/nashville-sex-trafficking-victim-speaks-out

http://www.dailyrecord.co.uk/news/editors-choice/2012/01/27/sex-trafficking-victims-reveal-horror-of-witchcraft-and-torture-being-used-to-enslave-women-in-scotland-86908-23722132/

http://homebrewedchristianity.com/2012/05/02/hell-on-earth-a-sex-trafficking-survivors-story/

http://communities.washingtontimes.com/neighborhood/world-view/2012/apr/27/breaking-silence-personal-story-sex-traficking/

http://www.asafeworldforwomen.org/trafficking/europe.html

APPENDIX B: VICTIMS' STORIES IN BOOKS

Bales, K. (2004). *Disposable people*. Berkeley, CA: University of California Press.

Bales, K., & Soodalter, R. (2009). *The slave next door*. Berkeley, CA: University of California Press.

Bales, K., & Trodd, Z. (2008). *To plead our own cause: Personal stories by today's slaves*. Ithaca, NY: Cornell University Press.

Batstone, D. (2007). *Not for sale: The return of the global slave trade and how we can fight it*. NY: Harper Collins.

Kara, S. (2009). *Sex trafficking: Inside the business of modern slavery*. New York, NY: Columbia University Press.

Lloyd, R. (2011). *Girls like us*. New York, NY: Harper-Collins.

Mam, S. (2009). *The road of lost innocence*. NY: Spiegel and Grau.

Muhsen, Z. (1994). *Sold*. London, UK: Little, Brown.

Sage, J., & Kasten, L. (2008). *Enslaved*. New York, NY: Palgrave MacMillan.

Shannon, L. (2011). *A thousand sisters: My journey into the worst place on earth to be a woman*. Berkeley, CA: Seal Press.

Skinner, E. B. (2008). *A crime so monstrous*. New York, NY: Free Press.

Smith, L. (2007). *From Congress to the brothel: A journey of hope, healing, and restoration*. Vancouver, WA: Shared Hope International.

Smith, L. (2009). *Renting Lacy: A story of America's prostituted children*. Vancouver, WA: Shared Hope International.

CHAPTER 10

Health Issues and Interactions With Adult Survivors

DONNA SABELLA

*M*imi was adopted at age 5 and brought to the United States by a family who had high hopes and expectations for her. A darling little girl with shockingly deep blue eyes and thick blond hair, she seemed to adjust well to her new country and family for the next 8 years. However, during her early teens she rebelled and started taking to the streets. By her mid-teens, thanks to the Internet, she connected with a "boyfriend" several states away who agreed to pay her way to join him where he and his family encouraged her to help them out with the rent. She felt excited to be out on her own in a new place with someone who professed love for her and where she could do what she wanted, unlike most of her 15-year-old friends she'd left behind. These people were taking care of her and treating her like family so the least she could do was bring in her fair share of the rent. The first time was the hardest, but after a few more "dates" she learned to take herself somewhere else during the time it took her to satisfy each customer. Within a month, she and her "boyfriend" had broken up and the next leg of her journey took her to the opposite side of the country. In Las Vegas, she managed to connect with several "boyfriends," each of whom told her what to do and how to do it. Over the next 5 years Mimi was a fixture on the Vegas Strip. She reported that she enjoyed what she was doing and that she felt loved and excited that men would pay to be with her. With her exotic accent and good looks, she was a financial asset to whomever she ended up working for. Although she had just turned 20, she was a true professional who could walk the walk and talk the talk with the best of them. But Mimi grew tired of the lifestyle, of the beatings from boyfriends and customers, the arrests, the uncertainty of what was around the next corner. The thrill was gone and after being beaten and told to get lost by her last "boyfriend," Mimi retraced her steps back home where she hoped to start anew.

After a few slip ups, with the help of some service providers who genuinely cared about her, Mimi finally seemed to be making progress. She found work at a convenience store, had a real boyfriend and appeared to be settling into a comfortable, safe, and routine lifestyle. It was therefore a surprise to all who knew Mimi when the call came in that she was dead at age 21, and perhaps by her own hand.

Little was known about Mimi's background prior to being adopted but it is safe to say that her hard-lived life in her new country undoubtedly played a role in her death. The impact of being exposed to the dark side of human desires and behaviors is difficult at any age, but especially traumatizing both physically and emotionally for those who start young. Although she professed her enjoyment over what she was doing, Mimi was clearly a victim of sex trafficking. The boyfriends who played a role in moving her across the country were all pimps and traffickers who took every advantage possible of a young, trusting, and loving girl from her teenage into her early adult years. With the news of her death came the question on everyone's mind who had worked with Mimi: Could anything have been done to have helped change the ending of Mimi's story? What sort of treatments and interactions may have made a difference for her and all the thousands of other young girls and boys and adults who are victims of sex trafficking here and abroad?

Service providers may often work with or have contact with victims of all forms of human trafficking. Chief among those who may be called upon to render care to this vulnerable population are nurses, who can make a world of difference by what they do or do not do. What do nurses need to know to offer the best care possible in working with victims of sex trafficking and hopefully make a difference in helping that person heal and recover? This chapter will offer an overview of what human trafficking is, followed by a discussion of the medical, physical, and mental health issues and consequences of victimization. The chapter concludes with a discussion regarding how nurses can best interact with survivors and provide care that is meaningful and appropriate.

HUMAN TRAFFICKING

Human trafficking is often referred to as modern day slavery and happens here as well as all over the world. According to Article 3, paragraph (a) of the Protocol to Prevent, Suppress and Punish Trafficking in Persons (United Nations, 2000) trafficking in persons is defined as follows:

> Trafficking in Persons [involves] the recruitment, transportation, transfer, harbouring or receipt of persons, by means of the threat or use of force or other forms of coercion, of abduction, of fraud, of deception, of the abuse of power or of a position of vulnerability or of the giving or receiving of payments or benefits to achieve the consent of a person having control over another person, for the purpose of exploitation. Exploitation shall include, at a minimum, the exploitation of the prostitution of others or other forms

of sexual exploitation, forced labour or services, slavery or practices similar to slavery, servitude or the removal of organs.

Quite simply, then, human trafficking involves a person or persons, typically referred to as traffickers, using force, fraud, and/or coercion to recruit, transport, or harbor other people, often referred to as victims, in order to exploit them for financial gain. Within the broader heading of human trafficking, the categories include sex trafficking, labor trafficking (including debt bondage, forced labor, and indentured servitude), and trafficking in child soldiers (U.S. Department of State, 2010). A given country can be a labeled as a country of origin, transit, or destination, or any combination of the three (United Nations Office on Drugs and Crime, 2012). According to the 2011 Trafficking in Persons Report (U.S. Department of State, 2011), a report issued yearly that ranks countries according to how well they combat human trafficking on their own soil, the United States is a source, transit, and destination country for men, women, and children subjected to forced labor, debt bondage, domestic servitude, and sex trafficking.

Although this volume focuses on sex trafficking, it is important for nurses to have some general background information about all types of trafficking to have a fuller picture of the scope of trafficking and to realize that victims can be trafficked in several different categories simultaneously. Human trafficking is a worldwide phenomenon that occurs everywhere, in towns, cities, and nations both large and small, and counts among its victims children, girls, boys, men, and women. Owing to the illegal and clandestine nature of human trafficking, exact numbers of victims are difficult to come by, and indeed there is some controversy regarding the actual number of victims, calling for more up-to-date and accurate figures (U.S. Government Accountability Office, 2006; Wyler & Siskin, 2010). The *2011 Trafficking in Persons Report* (U.S. Department of State) estimates that there are approximately some 27 million trafficking victims worldwide. Other figures from earlier reports placed the international numbers at 600,000 to 800,000 (U.S. Department of State, 2004, 2006).

In their report on estimating the number of trafficking victims in the United States, Clawson, Layne, and Small (2006) state the following:

The United States is widely regarded as a destination country for trafficking in persons, yet the exact number of human trafficking victims within the United States has remained largely undetermined since passage of the Trafficking Victims Protection Act (TVPA) in 2000. Initial estimates cited in the TVPA suggested that approximately 50,000 individuals are trafficked into the United States each year. This number was reduced to 18,000–20,000 in the U.S. Department of State's June 2003 *Trafficking in Persons Report*. In its 2005 report, the Department of State's Office to Monitor and Combat Trafficking in Persons cites 14,500–17,500 individuals annually. These shifting figures call into question the reliability of estimates and have potential consequences for the availability of resources to prevent human trafficking, prosecute traffickers, and protect and serve victims of this crime. (p. 2)

Regardless of the exact numbers, human trafficking is recognized as a growing problem both here and abroad. As mentioned above, there are several different categories of human trafficking. Basically, trafficking can be divided into the categories of labor trafficking and sex trafficking.

Labor Trafficking

Labor trafficking is defined by law as "the recruitment, harboring, transportation, provision, or obtaining a person for labor or services, through the use of force, fraud or coercion for the purpose of subjection to involuntary servitude, peonage, debt bondage or slavery" (U.S. Congress, 2000, p. 8). The various forms of labor trafficking include child labor, bonded labor, and forced labor (U.S. Department of Health and Human Services, *Labor trafficking,* n.d.). As the label implies, child labor goes beyond having children work what is considered to be a reasonable number of hours and type of work based on their age. It involves their being involved in any form of labor that is harmful to their mental and physical health, and spiritual, social, moral, and educational development and well-being. Children can and are pressed into service in any activities that their adult counterparts can be found in such as prostitution, drug trade, forced combat as child soldiers, and working as domestics or farm hands. Bonded labor, also known as debt bondage, occurs when a trafficking victim is required to pay back various charges trumped up by the trafficker as part of the fees the victim incurs, in essence for being trafficked. In such cases, a trafficking victim may be charged for room and board, transportation, and clothing, and be required to pay off the charges by working for the trafficker while at the same time incurring more fees. Finally, as the name implies, forced labor is any type of work the victim is mandated to perform against his or her will. Victims are often threatened, beaten, and/or held captive as means of getting them to work. Examples of forced labor include working in construction, hotels, restaurants, or as farm workers, nannies, or housekeepers (U.S. Department of Health and Human Services, *Labor trafficking,* n.d.).

An especially horrific form of labor trafficking involves the use of children in armed conflicts. According to the United Nations, approximately 300,000 children under the age of 18 are involved in 30 conflicts worldwide (UNICEF *Fact Sheet: Child Soldiers,* n.d.). Children, both male and female, are forced into becoming soldiers and doing battle through threats or actual physical force, and are made to engage in dangerous activities. During their time as child soldiers, they live in unhealthy and unsafe conditions and are brutalized, abused, and subjected to severe punishment for any infraction. Female child soldiers are often sexually abused and raped, and both boys and girls can be killed by those in charge of them for any number of reasons (Child Soldiers International, n.d.). For an overview of the recruitment and use of child soldiers in 197 countries, readers are referred to *Child Soldiers: Global Report (2008)*.

Sex Trafficking

According to the 2009 Global Report on Trafficking in Persons (United Nations Office on Drugs and Crime, n.d.) and other sources, the most commonly identified and recognized form of human trafficking is that of sex trafficking followed by that of forced labor (Barrows & Finger, 2008). The report acknowledges that this could be due to the result of statistical bias in reporting trafficking, with sex trafficking and sexual exploitation simply reported at much higher levels than all other forms combined. Regardless of the numbers, one can argue with confidence that sex trafficking occurs worldwide in great numbers.

Sex trafficking is any commercial sex act induced by force, fraud, or coercion, or in which the person performing the act is under the age of 18. Examples of force include beatings, rape, physical constraint, or confining someone against his or her will. Fraud requires some measure of deception or misrepresentation, and coercion involves threatening to do harm to someone or restrain them against their will. The legal definition of sex trafficking reads as follows: "Sex trafficking" means the recruitment, harboring, transportation, provision, or obtaining of a person for the purpose of a commercial sex act (U.S. Congress, 2000). When a minor is involved, the activity becomes a severe form of sex trafficking, defined as follows: "The recruitment, harboring, transportation, provision or obtaining of a person for the purpose of a commercial sex act, in which a commercial sex act is induced by force, fraud or coercion, or in which the person forced to perform such an act is under the age of 18 years" (U.S. Congress, 2000, p. 8). The commercial sexual exploitation of American children or children who are permanent residents is referred to as domestic minor sex trafficking (DSMT) and like other forms of human trafficking, exact numbers of victims are difficult to ascertain (Reid, 2010).

While victims of sex trafficking can be men, women, girls, and boys, the majority are girls and women (U.S. Department of State, 2007, 2009; U.S. Department of Health and Human Services, *Sex trafficking*, n.d.). They can be found working in brothels, pornography, massage parlors, and truck stops. Victims can also be found involved in street-level prostitution as well as escort services, in strip clubs, and gentlemen's clubs. In addition, the Internet serves as a medium through which sexual encounters can be arranged at private homes, apartments, and hotel rooms. In one case I am familiar with, a woman's trafficker owned a taxi-cab and would drive the woman to pick up the customer with whom she would then engage in sex while being driven around in the cab.

As with human trafficking in general, as pointed out above, reliable numbers of victims are hard to come by. What we do know, however, is that sex trafficking is the most common form of human trafficking of American citizens (U.S. Department of State, 2010). In a report on the characteristics of 2,515 human trafficking incidents within the United States from January 1,

2008 to June 30, 2010, approximately 82% of incidents were classified as sex trafficking, 1,200 of which involved allegations of adult sex trafficking and 1,000 of which were alleged to involve prostitution or sexual exploitation of a minor. Furthermore, 83% of the confirmed victims of sex trafficking incidents turned out to be U.S. citizens (Banks & Kyckelhahn, 2011).

In working with victims of sex trafficking, it is important for nurses to understand the basics related to the *who, what, when, where, why,* and *how* of this phenomenon. The "what" of human trafficking in terms of what it is and the types of trafficking that exist have been detailed and defined above. Regarding the "who," as stated above, in the United States the majority of trafficking victims between 2008 and 2010 were American citizens. However, other victims come from anywhere. At any given point in time we have people trafficked from such locations as Africa, Asia, South America, Canada, and Russia (Center for Problem-Oriented Policing, n.d.). We also know that in terms of who gets trafficked for sexual exploitation, the majority of those victims are women and girls (U.S. Department of State, 2010). Victims are often, although not always, from lower socioeconomic backgrounds. Sex trafficking occurs everywhere in the world, and is particularly widespread near military installations and bases, at sporting events such as Super Bowls, World Series, and Olympic Games, at conventions, and anywhere there tends to be large numbers of people, especially men, gathered for any period of time. In fact, traffickers and pimps will travel to any location with their victims to meet the demand of any given event. For example, for the 2012 Super Bowl XLVI in Indianapolis, Indiana, Governor Mitch Daniels urged Indiana lawmakers to tighten the state's already existing antitrafficking law in anticipation of increased prostitution activity connected to the sporting event (Clark, 2012).

In terms of why and how people get trafficked, there is no one simple or single answer. In asking why sex trafficking flourishes in Southeast Asia, Batstone (2007) provided four answers that ring true regardless of location: devastating poverty, armed conflicts, rapid industrialization, and an exploding population growth. Trafficking is often associated with poverty and economic hardships. People want to work and be able to take care of themselves (Kara, 2009). Where there are no jobs or means to support oneself, victims are willing to seek work elsewhere. Promises of a better life somewhere else made by traffickers are, in many cases, too good to pass up. Victims are tricked with fraudulent promises of getting a better education, learning a trade, finding well-paying jobs, or even promises of marriage to the trafficker who pretends to be in love with the victim (U.S. Department of Health and Human Services, *Sex trafficking,* n.d.). At times, traffickers promise parents to send their child to another country where that child will have many more advantages than he or she has in their homeland with no intention of following through. Instead the victims are forced into sex work with no recourse or way out. Aside from fraudulent approaches to recruiting victims for the purpose of sexual exploitation, at times women and girls are kidnapped and taken by force. Other factors driving trafficking include the subordination of women, viewing girls and women as sex objects, the feminization of poverty, economic deprivation, and financial burdens (Gajic-Veljanoski & Stewart, 2007). Sex trafficking is also motivated by a high demand for sexual services and not all traffickers are strangers to their victims. There are numerous accounts where victims have been trafficked by their own family members, trusted members of their communities, or people with whom they are romantically involved. One woman rescued from her trafficker in an outreach I was involved in Phoenix, Arizona, had been brought to the United States from South America by her boyfriend who promptly put her to work selling sex on the Internet and street. As evidenced by Mimi's experience, the woman rescued in Phoenix is not alone in how she ended up a sex trafficking victim at the hands of a "boyfriend."

CONSEQUENCES: PHYSICAL AND MENTAL HEALTH ISSUES

All victims of sex trafficking, regardless of age or gender, are impacted both physically as well as emotionally by their experiences, and there is little doubt regarding the importance of health care in aiding in the recovery of those who have been trafficked (Family Violence Prevention Fund, 2005). In a study of 192 trafficked women who were interviewed within 2 weeks of their entry into posttrafficking services, 95% reported being subjected to physical or sexual violence while trafficked and 59% reported pretrafficking abuse (Zimmerman et al., 2008). Among this population the mortality rate is increased as compared to women not involved in sex work (Potterat et al., 2004). One study found that those involved in sex work have a homicide rate 17 times higher than the rate for age-matched women in the general population (Shively et al., 2010). There is no doubt that human trafficking, regardless of the type, is indeed a health issue. The consequences can be severe, chronic, and life threatening. Some of the women I have worked with have stated that at times they welcomed death and prayed that they would die before they had to endure another day living the life they were living. It mattered little to them if death came at the hands of their customer or an intentional drug overdose. They just wanted things to be over. The majority of the women I have worked with also stated that the physical consequences, while serious and life threatening at times, were much easier to deal with and overcome than were the psychological consequences of having been involved in sex work.

It is important for nurses to be aware of some of the more common physical and emotional problems. Among sex trafficking victims we can expect to see any number of medical and physical health problems. Broken bones, bite and burn marks, black eyes, and bald spots where hair has been pulled out by customers, are some examples of injuries sustained by victims with whom I have worked. Traumatic brain injury and associated headaches and dizziness, concussions, and memory loss may also be observed in this population, as well as complaints of stomach aches, vision problems, head injuries, back pain, jaw problems, fatigue, memory problems, and dental problems (Cwikel, Ilan, & Chudakov, 2003; Zimmerman & Borland, 2009).

As customers tend to prefer sex without using condoms, it is not unusual for women to contract sexually transmitted infections (STIs). Beyrer and Stachowiak (2003) talk about the direct health consequences of commercial sex as having increased risk of being exposed to STIs, HIV, and sexual trauma with the long-term consequences of such including infertility, ectopic pregnancies, cervical cancer, and AIDS. They may also develop urinary tract infections (UTIs) and complain of menstrual problems. Rough and violent sex, often the case for this population, can result in vaginal, anal, and genital lacerations and trauma. Some victims are encouraged to use drugs and alcohol, in which case there are problems associated with being addicted. Nutritional problems are also common in this population, as eating properly is not on the menu. Dental care is limited so dentition may be adversely affected.

In a study on the health problems of trafficked women and adolescent girls, the women reported a number of problems including gastrointestinal problems, pelvic pain, complications from abortions, and various skin problems such as lice, rashes, and scabies (Zimmerman et al., 2003). Aside from HIV/AIDS, sex trafficking victims are also at higher risk for a variety of infectious diseases such as tuberculosis, hepatitis, and pneumonia (U.S. Department of Health and Human Services, *Sex trafficking*, n.d.). As is often the case, victims have limited, if any, access to health care and must depend on their traffickers whether or not they receive treatment (Beyrer & Stachowiak, 2003). Delay in getting treatment can result in worsened conditions or, in some cases, death (Barrows & Finger, 2008).

Far worse, however, for many of the sex trafficking victims, are the dire emotional and psychological consequences they are left with (Yakushko, 2009). It is believed that all victims of human trafficking experience trauma (Clawson, Dutch, Solomon, & Grace, 2009). Much of the research examining the mental health consequences of human trafficking, in particular sex trafficking, notes the high prevalence of posttraumatic stress disorder (PTSD) among this population (Williamson, Dutch, & Clawson, 2010). In a nine-country study, which included the United States, 67% of prostituted women met criteria for a diagnosis for PTSD (Farley et al., 2003). In a study carried out comparing two groups of trafficked women in Nepal the group trafficked for sex work showed higher rates of anxiety, depression, and PTSD than did the group of women trafficked for labor and not for sex work (Tsutsumi, Izutsu, Poudyal, Kato, & Marui, 2008). Findings from a study of 204 girls and women trafficked for sexual exploitation also found high levels of PTSD, depression, and anxiety among the participants (Hossain, Zimmerman, Abas, Light, & Watts, 2010). In order to develop PTSD one needs to experience, either directly or indirectly, a traumatic event that makes one fear for one's life, well-being, or safety, or the life, well-being, or safety of others. One experiences fear and helplessness. While everyone will react differently, the three main types of symptoms experienced can include intrusive reexperiencing of the traumatic event, avoiding reminders of the trauma, and experiencing increased anxiety and hyperarousal (American Psychiatric Association, 2000). Victims can develop the disorder anywhere from days to years after the precipitating trauma and treatment usually consists of therapy in combination with medication (Sabella, 2012).

Aside from PTSD, other common psychological and behavorial conditions among this population include major depressive disorder, believed to be the most common mood disorder experienced by victims (Williamson et al., 2010). In addition, sex trafficking victims report problems with substance abuse, dissociative identity disorder, anxiety disorders, obsessive–compulsive disorders and eating disorders (Clawson, Salomon, & Grace, 2008; Williamson et al., 2010; Zimmerman et al., 2003, 2006). There is also poor self-esteem, self-blame and loathing, fear that others will find out that they have been trafficked, suicidal ideation, and instances of suicide (U.S. Department of Health and Human Services, *Sex trafficking*, n.d.).

In a report on trafficked women from the Ukraine, women returning home from having been trafficked reported feelings such as fear, guilt, rage, betrayal, suspicion, shock, and helplessness (Bezpalcha, 2003). Likewise, a survey of 159 U.S.-based service providers and a focus group of trafficking victims revealed that compared to domestic violence victims, trafficking victims were less stable, more isolated and fearful, and had more severe and extreme mental health needs (Clawson, Small, Go, & Myles, 2003). In another study of women involved in sex trafficking, over 85% acknowledged feeling depressed and sad even years after they had been able to exit (Raymond & Hughes, 2001). For many victims, the experiences of having been trafficked for sexual exploitation can take years and even a lifetime to recover from. Unfortunately for some the only way out is suicide.

Interactions

It has been reported that after Germany, the United States ranks as the second largest destination for women and children trafficked for commercial sexual exploitation (Mizus, Moody, Privado, & Douglas, 2003). We know that sex trafficking occurs in the United States, yet unfortunately we do not always recognize a victim even when she is directly in front of us. In a study of 21 foreign nationals trafficked to the United States, 28% of those interviewed reported having been taken to a health care provider while they were trafficked, yet none of the health care providers they came in contact with recognized that the patient they were working with was also a trafficking victim (Family Violence Prevention Fund, 2005). Before health care providers can intervene and make a difference, it is important that they be trained in what to look for in terms of who may possibly be a victim (Barrows & Finger, 2008; Williamson, Dutch, & Clawson, 2009). Nurses occupy a front row seat in working with patients in a variety of contexts and health care settings and can indeed play an important role in combating human trafficking and advocating for victims (Sabella, 2011). While no one health care professional needs to work alone, and indeed treating sex trafficking victims requires the skills and knowledge of a variety of disciplines including law enforcement, social work, lawyers, counselors, interpreters, and religion, housing and benefits specialists, it is important to at least have a basic under-standing of some of the possible signs to be aware of. According to the United Nations Office on Drugs and Crime (n.d.), those who have been trafficked may give evidence of some of the following:

- Believe that they must work against their will
- Be unable to leave their work environment
- Show signs that their movements are being controlled and be accompanied by someone who speaks for them
- Feel that they cannot leave
- Show fear or anxiety
- Be subjected to violence or threats of violence against themselves or against their family members and loved ones
- Suffer injuries that appear to be the result of an assault
- Suffer injuries or impairments typical of certain jobs or control measures
- Be distrustful of the authorities
- Not be in possession of their passports or other travel or identity documents, as those documents are being held by someone else
- Be found in or connected to a type of location likely to be used for exploiting people
- Be unfamiliar with the local language
- Not know their home or work address
- Allow others to speak for them when addressed directly

No one expects nurses to make a determination that someone is actually being trafficked. There are a number of factors that make identifying victims dif-ficult, including being misclassified as a domestic abuse case if a victim is roman-tically involved with her trafficker or lack of knowledge on professionals' parts regarding what human trafficking is (Williamson et al., 2009). Following are some questions a nurse might ask to further assess the possibility that the person is a trafficking victim, although they are in no way definitive or prove that someone is indeed a victim (U.S. Department of State, 2009):

- Where are you from?
- What brings you to the United States?
- How did you get here?
- What type of work do you do? Do you have a set schedule?
- Are you paid for your work? How much do you earn?
- Have you been threatened with violence or harm if you decide you want to leave your job?
- Do you have identification (ID) on you? If not, why not? Who has your ID or other documents?
- Do you have to ask permission to eat, sleep, go to the bathroom, or talk with others?
- Are you being forced to do what you're doing?

- Are you allowed to go out on your own?
- Where and with whom do you live? Are there locks on the doors and windows so that you can't get out?

Of utmost importance is to ensure the physical safety and to assess the medical condition of the person you are working with. Life-threatening conditions need to be treated immediately, while at the same time it is important to make sure that the individual is safe, both physically and emotionally (Yakushko, 2009). Once the above concerns are addressed, that is the time to begin questioning, while keeping the following in mind:

- Separate the patient from the person or persons who transported her there for questioning.
- Question the individual in her native language and dialect using someone other than the person who brought her to the facility.
- Be mindful that the individual may be reluctant to speak to you as she may have been threatened if she does so or she may mistrust authority.
- While the majority of those forced into sex trafficking are women, men and boys are as well. Be aware that the male victim in front of you could also be a sex trafficking victim.
- The information presented in this chapter focuses more on working with victims in their late teens and older. In working with adolescents and children, it is essential to bring in professionals who have experience working with those who are minors and younger. They tend to have different needs and require different interventions from teenagers and adults.
- Some may not know what trafficking means, so avoid asking if they think they have been trafficked. Use questions more like those provided above.
- While the desire to help the victim is great, as in domestic violence cases, we need to honor the wishes of the individual. Unless we are mandated to report, as in the case of working with a suspected minor victim, if the person is over 18 it is usually best to work with her in determining what she would like done and how. At times, reporting the abuse or forcing the individual to report her situation can make things worse. Judgment and action need to be applied on a case-by-case basis.
- If a suspected victim refuses to act or turns down offers of help, ask if you can give her some information in case she changes her mind later. At the very least, offer her the National Human Trafficking Resource Center (NHTRC) hotline number: 1-888-3737-888.

We also need to keep in mind that there are a number of obstacles in meeting the needs of trafficking victims, including limited availability and access to appropriate services, especially mental health services that are culturally appropriate; finding providers who are culturally competent, knowledgeable about human trafficking, and who speak the same language and dialect as victims; expecting victims to trust us after what they have been through, sometimes at the hands of other authorities; and realizing that in some cases, mandated treatment may be counterproductive (Clawson et al., 2008).

CONCLUSION

In their chapter on the needs of and services for international survivors of sex trafficking into the United States, which can be adapted and applied to domestic survivors of sex trafficking as well, authors Macy and Johns (2011) suggest the following as survivors' most immediate needs: immediate safety, emergency shelter, basic necessities, language interpretation, emergency medical care, and legal advocacy. Once the above needs are addressed, then survivors can begin to focus on taking care of a number of other needs including their physical and mental health, substance abuse problems, education and life training, legal issues, permanent housing, and language skills if English is not their first language. Furthermore, the authors emphasize the importance in working with this population of conducting a comprehensive and thorough needs assessment, ensuring their safety and confidentiality, providing comprehensive case management, and providing culturally appropriate and trauma-informed care. Likewise, it is important to provide care that is respectful, to obtain informed consent for treatment, to respect the choices made by each individual, to provide information that is at the level of understanding of each individual, and to avoid calling the authorities unless given consent to do so by the victim (Zimmerman & Borland, 2009).

It is also important that nurses realize that when victims are ready to talk, we need to be ready to listen. Some of what we may hear from victims may be horrific, shocking, and beyond many of our own life experiences. Such is the nature of human trafficking. It is vitally important in working with victims that we are able to "listen dangerously" and not appear shocked or repelled by what they share with us. The moment a victim sees the listener's jaw drop, the opportunity for the victim to continue is often lost. Not wanting to traumatize the listener, the victim will stop narrating her story. As a profession in the trenches we will often be the first contact a victim has as a possible way out. It is important that we listen to the victims' stories, even though we may be afraid of what we may hear. To be unable to hear what they need to share with us with comfort and strength robs the victim of her comfort and strength to continue the telling. Listening can be dangerous, but it is necessary even when we are afraid of what we might hear (Rymes, 2001). In my experience one of the most important things I have offered the women I have worked with is to be able to listen dangerously to what they have told me. In looking back on Mimi, I wonder if anything more could have been done to help her. I and those who knew or worked with her have little doubt that her involvement in sex trafficking played a major role in her death. Hopefully as nurses become more aware and better informed about all aspects of human trafficking, the next Mimi will have a better outcome.

REFERENCES

American Psychiatric Association. (2000). *Diagnostic and statistical manual of mental disorders* (4th ed., text revision). Washington, DC: American Psychiatric Association.

Banks, D., & Kyckelhahn, T. (2011). *Special report: Characteristics of suspected human trafficking incidents* 2008–2010. U.S. Department of Justice Office of Justice Programs Bureau of Justice Statistics. Retrieved from http://bjs.ojp.usdoj.gov/content/pub/pdf/cshti0810.pdf

Barrows, J., & Finger, R. (2008). Human trafficking and the healthcare professional. *Southern Medical Journal, 101*(5), 521–524.

Batstone, D. (2007). *Not for sale: The return of the global slave trade and how we can fight back.* San Francisco, CA: Harper Collins Publishers.

Beyrer, C., & Stachowiak, J. (2003). Health consequences of trafficking women and girls in Southeast Asia. *Brown Journal of World Affairs, 10*(1), 105–117.

Bezpalcha, R. (2003). *Helping survivors of human trafficking: A practical guide.* Morrilton, AR: Winrock International. Retrieved 2/2/2012 from http://ukraine.winrock.org/DOS/publications/Blok_Eng.pdf

Center for Problem-Oriented Policing. Look beneath the surface: Role of health care providers in identifying and helping victims of human trafficking [PowerPoint presentation]. n.d. Retrieved from http://www.popcenter.org/problems/trafficked_women/PDFs/toolkit/Role_of_Health_Care_Providers.pdf

Child Soldiers: *Global Report 2008.* First published in 2008 by Coalition to Stop the Use of Child Soldiers, 9 Marshalsea Road (4th floor), London SE1 1EP United Kingdom www.child-soldiers.org. Copyright Coalition to Stop the Use of Child Soldiers. Retrieved from http://www.childsoldiersglobalreport.org/files/country_pdfs/FINAL_2008_Global_Report.pdf

Child Soldiers International Website. Retrieved from http://www.child-soldiers.org/home

Clark, M. (February 2012). Super Bowl prompts Indiana to rewrite human trafficking law Stateline Staff Writer. Retrieved from http://stateline.org/live/details/story?contentId=628677

Clawson, H. J., Dutch, N., Solomon, A., & Grace, L. G. (2009). *Human trafficking into and within the United States: A review of the literature.* Prepared for the Office of the Assistant Secretary for Planning and Evaluation (ASPE), U.S. Department of Health and Human Services. Retrieved from http://aspe.hhs.gov/hsp/07/HumanTrafficking/LitRev

Clawson, H. J., Layne, M., & Small, K. (2006). *Estimating human trafficking in the United States: Development of a methodology.* Fairfax, VA: Caliber, ICF International. Retrieved from https://www.ncjrs.gov/pdffiles1/nij/grants/215475.pdf

Clawson, H. J., Salomon, A., & Grace, L. G. (2008). *Treating the hidden wounds: Trauma treatment and mental health recovery for victims of human trafficking.* Prepared for the Office of the Assistant Secretary for Planning and Evaluation (ASPE), U.S. Department of Health and Human Services. Retrieved from http://aspe.hhs.gov/hsp/07/humantrafficking/Treating/ib.htm

Clawson, H. J., Small, K. M., Go, E. S., & Myles, B. W. (2003). *Needs assessment for service providers and trafficking victims.* Fairfax, VA: Caliber. Retrieved from https://www.ncjrs.gov/pdffiles1/nij/grants/202469.pdf

Cwikel, J., Ilan, K., & Chudakov, B. (2003). Women brothel workers and occupational health risks. *Journal of Epidemiological Community Health, 57*, 809–815.

Family Violence Prevention Fund, World Childhood Foundation. (2005). *Turning pain into power: Trafficking survivors' perspectives on early intervention strategies.* San Francisco, CA. Retrieved from http://www.futureswithoutviolence.org/user files/file/ImmigrantWomen/Turning%20Pain%20intoPower.pdf

Farley, M., Cotton, A., Lynne, J., Zumbeck, S., Spiwak, F., Reyes, M. et al. (2003). Prostitution and trafficking in nine countries: An update on violence and posttraumatic stress disorder. *Journal of Trauma Practice, 2*(3/4), 33–74.

Gajic-Veljanoski, O., & Stewart, D. E. (2007). Women trafficked into prostitution: Determinants, human rights and health needs. *Transcultural Psychiatry 44*(3), 338–358.

Hossain, M., Zimmerman, C., Abas, M., Light, M., & Watts, C. (2010). The relationship of trauma to mental disorders among trafficked and sexually exploited girls and women. *American Journal of Public Health, 100*(12), 2442–2449.

Kara, S. (2009). *Sex trafficking: Inside the business of modern slavery.* New York, NY: Columbia University Press.

Macy, R. J., & Johns, N. (2011). Aftercare services for international sex trafficking survivors: Informing U.S. service and program development in an emerging practice field. *Trauma Violence Abuse, 12*(2), 87–98.

Mizus, M., Moody, M., Privado, C., & Douglas, C. A. (2003). Germany, U.S. receive most sex-trafficked women. *Off Our Backs, 33*(7/8), 4.

Potterat, J. J., Brewer, D. D., Muth, S. Q., Rothenberg, R. B., Woodhouse, D. E., Muth, J. B. et al. (2004). Mortality in a long-term open cohort of prostitute women. *American Journal of Epidemiology, 159*(8),778–785. Retrieved from http://www.interscienti fic.net/reprints/AJE2004.pdf.

Raymond, J. G., & Hughes, D. M. (2001). *Sex trafficking of women in the United States: International and domestic trends.* U.S. Department of Justice. Retrieved from http://www.uri.edu/artsci/wms/hughes/sex_traff_us.pdf and https://www.ncjrs. gov/pdffiles1/nij/grants/187774.pdf

Reid, J. A. (2010). Doors wide shut: Barriers to the successful delivery of victim services for domestically trafficked minors in a Southern U.S. metropolitan area. *Women and Criminal Justice, 20*, 147–166.

Rymes, B. (2001). *Conversational borderlands: Language and identity in an alternative urban high school.* New York: Teachers College Press.

Sabella, D. (2011). The role of the nurse in combating human trafficking. *American Journal of Nursing, 111*(2), 28–39.

Sabella, D. (2012). *Trauma and posttraumatic stress disorder.* Manuscript submitted for publication.

Shively, M., McLaughlin, K., Durchslag, R., McDonough, H., Hunt, D., Kliorys, D. et al. (2010). *Developing a national action plan for eliminating sex trafficking: Final report.* Cambridge, MA: Abt Associates, Inc.

Tsutsumi, A., Izutsu, T., Poudyal, A., Kato, S., & Marui, E. (2008). Mental health of female survivors in human trafficking in Nepal. *Social Science and Medicine, 66*, 1841–1847.

UNICEF. *Fact Sheet: Child Soldiers.* (n.d.). Retrieved from http://www.unicef.org/emerg/ files/childsoldiers.pdf

United Nations. (2000). *Protocol to prevent, suppress and punish trafficking in persons, especially women and children, supplementing the United Nations Convention against transnational organized crime.* Retrieved from. http://www.uncjin.org/Documents/Conventions/dcatoc/final_documents_2/convention_%20traffeng.pdf

United Nations Office on Drugs and Crime. (2009). *Global report on trafficking in persons.* Retrieved from http://www.unodc.org/documents/Global_Report_on_TIP.pdf

United Nations Office on Drugs and Crime. (2012). *Human trafficking FAQs.* UNDOC. Retrieved from http://www.unodc.org/unodc/en/human-trafficking/faqs.html

United Nations Office on Drugs and Crime. (n.d.). *Human trafficking indicators:* http://www.unodc.org/pdf/HT_indicators_E_LOWRES.pdf

U.S. Congress. (2000). Public Law 106-386. *Victims of trafficking and violence protection act of 2000.* Retrieved from http://www.state.gov/documents/organization/10492.pdf

U.S. Department of Health and Human Services. (n.d.). *Sex trafficking fact sheet.* Administration for Children and Families, Campaign to Rescue and Restore Victims of Human Trafficking. Retrieved from http://www.acf.hhs.gov/trafficking/about/fact_sex.pdf.

U.S. Department of Health and Human Services. (n.d.). *Labor trafficking fact sheet.* Administration for Children and Families, Campaign to Rescue and Restore Victims of Human Trafficking. Retrieved from http:www.acf.hhs.govtraffickingaboutfact_labor.pdf

U.S. Department of State. (2009). *Report a trafficking victim* [fact sheet]. Washington, DC: U.S. Department of State. Retrieved from http://www.state.gov/g/tip/rls/fs/2009/106250.htm

U.S. Department of State. (2004). *Trafficking in persons report 2004.* Washington, DC: U.S. Department of State. Retrieved from http://www.state.gov/g/tip/rls/tiprpt/2004

U.S. Department of State. (2006). *Trafficking in persons report 2006.* Washington, DC: U.S. Department of State. Retrieved from http://www.state.gov/g/tip/rls/tiprpt/2006.

U.S. Department of State. (2007). *Trafficking in persons report 2007.* Washington, DC: U.S. Department of State. Retrieved from http://www.state.gov/g/tip/rls/tiprpt/2007.

U.S. Department of State. (2010). *Trafficking in persons report 2010.* Washington, DC: U.S. Department of State. http://www.state.gov/g/tip/rls/tiprpt/2010

U.S. Department of State. (2011). *Trafficking in persons report 2011.* Washington, DC: U.S. Department of State. http://www.state.gov/g/tip/rls/tiprpt/2011

U.S. Government Accountability Office (GAO). (2006). *Human trafficking: better data, strategy, and reporting needed to enhance U.S. Anti-trafficking efforts abroad.* (GAO-06-825). Retrieved from http://www.gao.gov/new.items/d06825.pdf.

Wyler, L. S., & Siskin, A(2010). *Trafficking in persons: U.S. policy and issues for Congress.* Washington, DC: Congressional Research Service, Library of Congress, RL34317. Retrieved from http://www.unhcr.org/refworld/docid/4cb429f62.html

Williamson, E., Dutch, N. M., & Clawson, H. J. (2009). *National symposium on the health needs of human trafficking victims: Post symposium brief.* Prepared for the Office of the Assistant Secretary for Planning and Evaluation (ASPE), U.S. Department of

Health and Human Services. Retrieved from http://aspe.hhs.gov/hsp/07/humantraf ficking/Symposium/ib.pdf

Williamson, E., Dutch, N. M., & Clawson, H. J. (2010). *Evidence-based mental health treatment for victims of human trafficking.* Prepared for the Office of the Assistant Secretary for Planning and Evaluation (ASPE), U.S. Department of Health and Human Services. Retrieved from http://aspe.hhs.gov/hsp/07/humantrafficking/Mental Health/index.pdf

Yakushko, O. (2009). Human trafficking: A review for mental health professionals. *International Journal for the Advancement of Counselling, 31,* 158–167.

Zimmerman, C., & Borland, R. (Eds.). (2009) *Caring for trafficked persons: guidance for health providers.* Geneva, Switzerland: IOM. 2009. Retrieved from http://publi cations.iom.int/bookstore/free/CT_Handbook.pdf.

Zimmerman, C., Hossain, M., Yun, K., Gajdadziev, V., Guzun, N., Tchomarova, M. et al. (2008). The health of trafficked women: A survey of women entering posttrafficking services in Europe. *American Journal of Public Health, 98*(1), 1–5.

Zimmerman, C., Hossain, M., Yun, K., Roche, B., Morison, L., & Watts, C. (2006). *Stolen smiles: A summary report on the physical and psychological health consequences of women and adolescents trafficked in Europe.* London, UK: London School of Hygiene and Tropical Medicine. Retrieved from http://www.humantrafficking.org/ uploads/publications/Stolen_Smiles_July_2006.pdf

Zimmerman, C., Yun, K., Shvab, I., Watts, C., Trappolin, L., Treppete, M. et al. (2003). *The health risks and consequences of trafficking in women and adolescents. Findings from a European study.* London, UK: London School of Hygiene & Tropical Medicine. Retrieved from ttp://www.lshtm.ac.uk/php/ghd/docs/traffickingfinal.pdf

CHAPTER 11

A Human Trafficking Toolkit for Nursing Intervention

PATRICIA CRANE

*T*he trafficking of humans is one of the fastest-growing crimes globally that violates human rights. However, limited research exists on the development of best practices for providing health care for trafficking victims. Review articles may address aspects of the experience of human trafficking, but are based on European, Asian, or African study findings, so health care professionals must generalize to the United States. The global nature of trafficking indicates that health care providers (HCP) in the United States will encounter trafficked persons in a variety of health care settings, and should be armed with clinical knowledge and resources to address their health care needs. No community is immune to the sex trafficking of minors and cases have been identified in all 50 states (McClain & Garrity, 2011). Frontline HCP may be in a key position to have the most critical impact with trafficking victims by identifying them and impacting their health and safety issues. The HCP may be one of few professionals likely to encounter a trafficking victim *while they are still in captivity.*

The challenge for clinicians is being aware of what trafficking victims look like. Since this is a condition of their life, and not a clinical diagnosis, persons who are trafficked may not have unique symptoms or evident physical findings. They are not likely to be identifiable at first glance. However, trafficking victims start out with existing vulnerabilities that differentiate them from others. Trafficking victims may already have been involved in the criminal justice or child protection systems and primarily they will be women and children. Countries or communities of origin may be impacted by severe poverty and marked with a recent history of strife and civil war. Big cites allow the trafficking to carry on virtually unnoticed, and traffickers can disappear in a moment (McClain & Garrity, 2011).

People who are trafficked start the vicious cycle of victimization by being drawn into work by means of force, fraud, or coercion, which is the key factor that differentiates them from persons who are smuggled. They make a choice to go and work for another person or organization, but often their choice is based on lies and trickery, not the truth. Frequently they are involved in domestic, sex, or farm work and other types of service jobs. In a clinical setting, as the patient history is revealed, the patient is unable to state demographic information and reproductive history. They are unclear and not able to answer questions routinely asked in a health screening history.

SEX TRAFFICKING

The constant demand for sex for purchase and the trafficking and purchase of women and girls for this purpose is reported to be the most rapidly growing form of organized crime and human rights abuse. Exact data on numbers of trafficking globally are difficult to assess due to the secretive nature of the illegal acts. Annually 27 million people are reported to be trafficked globally, 800,000 across national borders, with 80% being women and girls (TIP Report, 2011). It is estimated that as many as 17,500 per year are trafficked into the United States. Nearly all (95%) of the trafficked women and female adolescents report sexual and physical violence while in the trafficking situation; 76% reported physical abuse and 90% reported sexual abuse. In a national study in the United States on juvenile prostitution 14- to 17-year olds are the largest group involved (Mitchell, Finkelhor, & Wolak, 2010). When a young woman chooses to engage in sex work as a means of survival, she may think she is making a wise choice, and that it will be a temporary job. She may not realize that she is legally under the age of consent and it is not her choice and she may find it nearly impossible to leave, whether she is of age or not. At some point she will shoulder all the blame for being trafficked as have many who have been victimized do. Self-blame may continue even after she returns to her family or home community and others become aware that she was a sex worker and shun her.

Zimmerman et al. (2008) interviewed 200 women to gather information on their experience of trafficking. They followed the recommendations of the World Health Organization (WHO) to provide safe and secure interviews that were separate from routine clinical services (Zimmerman & Watts, 2003). The WHO advice is useful whether the clinicians are in domestic and international trafficking situations when the clinicians suspect trafficking. Safety of the patient or victim of human trafficking is of utmost importance.

Three Levels of Intervention in Stages of Trafficking

Zimmerman's seminal research (2008) recommends that with sex trafficking victims, health care interventions should be based on the stage of trafficking. Application of literature on trafficking victims is beneficial when the HCP cares for persons who are sex trafficking victims since, for the majority, it is a

1. Predeparture Stage

2. Travel and Transit Stage

3. Destination Stage

4. Detention, Deportation, Criminal Evidence Stage

5. Integration and Reintegration Stage

FIGURE 11.1 Stages of trafficking.
Source: Zimmerman, 2008.

coexisting situation. The HCP must be sensitive to the potential feelings, mental health needs, fear, anxiety, and other emotions while the person is in captivity and in the post-trafficking state. The services and health care needs of trafficking victims are similar to other vulnerable and exploited patients (Zimmerman et al., 2003).

Application of clinician tools during the stages of trafficking may help the HCP working with persons who are trafficked. Needs-based care is specifically beneficial as it depends on the most common biopsychosocial health care needs of the patient at the time (Figures 11.1 and 11.2).

Predeparture Stage

Persons are trafficked due to their poverty, personal history of violence, and living in broken homes. They are often lacking in simple knowledge about health care and diseases that may be encountered in the new life of opportunity they are seeking. Limitations in education also include the fact that education is

---

Primary prevention focuses on avoidance of the initial event related to a problem. A general plan of action is applied to a population or community. Primary prevention with human trafficking could include community education in the community of origin to increase awareness and ways to avoid buyers.

Secondary prevention focuses on prevention of repeat events. Secondary prevention with human trafficking could include the role of HCP in the country of arrival through identification of victims, providing a safety and recue net to interrupt the cycle of trafficking at that point of care.

Tertiary prevention is most intensive and focuses on reduction of the impact of an event. With human trafficking tertiary prevention could address care for mental and health issues that occurred as result of trafficking. It could also include intervention programs that address returning the victims to as normal a lifestyle as possible, whether in the community of origin if they can return or in a new life in the endpoint community.

FIGURE 11.2 Levels of prevention.
Adapted by Patricia Crane from material by the Polaris Project
(http://www.polarisproject.org/take-action).

not highly valued or pursued. Thus, there may be an unawareness of geography, where they are going compared to where they are, the topography of the land, distance, and travel time, which could actually portend how rigorous the transport will be. Very often the socio-political climate in the country of origin has left many people living in poverty, jobless or homeless. Those who are vulnerable to trafficking may not know where they are going but truly believe that it must be better than where they are. They are in dire need of opportunities to survive, and the trafficker takes advantage of this need or vulnerability. Also, the trafficking victim may already be a migrant alone in a culturally strange place far from home where job opportunities were thought to be more prolific.

Intervention
Primary prevention strategies must begin prior to the trafficking experience, in the country of origin, in the predeparture stage. Global citizens, including many HCPs, dedicate sincere efforts and donations of time, money, and knowledge in countries at risk for trafficking. Prevention efforts may include large public health education campaigns that educate citizens about health, safety, contraception, common diseases, and immunizations when migrating or traveling for work. Prevention may also be aimed at information regarding the laws and legal issues in the destiny country. However, small local efforts in vulnerable border communities also aim at the creation of work and education programs that empower those most at risk to migrate or be lured in by the traffickers, and become ensnared in the life of debt bondage with little chance of escape.

Risks and vulnerabilities are interconnected psychosocial factors, conditions in their lives, as well as economic factors. Researchers found that the vulnerabilities of trafficking victims are much the same as with victims of other interpersonal violent crimes (Zimmerman et al., 2003). Over half (59%) reported pretrafficking experiences of sexual and physical violence before 15 years of age. Assaults that were perpetrated by more than one person were reported by 26%, and many named the father or stepfather as perpetrator. Personal life experiences may lead them to want to leave home, but also it has conditioned them to tolerate abuse, work long hours without complaining, and to mentally separate themselves from the tough conditions of their lives. Leaving home and relocating to another location for work seems like a solution rather than the nightmare of torture and human rights abuse in which they find themselves. The actions taken to prevent human trafficking in the communities of origin should involve people from that community, and be sensitive to the cultural and linguistic facets when using an education and awareness campaign.

The primary prevention toolkit for clinicians and community workers at this point may not look very clinical. In the United States there are programs such as Free the Captives "Reducing the Demand Campaign" with youth and college students available at www.FreeTheCaptivesHouston.com. The focus is on reducing the demands of buyers who often have criminal records, are family members with children, know where to buy children for the sex slave industry, and ensure the continuation of the sex trafficking business. The web site includes a description of steps of an action plan and materials that can be used for a local community project.

Shared Hope International (2009) addresses domestic sex trafficking (DMST) through provision of a resource packet with curriculum, training videos, fact sheets, and more. Basic education tools for use in U.S. communities are essential for initiating prevention strategies. Too often children (individuals under the age of 18) are exploited through prostitution, pornography, and sexual entertainment as the victims. Labeled and treated as victims and sent to detention centers, the problem involves many public servants and HCPs who blame and punish the wrong party and fail to see the vulnerability and social context in which youth are drawn into selling sex for profit of pimp-controlled prostitution, family prostitution, and survival sex.

Another good tool was demonstrated by students interested in prevention activities with other students and getting community members involved. Educating and discussing the issue of human trafficking in their communities is effective as an education project. Films such as *Trade, The Dark Side of Chocolate*, or *Cargo: Innocence Lost* are easily ordered for rental or purchase. One student showed videos in class and at community gatherings (personal conversation with A. Gallegos, 2010). Students provide handouts with some definitions, and show a movie that emphasizes cases familiar to the audience, which sensitizes them to the issues. Citizens often need information that can help them understand that the law forbids children to have sex for the profit of another. It is not a choice and children are not the criminals but the buyers and sellers are.

Travel and Transit Stage

During the Travel and Transit Stage of trafficking, whether international or within national borders, victims may endure difficult travel conditions, being exposed to severe weather with little protection, scarce food and water, no sleep or toilet breaks. Traffickers often have time deadlines to transport a group to the destiny location. Traffickers have a lot to lose if they are late: loss of money, future business, or their own lives. The cargo is not considered human beings but a means to make a living. Transporters are seldom very high in the chain of command and may be more at risk of losing their lives than the cargo.

Zimmerman describes this stage as being from recruitment to reaching the final destination point. Multiple tactics are employed to maintain and sustain control of the victim. Usually the harmful behavior starts because the trafficker has a lot to lose if the cargo does not reach the final destination. A great deal is at stake, and he must maintain control over his charges. For this reason transit is the most dangerous stage, and it is the time that confinement, rape, and physical abuse are used as further means of control (Zimmerman, 2003).

While in transit to the destiny location, acts of violence may include but not be limited to sexual abuse, threats, or actual physical abuse. When they were most vulnerable due to the trauma, the trafficker offers them assistance, work, extra food or water, and special living quarters. Victims are lured further into the web of deceit by traffickers' attempts to play favorites among the victims, turning them against one another or at the very least preventing them from communicating with one another and ensuring further isolation, even within the group.

Myriad health problems related to the physical and sexual assaults that are used to control the victims may begin while in transit. While in the grasp of the control of the trafficker, there is no limit to the bullying and threatening tactics that may be used to maintain control of a group of women in transit. However, one of the greatest barriers to escaping is the psychological barrier of fear surrounding the victims when they first realize the mortal danger they are in, which Zimmerman (2003) refers to as the initial trauma. Further, the impact of such high anxiety psychological trauma often leads to dissociation, a type of denial that will prevent them from further harm. The psychological processing also leads to a selective memory of the event and hypervigilance to avoid future trauma.

Intervention

At the travel stage, interventions will be secondary interventions to prevent future trauma or reentering the trafficking cycle. The challenge to rescue at this stage is the altered memory state of the victims. To avoid total mental breakdown and devastation, victims often may claim they are safe and being taken care of and no abuse is taking place. Anxiety and fear lead to placid compliant victims. The second barrier at this stage is that the modes of travel vary greatly but seldom without armed guards or traffickers, who quell the interest of their fatigued victims to attempt a run for freedom.

There may be scant opportunities and difficulty getting a trafficker to allow stopping for medical care, healthy nutrition, and adequate hydration or sleep. Unless there is a life threat that could lead to the loss of cargo that would reduce delivery payment, a trafficker is unlikely to interrupt the journey for his victims. However should the victim be able to escape, or be running from the captors, then there is a possibility of finding themselves in a health care setting.

Interviewing newly escaped victims of human trafficking requires great care. Use of the WHO safety guidelines for interviewing victims should guide the health professionals' actions and are key items to have in the clinician's toolkit. Communication skills for emotionally, psychologically and physically traumatized patients are critical tools. As the most dangerous stage, the delicate mental state of victims makes them very fragile and physical trauma may be easier to deal with.

All tools for interviewing and gathering evidence with sexual assault victims may be useful for interactions with trafficking victims. Nurses and other health professionals who are experienced in dealing with victims of violence such as rape victims would be excellent resources to provide physical care at this time and possibly collect evidence and a sexual assault evidence kit.

Destination Stage

When they have reached the destiny location, it may be the first time they are told they have to work for the trafficker until the transport debt is paid in full. Essentially they are kept in bondage or enslaved. Over time, the food, clothing, room rental fees, and necessities of life are all deducted from wages, leaving them almost nothing to apply to the transport debt, much less send home to their family (Figure 11.3).

At the end of the transit stage, the human cargo may be sold; however, a human trafficking victim may be bought and sold repeatedly as they travel across borders of countries or states. Arrangements may have been made to meet with a buyer or to have transported a prearranged amount of women or adolescents or children. Women and children are more docile and easy to control and bring a high price in the sex trade industry. If they are already migrants and have endured a treacherous journey for the purpose of finding work in another country or state, then the end of the journey is a perfect point of vulnerability for a trafficker to sell a group of people, children included, taking them off the transporter's hands. The offer of work and survival to a group of extremely vulnerable people may seem like a miracle, but they are unaware of the debt bondage that awaits them and may entrap them for years to come. Reaching a destination for some may provide respite following a torturous trip replete with episodes of violence. For most, however, it is when the work begins. Various forms of physical, sexual, and mental trauma are endured by the women throughout the transit. At the endpoint when the final sale takes place, the work begins. Often the victims have to live in isolation, locked in close quarters with no access to toilets, food, or sunshine. Now the work begins, and the captors must keep their charges under control. Sadly, however the captives need to work to repay the constantly accumulating debt associated with their life of bondage.

---

1. Patient is accompanied by another person who seems controlling and answers questions directed at the patient.

2. Patient seems submissive or fearful.

3. Movements on and off the job are restricted.

4. Signs of physical abuse are present.

5. Person possesses no identification documents such as passport, birth certificate, visa.

6. Patient has difficulty communicating due to language or cultural barriers.

7. Patient suffers from health care problems experienced by trafficking victims.

FIGURE 11.3 Indicators of trafficking.
Adapted from Campaign to Rescue and Restore Victims of Human Trafficking.

Interventions

The most valuable tool for any clinician is the ability to build trust with therapeutic communication skills. Building trust is a slow process. After all they have endured, the victims may have a negative view toward health providers or anyone in authority, a sentiment that has been reiterated repeatedly by their captors or pimps to keep them from seeking help. Few interruptions, use of open-ended questions, and understanding the role of family and values may help to build rapport. What the HCP and legal professionals may label as "trafficking" is not so clear or obvious to the victims themselves. More often than not they would deny it or need to have a legal definition of their status as a "victim of human trafficking" explained to them. An example of a tool that may help the HCP is a set of screening questions. Avoiding confrontational directness with a set of simple focused questions can help confirm a strong clinical suspicion that the patient is likely involved in trafficking (Figure 11.4).

A wide array of health issues are likely with trafficking victims beyond what is normally expected for their age, sex, and country of origin (Barrows & Finger, 2008). It is not uncommon to see broken bones, contusions, trauma, dental problems, sexually transmitted infections, and gastrointestinal problems with the victim in a clinical setting. Medical care is not likely to be sought or granted to them when requested, so symptoms may exist for months until the victim's condition is much worse and requires hospitalization. Stress, poor living conditions and deprivation of basic food, water, and good hygiene can lead to a poor immune response to common illnesses resulting in worse health outcomes. Additionally the nature of the work they become engaged in while they are captive is hazardous to health and well-being.

Zimmerman (2003) reports that many women would say they decided not to seek care if they had to pay or miss hours at work, or that their identification papers had long ago been confiscated by a trafficker. Every tool in the clinician's tool box may be needed to break the bonds at this time due to the trafficker's controlling grasp. The victims know what awaits them if they speak or attempt to

---

Can you come and go at the job and your home as you please?
Have you been threatened if you try to leave your job?
Have you been physically harmed in any way?
What is it like where you work?
Where do you sleep and eat?
Do you sleep in a bed, on a cot, or on the floor?
Do you have to ask permission to eat, sleep, or go to the bathroom?
Have you ever been deprived of food, water, sleep, or medical care?
Are there locks on your doors and windows so you cannot get out?
Has anyone threatened your family?
Have your identification papers been taken from you?
Is anyone forcing you to do anything that you do not want to do?

FIGURE 11.4 Screening questions for health care providers.

run. The health care provider must use the approach to safe screening that would be used with any victim of domestic violence when the controlling partner is nearby. Any means of separating the victim from any male or female accompanying them allows the opportunity to question them about their safety, freedom, work conditions, and safe means of escape if they choose that. A sensitive and caring person in a safe environment may be able to reach through to the victim and determine their health and safety needs and their perceived danger due to the degree of threat and control being used (Figure 11.5).

The person who is trafficked may have myriad and diverse mental and physical health care needs, but most importantly safety needs. Trafficked persons suffer a wide variety of health problems beyond what would be expected given their age, gender, and country of residence. Health status is also based on the intimidation/indoctrination tactics used by the trafficker against the victim performing their work and the conditions trafficking victims are subjected to. They are likely to have had no access to health care while in transit because of the illegal nature of trafficking activities and secrecy in transport. And yet a number of their longer term medical problems were initiated during that time.

Victims of trafficking may be taken to a clinic at the completion of their transit for a variety of medical complaints. For all HCPs, the greatest asset is the skill of therapeutic communication and a nonbiased approach to each patient, and physical assessment skills (Figure 11.6).

The basic skills of every health care clinician include the observation and documentation of patient demeanor, avoidance behaviors, noticing discomfort

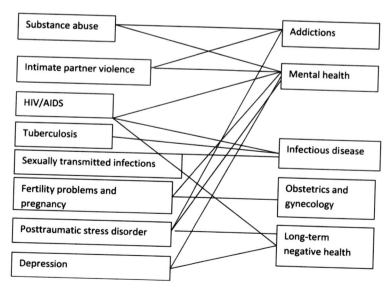

FIGURE 11.5 Health problems of human trafficking victims.

We are here to help you.

Our first priority is your safety.

We will give the medical care that you need.

We can find you a safe place to stay.

We want to make sure this does not happen to other people.

You are entitled to help and we can get assistance for you.

If you have been held against your will (trafficked), and cooperate you will not be deported and can receive help to stay safely in this country.

FIGURE 11.6 Trust-building messages.

and evasiveness in the look on the victims' faces that denotes something is not right. Clinicians should have a heightened index of suspicion when a patient has some indicators of a trafficking victim. A trafficking victim may be accompanied by a person who is very controlling and attempts to answer simple history questions for the patient. The patient may glance warily at the controlling person and appear submissive or fearful. A trafficking victim may not understand questions or be able to say where they are geographically or possess identification papers. They may be uncomfortable with direct eye contact and communicate poorly. Challenges in communication could be due to minimal or limited knowledge of the language used by the HCP, or fear of the person who accompanies them and remains present in the room. The victim may not have answers to the questions because they have only been given scant information by the captor to allow them to respond. With routine questions about demographic information, health assessment, and analysis of clinical symptoms, the victim appears confused and cannot provide the details for routine health questions. They have been in isolation and been told what to say, but the scant information is inadequate for the clinician.

Detention, Deportation, Criminal Evidence Stage

This is the phase described as the time when a victim may be in police custody for immigration violations or for cooperating with someone who is involved in illegal activities, such as the trafficker, pimp, or their abuser. The HCP is not the primary actor in this stage but the immigration, police, or legal official is.

When authorities come in contact with human trafficking victims it is often not a voluntary situation. Human trafficking victims and authorities come in contact because of a helping organization such as a nongovernmental organization (NGO) or local hotline worker. Additionally the legal authorities may make a raid on a brothel, due to more vigorous antiimmigrant government policies or aggressive treatment of undocumented persons. A pimp may drop off the victim at police headquarters because the victim is of no further value to them (due to illness or pregnancy) or they want to avoid paying the victims their wages.

Protections for victims of human trafficking are scanty but are notably underused. Internationally the programs and policies offer little support, and leave victims unprotected and open to further abuse by traffickers. Despite the deplorable conditions in transit and detention, once removed or rescued, they resent the action, and did not perceive their need for help. Pimps using underage girls for profit with prostitution have led them to have a criminal record, even though the definition of human sex trafficking identifies them as a victim.

Interventions

Zimmerman (2003) interviewed authorities who admitted that officers know that health needs must be taken care of when planning to interview a victim, and can verbalize what a mentally and physically abused woman may look like, but they also admit her abuse as a trafficking victim is a low priority. Dealing with her violation of the law is their priority. Different countries have different laws. In some countries contacting an advocacy agency for the victims may lead to getting health care needs met. Because of the legal violation, however, sex-trafficking victims are not treated as a victim in most countries but are treated coldly and like other criminals. Enduring extreme psychological and physical abuse, and then the legal abuse within the system that should protect them, is a barrier to accessing timely care even after the rescue has occurred. Limited services due to diminished financial resources invested in social services act as further barriers to care.

Health professionals can be instrumental in bringing education programs to the public and legal authorities about human trafficking and the need for policy changes and greater respect for human rights. Just as the clinician might do with educational interventions as prevention strategies, the educational component may sensitize authority figures. However little change is likely until country, state, and regional policies mandate changes in treatment to determine the status of women who are arrested for prostitution, whether or not they have a choice in the matter.

Deportation is the most common outcome and is usually planned rapidly after a person is picked up by immigration authorities. They are not medically evaluated, nor is there any coordination with an advocacy agency for their care. Upon deportation the return points are common places where previous traffickers meet them and begin the process again with the women. Added debt for relocation is added and with little money or resources for their health care, they continue to suffer from all maladies through all stages of trafficking.

In the United States, it is far more likely that a medical examination or a sexual assault forensic examination could be performed in the timeframe when women are incarcerated or awaiting deportation. Testing for sexually transmitted infections is required, but the routine health screening and immunizations needed by all age groups should be offered. In human trafficking summits and conferences with rape crisis services and addictions programs are highly involved in providing care for human trafficking victims.

Assistance may come from international migration officials or their local voluntary organization counterparts if they are present in the area. They may help the victims get medical needs met and find a safe place to stay. Often the temporary residence depends on helping police prosecute the buyers or traffickers. Turning in the traffickers is a very uncommon option for women for many reasons. They have just left the captive situation in which the only friend or protector was the captor or boyfriend/fiance, even though he was also abusive. Fear of harm to themselves and their families are always a threat. Often the women have little knowledge of the captor and his other illicit activities and thus the women are of little help to the legal authorities. Memories and details of the transit stage are difficult to recall since they were living in a heightened sense of survival mode.

While there is much literature about the therapeutic benefits of going to trial and facing the accused for crimes of abuse and sexual assault, they are not seeking rescue or escape. Victims of human trafficking are seldom prepared for such a trial and the threats incurred with such a bold action. Authorities often lack a true understanding of the psychological and emotional impact of rape trauma. Attorneys fail to prepare women for the grueling trial and the treatment the women are likely to receive in the legal system. Involvement of nursing and advocacy agencies is very much underutilized with this type of victim because they are usually involved in criminal activity.

Integration and Reintegration Stage

Starting life anew is the last stage in human trafficking, whether they are integrating into a new community in a different country or have been returned to their home country for reintegration. Few get assistance from any agency or individual to start life anew following life-altering circumstances (Zimmerman, 2003). Safe housing is their greatest need and an even greater challenge when LGBT sex trafficking victims need housing (Mitchell, Finkelhor, & Wolak, 2010).

Interventions
Long- and short-term health problems can be addressed at this time, but the limitations are overwhelming. Secondary and tertiary interventions are going to be needed for the rest of the survivor's life. Thus, while the primary prevention strategies must be ongoing and intensified, the majority of the clinician's work is over the long term after the initial event. Scant social and financial resources are available to allow for adequate mental and physical health care being sought. Immigrants are usually aid recipients and this often leads to a subordinate and disrespected treatment status within a health system.

Similar difficulties exist even when the survivor returns for reintegration in the country of origin. Family and community members will never see the victim as the same person if they know the truth. Living alone with the horror of their experience is easier than trying to explain to others. Access to health care services is very difficult and quality of care is poor. Health professionals who know little about the trafficking of human beings are insensitive to the issue and treat the survivors in a judgmental manner.

Nongovernmental service organizations are the sources through which many survivors seek care or assistance for anything. If agencies of health workers or social workers were the same groups seeing women while they were still captive, it provides some similarity of faces and continuity of care. Assistance into programs to assist with integration or reintegration are often tied to the survivor's agreement to participate in the legal proceedings.

The type of lifestyle they sought to escape is often the same as that they integrate or reintegrate into. Only the loss of respect, friends, and family makes the likelihood of returning to their pimp very common.

TOOLKIT

The novelty of human trafficking is a toolkit that should contain educational materials, referrals, and resources in addition to screening tools that may be of value in teaching other clinicians or in clinical settings. A toolkit should have items tailored for each user to fit human trafficking.

The primary element in every HCP toolkit is the bio-psycho-social knowledge that allows sensitivity and nonbiased communications with patients for whom they provide care. The second most critical element is the health assessment skills that allow the clinical history and physical examination of the patient to be individualized and focused on his or her unique health care needs. Additional toolkit contents may vary.

In all clinical settings there will be a standard intake form for documentation of demographics and medical history and physical findings. It is unlikely there will be questions needed to delve deeper into the experience of a trafficked patient (currently trafficked or recently rescued). In addition to indicators and clinician screening questions, these additional points may need to be added:

- Languages spoken
- Nationality/where was passport from
- Ethnicity
- Safe contact telephone number or person
- Date of leaving/escape/rescue
- Type of employment
- Primary employer
- Length of servitude
- How recruited and by whom
- Were you recruited in your country or after crossing the border
- Do you know where you have been
- Type of travel

- Cost of travel paid to transporter
- Were you required to pay off the debt
- How many times were you sold
- Documents withheld

This chapter contains items that may help educate the HCP, promote community awareness, and assist with patient management and referral, as well as resources or links that may contain additional or more specific content for the HCP to use or to share depending on the intention or purpose. For development of a toolkit, consider the range of individuals that will be targeted (age, profession, level of familiarity) and how they might be using information on human trafficking.

The toolkit for practicing HCPs might be more clinical in nature with a pretest and posttest to measure knowledge gained in an education session. It might include the videos mentioned previously or the video "Human Trafficking," Powerpoint presentations, free downloadable handouts available from the Rescue and Restore web site (www.acf.hhs.gov/trafficking/rescue_res tore/index.html) such as a profile of trafficking victims, specific focused screening questions, location and contact information for specific referrals, information on shelters and local HCPs who accept patients who are not able to pay for care, and laminated pocket screening and referral cards that can be ordered from the web site at no charge and handed out to professionals.

Other online educational resources for emergency health professionals may have what you prefer to use at www.humantraffickinged.com.

With a toolkit for the HCP, indicators, brief information, resources, web sites, and screening instruments or tools can be used to educate and quickly come to a decision on who to screen, precise questions to ask, and where to refer patients who were involved in trafficking in order to best meet their unique health care and legal needs. The clinician's toolkit might include other tools for the HCP to comprehend and address the needs of the trafficking victims as patients. This chapter focuses on the appropriate application of the clinician's toolkit for use, revision, and application for practice.

In order to document the types of abuse seen with many forensic patients, it may be beneficial to have rulers, camera, and body diagrams to document wounds or physical findings clearly that corroborate verbal information regarding abusive treatment. If the HCP is able to secure time alone with the patient and have good communication, then the interaction with the patient may follow the institutional guidelines of any forensic patient visit with proper documentation and evidence collection. It would be wise to have the evidence kit used by the hospital and forensic protocols in the toolkit.

SUMMARY

Currently, it is very popular to support health care professionals' ability to address health care management and education on a unique contemporary health care topic by developing a "toolkit" that enhances knowledge and competency in the area. With the information included in this chapter, it is likely the reader will have many more resources and documents to add to their toolkit for dealing primary, secondary, or tertiary interventions with human trafficking.

REFERENCES

Barrows, J., & Finger, R. (2008). Human trafficking and the health care professional. *Southern Medical Journal, 101*(5), 521–524.

Campaign to rescue and restore victims of human trafficking. Accessed May 30, 2012 at http://www.acf.hhs.gov/trafficking/campaign_kits/index.html. Website last updated Dec. 2008.

McClain, N., & Garrity, S. (2011). Sex trafficking and the exploitation of adolescents. *Journal of Obstetric, Gynecologic, and Neonatal Nursing, 40,* 243–252.

Mitchell, J., Finkelhor, D., & Wolak, J. (2010). Juvenile prostitution as child maltreatment: Findings from the national juvenile prostitution study. *Child Maltreatment, 15*(1), 18–36.

Polaris Project. (n.d.). Retrieved from http://www.polarisproject.org/take-action.

Shared Hope International. (2009). The national report on domestic minor sex trafficking: America's prostituted children. Accessed online May 30, 2012. http://www.share dhope.org/Resources/TheNationalReport.aspx

U.S. Department of State. (2010). *Trafficking in Persons Report (TIP).* Retrieved October 1, 2012 from http://www.state.gov/j/tip/rls/tiprpt/2010/

Zimmerman, C., & Watts, C. (2003). *WHO ethical and safety recommendations for interviewing trafficked women.* Geneva, Switzerland: World Health Organization.

Zimmerman, C. (2003). *WHO ethical and safety recommendations for interviewing trafficked women.* Geneva, Switzerland: World Health Organization. Retrieved October 1, 2012 from http://www.who.int/gender/documents/en/final%20recom mendations%2023%20oct.pdf

Zimmerman, C., Yun, K., Guzun, N., Ciarrocchi, M., Johansson, A., Kefurtova, A. et al. (2008). The health of trafficked women: a survey of women entering posttrafficking services in Europe. *American Journal of Public Health, 98*(1), 55–59.

Zimmerman, C., Yun, K., Schvab, I., Watts, C., Trappolin, L., Treppete, M. et al. (2003). *The health risks and consequences of trafficking in women and adolescents: Findings from a European study.* London: London School of Hygiene & Tropical Medicine (LSHTM).

CHAPTER 12

Malnutrition

NICOLE MARENO AND MARY DE CHESNAY

A common problem of victims of human trafficking is malnutrition. Globally, these victims tend to be poor with life histories of not having enough to eat, leaving them vulnerable to the traffickers who promise them a better life for themselves and their families. In the United States, though victims can come from any socioeconomic class, they quickly learn that their pimps will not place a high priority on proper diet. In fact, pimps usually keep them malnourished and sleep deprived as a means of control. As a reward for good behavior, pimps may take them out to breakfast at a fast-food restaurant. If the girls are given any of the money they earn for food, they are likely to spend it on snacks for a short-term energy boost.

Nurses who encounter victims prior to rescue can do little to help them reverse the effects of malnutrition, but once victims are in a safe space, they can be fed appropriately and taught better habits. In this chapter, the authors will explain some of the effects of malnutrition, explain how to assess deficiencies, and provide a nutritional teaching plan nurses can use with survivors.

BEST PRACTICES

Nutrition for Children and Adolescents

The healthiest diet for individuals over the age of 2 years is one that includes adequate amounts of fruits, vegetables, whole grains, low-fat or nonfat dairy products, beans, fish, and lean meats (American Heart Association et al., 2006). A nutritionally adequate diet should principally contain plant-based foods such as fruits, vegetables, beans, grains, nuts, and seeds, while simultaneously limiting saturated fats and cholesterol, which are found in animal products. The American Academy of Pediatrics endorses dietary strategies that encourage the reduction of saturated fats, cholesterol, added sugars, and added salt (American Heart Association et al., 2006).

Children and adolescents should consume a variety of fruits, vegetables, whole grains, low-fat or nonfat dairy products, beans, fish, and lean meats. This variety ensures an adequate amount of macronutrients and micronutrients necessary for proper growth and development. A sufficient consumption of fluids is also critical in order to maintain fluid balance and prevent dehydration. Failure to consume adequate amounts of fluids, macronutrients, and micronutrients can lead to undernutrition or malnutrition, and chronic health problems.

Ensuring satisfactory caloric consumption of healthful foods is a priority. For girls aged between 9 and 18 years, the American Heart Association and colleagues (2006) recommend a caloric consumption of 1,600 to 1,800 calories per day. The recommendation for boys aged between 9 and 18 years is 1,800 to 2,200 calories per day (American Heart Association et al., 2006). The preceding caloric recommendations are general, and do not account for variations in activity level or metabolic need. The recommendations should be used as a universal guideline, and adjusted based on an assessment of individual needs.

An acute or chronic deficiency in calories, macronutrients (protein, fats), and micronutrients leads to undernutrition or malnutrition (Voss, Tootell, & Gussler, 2006). For children and adolescents who fall victim to human traffickers, causes of poor nutrition include irregular eating patterns, lack of caloric intake (especially foods with substantive nutritional value), and lack of fluid intake. As Zimmerman, Hossain, and Watts (2011) note, human traffickers use economic exploitation or debt bondage to maintain control over trafficked persons, and this often includes withholding food.

Women who fall victim to human traffickers and are forced into sex work are at a high risk of poor nutrition due to food and fluid deprivation (Voss et al., 2006). Researchers who have studied street sex workers and individuals who abuse intravenous drugs have found a higher prevalence of underweight (Sæland et al., 2008) and an inadequate number of daily food servings (Baptiste, Hamlin, & Côté, 2009). Sæland and colleagues studied 72 female heroin users in Norway (38 of whom engaged in prostitution), reporting that the women averaged 2.7 food servings per day, and had low levels of hemoglobin, serum ferritin, and albumin levels, indicating malnutrition. Baptiste et al. interviewed 23 street sex workers in Canada, finding that high levels of intravenous drug use were associated with low food consumption levels (average of two or less meals per day). Baptiste and colleagues reported that when the women chose to consume foods, they opted for juice, chocolate, soft drinks, alcohol, or chips to supply quick energy.

The coerced or forced use of alcohol and drugs impacts nutrition and overall health. As Voss and colleagues note, drugs and alcohol can be used as a means of controlling the victim, as a method to prevent hunger, or as a way for the victim to cope with the trafficking situation. As past researchers have found, when drugs or alcohol are being used, the substance becomes the priority, while food consumption becomes less important to the user (Baptiste et al., 2009).

Victims of human trafficking are often starved or deprived of food, leading to decreased caloric consumption and low levels of nutrient dense foods and fluids. When food becomes available, it is often quick energy foods with little nutritional value. Furthermore, the concomitant use of alcohol or drugs causes deleterious effects on health. Once a victim is rescued from a human trafficking situation, the focus should be to provide an adequate number of calories from nutrient-dense foods in order to reverse undernutrition or malnutrition, enhance healthy weight gain, and facilitate healing from physical trauma.

Reversing Effects of Poor Nutrition/Starvation

Reversing the effects of poor nutrition or starvation has several foci: (1) bringing the body weight to a normal body mass index (BMI) for age, (2) improving the general eating pattern, (3) increasing total energy (calories), macronutrients, and micronutrients, and (4) increasing fluid intake. Addressing each of these areas will help to enhance health and facilitate healing from physical trauma.

The recovery plan lasts several weeks and should begin with a thorough assessment of nutritional needs. According to the World Health Organization (1999) the first 3 days of treatment involve correcting hypoglycemia and dehydration. The initial 6 weeks of therapy should include correction of electrolyte imbalances and micronutrient deficiencies. Depending on the level of severity, during the first 7 days of micronutrient replacement, iron should not be included. Iron can be added after the first 7 days if severe anemia is resolved. Feeding can begin immediately. In severe cases of malnutrition, formula feeding or total parenteral nutrition that is high in carbohydrate content and low in dietary protein, fat, and sodium is used because these nutrients may not be tolerated initially (World Health Organization, 1999).

After fluid, electrolyte, and micronutrient deficiencies are corrected, the focus should be on normalizing the body weight, improving the general eating pattern with nutrient-dense foods, increasing the total calories, increasing macronutrients/micronutrients, and increasing fluid intake. Depending on the level of physical trauma, treatments to heal wounds or infections may be given concomitantly during the recovery phase. Attention to psychosocial needs is also warranted during the initial recovery period, as mood levels, depression, or anxiety have an impact on appetite (Scott, 2008).

The first step in the process of reversing the effects of poor nutrition is to complete an individualized assessment of nutritional needs. One example of a brief nutritional screening tool useful in clinical practice is the Malnutrition Universal Screening Tool (MUST) (British Association for Parenteral and Enteral Nutrition, 2003). The MUST estimates nutritional risk by allowing the clinician to input height and weight (to calculate BMI), percentage of unintended weight loss, and an estimate of the effect of illness on nutritional intake. A higher score on the MUST indicates a greater level of nutritional impairment.

Once the level of nutritional impairment has been established, the first goal is to bring the body weight to a normal BMI for age. Scott (2008) emphasizes that there are three possible aims related to body weight when treating undernutrition or malnutrition: weight gain, weight maintenance, or the prevention of further weight loss. Body weight goals should be established after assessing the individual's situation, perception of ideal body weight, current BMI, and percentage of unintended weight loss.

After an individual is able to tolerate whole foods, the second goal is to improve the general eating pattern. Prior to initiating an eating plan, assessment of an individual's food likes/dislikes, time of day when the appetite is the most robust, and cultural preferences related to food intake is warranted. Scott (2008) suggests a goal of three small/light meals and three small snacks daily customized to an individual's food preferences and appetite patterns. Associated with nutrition is adequate hydration, normally eight, 8-oz glasses of fluids per day.

CASE STUDY: KATERINA

Katerina is a 20-year-old from Moldova who was trafficked to New York at the age of 18 and held in a brothel where she was handcuffed to an iron bed with a thin mattress and repeatedly raped. The bed was in a cubicle with many others in a large warehouse, which had been converted to a brothel. There were no windows in her area and she was not able to exercise. Once a day she was given a ration of thin potato soup with unidentifiable vegetables. She was rescued when the police raided the brothel and taken to a hospital barely alive where she received fluids intravenously for a week until she could take in food. She received physical therapy to exercise so that she could walk again. Her numerous injuries (from repeated rape, sodomy, and beatings) were treated and she was allowed a T Visa (available to people who have been trafficked) and discharged to a shelter. As a nurse who volunteers at the shelter, you consult with the staff to draw up a nutritional plan for Katerina and you meet with her for nutritional counseling.

Katerina's case is not uncommon for women who have been trafficked from the Eastern bloc countries under conditions of extreme deprivation and trauma. Although barely alive when rescued, she is young enough to recover with good nutrition, therapy, skills training, and care. The following care plan might be implemented.

Assessment
Katerina weighs 100 pounds and is 5 feet 6 inches tall. She reports weighing 121 prior to 18 when she was trafficked. Her BMI is 16.6 and her triceps measurement is 10 mm (less than 13 is normal for a female). She presents with pale skin, looks

fatigued, and her temperature is 97.2. Serum albumin is 3.0 (normal is 3.4–4.8) and her serum cholesterol is 118 (normal is 150–200 mg/dL).

Nursing Diagnoses

1. Protein-calorie malnutrition.
2. Imbalanced nutrition related to low caloric intake.
3. Risk of infection related to malnutrition.
4. Impaired appetite related to consistent abuse over time.
5. Impaired social interaction, related to isolation over time.

Expected Outcomes

1. Gain 1–1/12 pounds per week until target weight of 120 is reached.
2. Blood values have improved to normal limits.
3. Verbalize understanding of healthy nutrition choices as discussed with the nurse.
4. Make healthy eating choices when shopping for own food.
5. Remain infection-free as evidenced by normal range of vital signs and blood values.
6. Increase social interaction by participating in survivor's groups and developing new skills.

Plan and Implementation

1. Weigh weekly at consistent time to chart progress.
2. Develop a teaching plan for simple concepts related to nutrition and how to make healthy choices.
3. Develop schedule for five small meals per day to balance intake over time.
4. Encourage to chart progress by keeping a food journal.
5. Provide exercises that will strengthen muscle tone and endurance.

Evaluation

1. At end of first month, Katerina's weight is 105 and she feels more energized.
2. At end of first month, her journal is detailed and she has noted questions to ask.
3. At end of first month, she has participated in shopping for the shelter and she can distinguish between healthy and unhealthy choices.
4. She has participated in the cooking classes offered at the shelter and mentored new arrivals in how to learn to make healthy food choices.

NUTRITION PLAN FOR HEALTHY LIVING

We recognize that shelters have food preparation procedures that may differ from the kind of food survivors will prepare once they are living independently.

The needs of institutions with limited budgets and resources will dictate food choices. However, teaching survivors to make healthy food choices when they are on their own will reverse the malnourished states in which they come to the shelter. The following teaching plan can be used by shelter staff to provide healthy nutrition information to clients who are beyond the medical emergency of malnutrition. A bonus of teaching healthy nutrition is that cooking is fun and can be a therapeutic strategy to teach survivors new life skills. Television shows, magazines, and the Internet are full of information presented in an entertaining way while teaching viewers or readers how to improve their skills and standard of living.

A Well-Stocked Pantry

A major goal of helping survivors to reintegrate into independent life is to teach them how to prepare nutritious meals in a cost-effective way. Keeping basic

TABLE 12.1   Foods to Keep on Hand

Pantry	Refrigerator	Freezer
SPICES: kosher salt or sea salt, black pepper, red pepper flakes, cinnamon, nutmeg, thyme, rosemary, basil, bay leaves, oregano	DAIRY: butter, cheese, milk, buttermilk	NUTS: pecans, walnuts, pine nuts
GRAINS: rice, cereal, oatmeal, flour, wheat flour		MEALS: Many meals prepared ahead can be frozen in small containers – label and date these. Soups freeze well if they do not contain milk.
CANNED: red beans, white beans, black beans, tuna, chicken, salmon, tomato sauce, tomato paste, soup, low-sodium broths	FRUIT: lemons, limes, apples	DAIRY: cheddar, Swiss, mozzarella, parmesan, butter
PASTA: spaghetti, macaroni, penne, bowties	VEGETABLES: lettuce, cucumber, broccoli, cauliflower, scallions	VEGETABLES: many vegetables such as corn, peas, and pearl onions are flash frozen without additives, retain nutrients, and taste almost as good as fresh
OTHER: potatoes, onions, garlic, tomatoes, sugar, honey, coffee, tea	CONDIMENTS: mustard, ketchup, olives, pickles, tomato paste in tube, garlic paste in jar	

spices, proteins, grains, cooking oils, and canned goods on hand in pantry, refrigerator, and freezer is costeffective and convenient. With a few essential ingredients, such as pastas and beans, one can supplement with fresh vegetables and fruits and quickly prepare healthy meals for a fraction of the cost of fast foods. Table 12.1 is a general guide developed by the authors and can be modified to taste. Multivitamins might be helpful but are not a substitute for proper nutrition.

A Healthy Plate

A helpful hint to follow for healthier eating is the *myplate* icon on the USDA (U.S. Department of Agriculture) website (USDA, 2012). This tip eliminates the need to memorize all the confusing information about food content and simply use a formula when preparing food. Their new *myplate* icon replaces the pyramid of foods that was popular in past decades. The USDA recommends that we fill half the plate with fruits and vegetables, one-fourth with healthy grains, and one-fourth with protein. Download materials from the website at myplate.gov to obtain full details and many helpful hints on cutting food costs while maintaining good nutrition.

SUMMARY

In this chapter, the authors have addressed the key issue of malnutrition which must be reversed in survivors as they progress in learning to adapt to the outside world. It would be rare to find survivors who are well-nourished at the point in which they are just making the choice to escape "the life." Shelter staff and the other professionals who are engaged to help survivors are in a unique position not only to reverse the effects of malnutrition and dehydration, but also to teach skills that can help survivors become successful through the rest of their lives.

REFERENCES

American Heart AssociationGidding, S. S., Dennison, B. A., Birch, L. L., Daniels, S. R., Gilman, M. W. et al. (2006). Dietary recommendations for children and adolescents: A guide for practitioners. *Pediatrics, 117*, 544–559.

Baptiste, F., Hamlin, A., & Côté, F. (2009). Drugs and diet among women street sex workers and injection drug users in Quebec City. *Canadian Journal of Urban Research, 18*, 78–95.

British Association for Parenteral and Enteral Nutrition. (2003). The "MUST" explanatory booklet: A guide to the "Malnutrition Universal Screening Tool" ("MUST") for adults. Retrieved March 14, 2012, from: http://www.bapen.org.uk/pdfs/must/must_explan.pdf

Sæland, M., Hausen, M., Eriksen, F.-L., Smehaugen, A., Wandel, M., Böhmer, T., & Oshaug, A. (2008). Living as a drug addict in Oslo, Norway—A study focusing on nutrition and health. *Public Health Nutrition, 12,* 630–636.

Scott, A. (2008). Acting on screening results: A guide to treating malnutrition in the community. *British Journal of Community Nursing, 13,* 450–456.

U.S. Department of Agriculture (USDA). (2012). Getting started with myplate. Retrieved March 22, 2012 from http://www.cnpp.usda.gov/Publications/MyPlate/GettingStar tedWithMyPlate.pdf

Voss, A. C., Tootell, M., & Gussler, J. D. (2006). *Malnutrition: A hidden cost in health care.* Columbus, OH: Ross Products, Division, Abbott Laboratories.

World Health Organization. (1999). *Management of severe malnutrition: A manual for physicians and other senior health care workers.* Retrieved March 15, 2012, from: http://whqlibdoc.who.int/hq/1999/a57361.pdf

Zimmerman, C., Hossain, M., & Watts, C. (2011). Human trafficking and health: A conceptual model to inform policy, intervention and research. *Social Science & Medicine, 73,* 327–335.

CHAPTER 13

Pregnancy and Termination of Pregnancy

MARY DE CHESNAY AND LACIE SZEKES

*I*n this chapter, the authors present special considerations of pregnancy with commercial sexual exploitation of children (CSEC) victims. Since CSEC by definition involves children, the focus and examples will be on adolescents though the principles of treatment applicable to pregnant adults as well. Of particular relevance to CSEC victims are normal pregnancy, ectopic pregnancy, and complications from unsafe abortions.

Some women who work as prostitutes are not enslaved and have more control over their lives than women who are held by traffickers. They might keep their children and work toward the goal of leaving the life, but have no other way to earn a living (Sloss & Harper, 2004). Some work in brothels but manage to keep their children or send them to family members in the country (Pardeshi & Bhattacharya, 2006). Women who are not held as sex slaves and who become pregnant have options victims do not have. Although they may have similar risks, by law they have the right to terminate the pregnancy or carry to term and either keep or adopt their infants. They can expect reasonable medical care for complications, such as ectopic pregnancy. They are at lower risk for complications from abortion because they do not have to resort to unsafe abortion.

Although CSEC victims have the same rights, they usually are not aware of their rights or are denied help by their exploiters, who control their schedules, transportation, and money. The focus of this chapter is on pregnancy and the associated conditions of unsafe abortion and ectopic pregnancy. These conditions are particularly risky for girls who are trafficked because they have less control over their lives than girls who face pregnancy but who have supportive friends or family. Even if no supportive family, they at least have control over their schedules and money.

UNCOMPLICATED ADOLESCENT PREGNANCY

Prevention programs for adolescent pregnancy tend to focus on abstinence, safe sex, limited partners, and contraception (Nitz, 1999; Sieving et al., 2011), none of which are feasible for CSEC victims. There is an assumption in primary prevention of pregnancy that children can control with whom they have sex and if they just say "no" they will not get pregnant. That approach is not the case in CSEC in which children are controlled by pimps or handlers, who decide not only with whom and when they will have sex, but also what they eat, where they sleep, and with whom they can associate. First-person stories by survivors indicate that they are forced to service 15 to 25 men per night or they risk beatings, burns, food and sleep deprivation, and other forms of torture (Lloyd, 2011; Mam, 2009). Rape is common, both initially as a means of control and later by violent "johns." In one study by Farley and Barken (1998), prostituted women reported they had been raped multiple times:

- 68% reported rape
- 48% were raped more than 5 times
- 46% rapes were by customers

The trauma induced by one rape can destroy the spirit. Enduring multiple rapes with resulting pregnancy takes a strength most women do not possess.

The best practices in pregnancy to deliver a healthy infant with positive maternal outcomes include adequate rest, nutrition, and frequent monitoring. Early pregnant adolescents who engage in consensual sex and who have immature bodies are a high-risk group (Sarri & Phillips, 2004), but prostituted children who become pregnant are deprived not only of adequate prenatal care but also of the basics—food and sleep (McClain & Garrity, 2011). Malnutrition is common among trafficking victims and restoring a positive nutrition state is critical to promote the best pregnancy outcomes. For example, in healthy women, folic acid is the only supplement recommended to be taken during pregnancy, while iron, calcium, iodine, and zinc can usually be supplied through a good diet (Collins, Arulkumaran, Hayes, Jackson, & Impey, 2008). However, prostituted women do not have access to adequate nutrition. Deprivation of food and sleep are pimps' means of control.

Even in good circumstances, a prenatal vitamin is recommended in order to receive the nutrients essential for a pregnancy. An adolescent not only needs nutrients for the growth of the baby, but also her own growth, especially younger adolescents aged 13 to 15 (Davidson, 2002; Davidson et al., 2007). Low weight and malnutrition increase risk of perinatal mortality or low birth weight babies, possibly because with malnutrition and low weight, women probably have irregular periods, which makes using history of last menstrual period not reliable in determining age of gestation.

For any pregnant woman, it is important to determine her Rh status. A woman who is Rh negative and carries an Rh positive baby will form antibodies that attack the baby's blood if that blood crosses the placental membrane. Theoretically, the mother's and baby's circulations are separate, closed systems, but it is not uncommon for small particles to cross the membrane. The danger to the fetus is hemolytic disease of the newborn, manifested by mental retardation, cardiac disease, or jaundice. RhoGAM is the treatment of choice (Ward & Hisley, 2009). Given as an intramuscular injection usually at 28 days gestation but at least 72 hours before birth, RhoGAM coats and destroys fetal blood cells in the maternal circulation.

While pregnancy is common among prostituted women, we could find no literature that addressed how to treat these specific women, and what little literature is available speaks to broad concepts of promoting positive outcomes in any pregnancy. The complication of vaginal fistula due to early pregnancy in child brides or rape trauma is discussed in the chapter on physical trauma. There were a few sources that spoke to childhood pregnancy in cases of child sexual abuse and early marriage (Kenney, Reinholtz, & Angelini, 1997; Stechna, 2011). Stechna (2011) presented a case study of an incest victim and described the complex nature of meeting the child's medical and psychosocial needs, as well as interacting with the criminal justice system. Thompson (2010) describes a teen pregnancy clinic in Great Britain, run by midwives. This project has a high rate of success but does not specifically address the special needs of girls in the sex trade.

A factor that specifically complicates the pregnancy of a prostituted woman is the choice of keeping, aborting, or carrying to term, and adopting. For any other pregnant woman, even adolescents who live with nonsupportive families, the final choice is hers, hopefully with the guidance of supportive family members. In the case of slaves, the traffickers control the outcome of pregnancy and all decisions related to the woman's progress and outcome. If the pimp has deliberately impregnated the girl to bind her to him, he may allow her to keep the baby, who then gets raised in the pimp's "family." He would threaten to remove the child if the girl steps out of line.

If the pimp allows her to keep the child, he may or may not give her time off to have the child. One client told me she was delivered by one of the other girls, cleaned up, and out on the street the next day while the others looked after the infant. She developed an infection and was hospitalized at which time she was able to accept help to escape.

An additional source of revenue for the traffickers is "baby farming." "Baby farming" is a term used in the late 18th century and early 19th century to describe the practice of selling infants from unwanted pregnancies (Broder, 1988; The Adoption History Project, n.d.). The modern version is literally to hold girls in locked quarters, rape them, and sell the infants. In a series of arrests in Nigeria, 32 pregnant girls were rescued and told stories of being drugged, then raped by the doctor. When their babies were born they were removed and sold in lucrative black-market adoptions. One young woman had been held captive and bred continuously for 3 years (Babies bred for sale in Nigeria, 2008).

UNCOMPLICATED PREGNANCY CASE

Nina is a pregnant 15-year-old Latina girl coming in to the local health department for a prenatal visit. Gestational age was determined to be between 30 and 32 weeks. Nina is accompanied by another pregnant girl who states that she is her older sister, 16-year-old Ana, and an older man who states that he is their Uncle Juan. Juan states that the two girls are his brother's children and that they are living with him and working on his farm while they earn enough money to bring their parents to this country. The girls speak very little English, and their uncle states that he can answer the nurse's questions because they are very close. After an assessment was performed by the nurse, it was determined that both Nina and Ana are underweight for their age, height, and stage of pregnancy. The nurse asks the girls if this is their first pregnancy and determines that it is Nina's first and Ana's third. Nina seems anxious about her pregnancy and tells the nurse that she hopes it is a boy because that would please her boyfriend. When the nurse begins to ask more about the child's father, she is abruptly cut off by Juan. Ana is more reserved and reluctant to speak to the nurse about her pregnancy. She is in her 34th week, and appears emaciated and weak. Her uncle states that her other two children were given up to family members and that this next one will likely be the same.

Although this case is presented as uncomplicated pregnancy, several problems are clear. Their ages are certainly problematic but the fact that they are emaciated is a major indicator of poor nutrition perhaps from a forced work environment. Chances are good that if they work on a farm they work long hours without proper food and rest and are likely forced to have sex after the farm work is over for the day.

The following care plan is only one of many models that can be used. Key points are listed under each phase. Preparation for assessment: separate the three family members. Nina is the presenting patient, but Ana should also be considered a patient. Divert Juan by telling him it is hospital policy to examine each person privately. Since the girls' English is not good and we are assuming the nurse or physician does not speak Spanish, obtain a hospital interpreter to assist. (Seek another nurse, a staff member, or a person on call for this purpose.) You, the nurse, and the obstetric resident examine Nina while her sister is examined in another room. You make a point of being nonjudgmental and stress that you are there to help her and her baby. You explain that young girls' bodies are not matured fully and that childbirth can be difficult for someone of her age. It is difficult to maintain a kind, nonjudgmental attitude in the face of the information given so far, but save the anger and distress you feel for a team meeting and do not burden Nina with overwhelming sympathy, which is likely to make her feel worse at distressing you.

You have rightly concluded that the girls are possible trafficking victims by virtue of their emaciated states, domineering "uncle," and submissive demeanor. The supervisor calls protective services for both underage girls and the police who take charge of the "uncle." You and the physician conduct a comprehensive physical exam, including blood levels. It is critical to obtain an adequate prenatal lab workup but, if possible, keep intrusive measures to a minimum. For example, gonorrhea and chlamydia can appear in urine eliminating the need for excessive blood work. Obviously, if drugs are suspected, more lab work might be necessary. Refer to the chapter on substance abuse.

Findings are that Nina is malnourished, has low iron, and her electrolytes are outside normal range. Adolescents are at risk for preeclampsia, so a plan for monitoring blood pressure is essential. A prenatal plan for a safe delivery is devised with the social worker from protective services and you and the social worker explain to both Nina and Ana what medical and social services are available to them.

The medical plan for maximizing the chance of a healthy outcome for both mothers and their infants would include nutritious diet high in protein, fruits and vegetables, folic acid, iron, and other vitamins to reverse the effects of poor diet early in pregnancy, and adequate fluid intake. If possible, refer the women to a registered dietician for a dietary plan and monitor adequate weight gain. The American Dietetic Association (Kaiser & Allen, 2008) also cautions that low birth weight with the associated infant development problems is a particular risk of young pregnant adolescents.

ECTOPIC PREGNANCY

Ectopic pregnancy, a potentially life-threatening condition, occurs when the fertilized ovum is implanted outside the endometrial cavity (Barnhardt, 2009). Although having multiple sex partners is one risk factor, as are smoking and chlamydia, half of women with ectopic pregnancy do not show evidence of risk factors (Barnhardt et al., 2006; Hillis, Owens, Marchbanks, Amsterdam, & MacKenzie, 1997). Women with untreated sexually transmitted infections (STIs) are likely to develop chronic pelvic inflammatory disease (PID) that can result in ectopic pregnancy and eventual need for hysterectomy (Willis & Levy, 2002). Most ectopic pregnancies occur in a Fallopian tube but the ovum can also implant in the cervix, scar tissue from a caesarian section, an ovary, or in the abdomen. These are harder to diagnose and mortality is higher (Barnhardt, 2009). First-trimester bleeding and pelvic pain are early warning signs for which ectopic pregnancy should be ruled out. Comorbid appendicitis with ruptured ectopic pregnancy should also be considered (Riggs, Schiavello, & Fixler, 2002). Patients with ruptured ectopic pregnancy, an emergency condition, present with signs of shock, such as hypotension, tachycardia, and fainting in addition to rebound tenderness (Barnhardt, 2009; Hillis et al., 1997). However, it is recommended that any woman of child-bearing age who presents with the triad symptoms of lower abdominal pain (particularly one-sided), vaginal bleeding, and amenorrhea, should be examined for ectopic pregnancy (Wong & Suat, 2000).

The diagnosis of ectopic pregnancy is effectively made through transvaginal ultrasound (due to its low radioactivity) and measurement of beta-human chorionic gonadotropic (beta-HCG) hormone (Kruszka & Kruszka, 2010; Wong & Suat, 2000). Although these tests are not always definitive, they are the standard method to date. Ectopic pregnancy should be ruled out in any woman of child-bearing age with abdominal pain. Differential diagnosis would also rule out other abdominal issues such as appendicitis, ovarian cyst, PID, and so on. Ultrasound and laparoscopy are used to diagnose ectopic pregnancy and beta-HCG at low levels with empty uterus is a key indicator.

ECTOPIC PREGNANCY CASE

Luisa is an 11-year-old Mexican American girl who lives with her father and four brothers in a mobile home on the outskirts of a large, Southwestern U.S. city. She presents in the emergency department with abdominal tenderness, dizziness, shoulder pain, vaginal bleeding, and fatigue. She reports that symptoms have gotten worse during the past 8 weeks. She considers the vaginal bleeding an aberrant menstrual period and she tells you that the vaginal bleeding means "something is wrong with my period." Upon physical examination, the resident informs you that Luisa is experiencing an ectopic pregnancy. When she is told her diagnosis and asked who the father is, she tells you she doesn't know because she is forced to have sex with her father and brothers and they rent her to their friends on a regular basis for money. She is referred to an attending in Obstetrics and Gynecology and treated with single dose methotrexate, then evaluated for the necessity of laparoscopy. It was determined that the single dose was effective and that there was no need for surgical intervention. Luisa was placed in a shelter that serves exploited children and provided with follow-up counseling and other appropriate after-care services.

Treatment

Special considerations:

- She is under 15, the age of sexual consent in her state
- She is in imminent danger of being abused again
- She has had multiple sex partners
- She has a history of chlamydia from long-term sexual abuse

Luisa was removed from her home and placed under protective services, whose responsibility it would be to follow-up with the father and brothers.

In terms of the medical treatment, Luisa recovered fully and was given trauma-focused psychotherapy.

UNSAFE ABORTION

Abortion is legal in the United States and many countries, but some countries continue to prohibit abortion. Whatever the nurse's personal feelings about abortion, we have an ethical responsibility to care for all sick and injured and it is necessary to educate ourselves about the unsafe abortion practices prevalent in many areas of the world and some areas of the United States. Though abortion is legal here, it may cost more than a girl can pay. Prostituted women and children do not generally have access to medical insurance. Her pimp may not allow her to have an abortion, especially if he has deliberately impregnated her as a means of binding her to him, holding out hope of a future as "a real family." Finally some pimps save the money by the do-it-yourself method. In one source, Jill relates the story of having her pimp suspend her from the ceiling with her legs spread so that he could perform an abortion with a broken long-necked beer bottle. The abortion failed and she nearly died (Sage, 2006).

Between 1 million and 10 million children around the world are prostituted, resulting in high prevalence of pregnancy, unsafe abortion, and medical and mental health consequences of unsafe abortion (Willis & Levy, 2002). Unsafe abortion is common in developing countries among women who do not have access to safe abortion or live in countries where abortion is still not legal. In ancient times, abortions were performed by a host of methods we would consider frightening today and many are still used, including detergents, solvents, turpentine, teas, bleach, and animal dung (Grimes et al., 2006). Current methods can be classified into the following categories:

- Oral or injectable medicines
- Vaginal preparations
- Intrauterine foreign bodies
- Trauma to the abdomen

Every year, about 42 million women with unintended pregnancies have abortions and approximately half of these, or 21 million abortions, are unsafe. Of these, about 68,000 women die, and of those who survive, about 5 million suffer long-term complications such as hemorrhage and sepsis (Haddad & Nour, 2009). Fistula is discussed in the chapter on trauma, but poor wound healing, infertility, and internal organ damage are common. Kidney damage resulting in death was reported in two studies in Thailand in which intrauterine chemical injection was the method of abortion (Srinil, 2011; Srinil & Panaput, 2011).

Both suction curettage and pharmacological abortion are safe in early pregnancy. There is evidence that misoprostol alone is effective (Dahiya, Madan, Hooda, Sangwan, & Khosla, 2005; Grimes, 2003). These methods are for trained practitioners, who provide a clean setting and appropriate post-abortion care.

UNSAFE ABORTION CASE

Cindy is a 21-year-old Caucasian woman entering the emergency department after an alleged botched abortion and is accompanied by her boyfriend Marco. Cindy looks to be severely malnourished and has bruises covering her arms and legs. The nurse notices that Cindy's arms are covered in bulging bluish colored veins and areas of blackened, necrotic skin with multiple puncture sites; a telltale sign of IV drug use. Cindy's boyfriend, Marco, seems much older than Cindy, and is acting angry and hostile toward the medical staff. He refuses to leave the room, and answers all of the questions while Cindy floats in and out of consciousness. Finally he admits that she has had a botched abortion attempt but claims she did it herself with a knitting needle while he was out. Her exam reveals severe trauma to the vaginal wall, with tearing and multiple lacerations to the perineum. Lab work is done, including Rh factor to determine if RhoGAM is needed. The ED doctor refers her to Gynecology for immediate repair under anesthetic.

Once the surgery is complete and she is discharged from recovery to a room, she tells the nurse that she is "a whore" and admits that it was her pimp who tried to abort with a knitting needle, but insists she does not want help leaving the life. She explains that her "man" is going to take care of her and that she just has to hold on and things will be better. The nurse responds: "You know if you go back to him he will kill you." She is silent for a few moments and then says: "You don't understand. I pray every day that he will."

Cindy's sense of hopelessness paralyzes her to the point where she cannot take action to leave her pimp even when an escape route is offered to her. The Stages of Change Model provides a useful framework to understand readiness to change, despair, and relapse. Prochaska and DiClemente (1983) studied 872 subjects to determine how they progressed in their own efforts to stop smoking. They identified five stages in the process. Their model was refined over time to eight stages and currently, the Stages of Change Model has broad applicability to a variety of behaviors (Connors, Donovan, & DiClemente, 2001; DiClemente & Prochaska, 1998). Corcoran (2002) worked with nonoffending parents of children who had been sexually abused. These mothers experienced ambivalence over whether to support the child or the offending parent.

The Stages of Change are:

- Precontemplation—not ready to acknowledge the problem (may deny feelings or defend current lifestyle)
- Contemplation—acknowledging that there is a problem but not yet ready to change (a major change would be to allow others to help)

- Preparation/Determination—preparing to change (finding courage)
- Action/Willpower—actually making some change (may not be major changes but small steps)
- Maintenance—maintain the changes (stays away from pimp)
- Relapse—returning to old patterns (examples are returning to pimp or resuming prostitution on own from fear of success)

Because Cindy is an adult, she has the right to make her own choice and she is clearly in the precontemplation stage in which she is not ready to consider alternatives. This stage is particularly frustrating to nurses and doctors who want so much to "save her," but rescuing her against her will is not only disrespectful to her but counterproductive since the chances that she would return to her pimp are high. Providing antidepressants in the hospital might help her to feel strong enough to consider other options than staying with her pimp, but may not help. Logical arguments almost certainly will not sway her. In fact, if one argues with her, she is likely to shut down.

Sometimes, all that one can do is to leave the door open in the hope that someday soon she will be ready to consider a different life. In Cindy's case, perhaps asking her to make follow-up appointments for postabortion medical care might enable the staff to develop a relationship with her. Unfortunately, it is more likely her pimp will move her to another city to avoid this possibility.

SUMMARY

This chapter has presented information on pregnancy, ectopic pregnancy, and unsafe abortion. Pregnancy is one of the highest risk health issues experienced by prostituted children. Pimps do not allow condoms if they can get more money. Prenatal care is nonexistent for these girls. Sometimes the baby is welcomed by the mother because she believes that she will have a vacation during pregnancy, but this is rarely the case. Pimps force girls to work through pregnancy and when the girl is off for giving birth, she has to make up the money missed.

REFERENCES

Babies bred for sale in Nigeria. (November 29, 2008). *Mail and guardian: Africa's best read*. Retrieved July 10, 2012, from http://www.mg.co.za/article/2008-11-09-babies-bred-for-sale-in-nigeria.

Barnhardt, K. (2009). Ectopic pregnancy. *New England Journal of Medicine, 361*, 379–387.

Broder, S. (1988). Child care or child neglect: Baby farming in late nineteenth century Philadelphia. *Gender and Society, 2*(2), 128–148.

Collins, S., Arulkumaran, S., Hayes, K., Jackson, S., & Impey, L. (2008). *Oxford handbook of obstetrics and gynaecology*, New York: Oxford University Press.

Connors, G., Donovan, D., & DiClemente, C. (2001). *Substance abuse treatment and the stages of change: Selecting and planning interventions.* New York: Guilford Press.

Corcoran, J. (2002). The Transtheoretical Stages of Change Model and motivational interviewing for building maternal supportiveness in cases of sexual abuse. *Journal of Child Sexual Abuse, 11*(3), 1–17.

Davidson, C. J. (2002). The transtheoretical stages of change model and motivational interviewing for building maternal supportiveness in cases of sexual abuse. *Journal of Child Sexual Abuse, 11*(3), 1–17.

Davidson, M., London, M., Ladewig, P., & Olds, S. (2007). *Olds' maternal-newborn nursing & women's health across the lifespan* (8th ed.). Philadelphia: Prentice-Hall.

Dahiya, K., Madan, S., Hooda, R., Sangwan, K., & Khosla, A. (2005). Evaluation of the efficacy of mifrepristone/misopristol and methotrexate/misopristol for medical abortion. *Indian Journal of Medical Sciences, 59*(7), 301–306.

DiClemente, C., & Prochaska, J. (1998). Toward a comprehensive, transtheoretical model of change: Stages of change and addictive behaviors. In W. R. Miller, & N. Heather (Eds.) , *Treating addictive behaviors* (2nd ed., pp. 3–24). New York: Plenum.

Farley, M., & Barken, H. (1998). Prostitution, violence and post-traumatic stress disorder. *Women & Health, 27*(3), 37–49.

Grimes, D. (2003). Unsafe abortion: The silent scourge. *British Medical Bulletin, 67,* 99–113.

Grimes, D., Benson, J., Singh, S., Romero, M., Ganatra, B., Okonofua, F. et al. (2006). Unsafe abortion: The preventable pandemic. Retrieved April 12, 2012, fromhttp://www.who.int/reproductivehealth/publications/general/lancet_4.pdf.

Haddad, L., & Nour, N. (2009). Unsafe abortion: Unnecessary maternal mortality. *Reviews in Obstetrics and Gynecology, 2*(2), 122–126.

Hillis, S., Owens, L., Marchbanks, P., Amsterdam, L., & MacKenzie, W. (1997). Recurrent chlamydial infections increase the risks of hospitalization for ectopic pregnancy and pelvic inflammatory disease. *American Journal of Obstetrics and Gynecology, 176,* 103–107.

Kaiser, L., & Allen, L. (2008). Position of the American Dietetic Association: Nutrition and lifestyle for a healthy pregnancy outcome. *Journal of the American Dietetic Association, 108*(3), 553–560.

Kenney, J. W., Reinholtz, C., & Angelini, P. (1997). Ethnic differences in childhood and adolescent sexual abuse and teenage pregnancy. *Journal of Adolescent Health, 21*(1), 3–10.

Kruszka, P., & Kruszka, S. (2010). Evaluation of acute pelvic pain in women. *American Family Physician, 82*(2), 141–147.

Lloyd, R. (2011). *Girls like us.* New York, NY: Harper-Collins.

Mam, S. (2009). *The road of lost innocence.* New York, NY: Spiegel and Grau.

McClain, N., & Garrity, S. (2011). Sex trafficking and the exploitation of adolescents. *Journal of Obstetric, Gynecologic, and Neonatal Nursing, 40,* 243–252.

Nitz, K. (1999). Adolescent pregnancy prevention: A review of interventions and programs. *Clinical Psychology Review, 19*(4), 457–471.

Pardeshi, G., & Bhattacharya, S. (2006). Child-rearing practices amongst brothel-based commercial sex workers. *Indian Journal of Medical Sciences, 60*(7), 288–295.

Prochaska, J., & DiClemente, C. (1983). Stages and processes of self-change of smoking: Toward an integrative model of change. *Journal of Consulting and Clinical Psychology, 51*(3), 390–395.

Riggs, J., Schiavello, H., & Fixler, R. (2002). Concurrent appendicitis and ectopic pregnancy: A case report. *The Journal of Reproductive Medicine, 47*(6), 510–514.

Sage, J. (2006). *Enslaved: True stories of modern day slavery.* New York: Palgrave Macmillan.

Sarri, R., & Phillips, A. (2004). Health and social services for pregnant and parenting high-risk teens. *Children and Youth Services Review, 26,* 537–560.

Sieving, R., Resnick, M., Garwick, A., Bearinger, L., Beckman, K., Oliphant, J. et al. (2011). A clinic-based, youth development approach to teen pregnancy prevention. *American Journal of Health Behavior, 35*(3), 346–358.

Sloss, C., & Harper, G. (2004). When street sex workers are mothers. *Archives of Sexual Behavior, 33*(4), 329–341.

Srinil, S. (2011). Factors associated with severe complications in unsafe abortion. *Journal of the Medical Association of Thailand, 94*(4), 408–413.

Srinil, S., & Panaput, T. (2011). Acute kidney injury complicating septic unsafe abortion: Clinical course and treatment outcomes of 44 cases. *Journal of Obstetrics and Gynecology Research, 37*(11), 1525–1531.

Stechna, S. (2011). Childhood pregnancy as a result of incest: A case report and literature review with suggested management strategies. *Journal of Pediatric Adolescent Gynecology, 24*(3), 83–86.

The Adoption History Project. (n.d.). *Baby farming.* Retrieved July 2, 2012, from http://pages.uoregon.edu/adoption/topics/babyfarming.html

Thompson, S. (2010). The complexities of supporting teenagers in pregnancy. *British Journal of Midwifery, 18*(6), 368–372.

Ward, S., & Hisley, S. (2009). Chapter 11: Caring for the woman experiencing complications during pregnancy. *Maternal-child nursing care: Optimizing outcomes for mothers, children & families* (pp. 291–351). Philadelphia: F.A. Davis Company.

Willis, B., & Levy, B. (2002). Child prostitution: Global health burden, research needs, and interventions. *The Lancet, 359,* 1417–1422.

Wong, E., & Suat, S. (2000). Ectopic pregnancy—A diagnostic challenge in the emergency department. *European Journal of Emergency Medicine, 7*(3), 189–194.

CHAPTER 14

Drug-Abused Women and Children

KIMBERLY GROOT

*T*his chapter is written for nurses as an introduction to three main addiction substances that sex trafficking victims are most likely to experience: heroin, cocaine, and alcohol. Any contact a nurse has with women and children who abuse substances is an opportunity to refer a possible victim for treatment. Nurses will find useful resources to deliver effective care based on current evidence, and practical suggestions are given for caring for drug-addicted patients who are victims of sex trafficking.

Nurses have a significant role in screening for substance abuse and related problems. Basic assessment can uncover multiple problems (Clancy, Coyne, & Wright, 1997). The drugs used in trafficking are a form of control and intimidation by traffickers to remind women and children "who is in command." Many victims have found ways to survive violence by using drugs. Drug addictions keep the trafficking business profitable by adding a second source of revenue.

The words "drug" and "substance" will be used interchangeably and are related to both legal and illegal forms. Drug addiction is considered a multifactorial health disorder that follows the course of relapsing and remitting chronic disease. The *Diagnostic and Statistical Manual of Mental Disorders (DSM)* is the leading classification system used for all categories of addiction. For this chapter, the *DSM-IV* (2004) is referenced.

It is a challenge to care for people who have both mental illness and substance use disorders (SUDs). These co-occurring illnesses complicate assessment, care, and treatment of victims. In many societies, drug addiction is not recognized as an illness and many women, adolescents, and children are stigmatized. Unfortunately, some nurses share this view, complicating their ability to establish rapport with people who abuse drugs. Another barrier to identifying victims of sex trafficking and substance abuse is that women and children initially may resent intervention because they do not always know they need to be rescued (Clawson, Small, Go, & Myles, 2003). It is important to understand the challenges and barriers these clients face.

The chapter will address aspects of cocaine, heroin, and alcohol addiction and treatment practices to help women and children in their recovery, and will:

- Educate nurses with general information to meet the physical, emotional, and safety needs of drug-abused women and children
- Provide nurses with practical guidance and assessment skills to identify victims
- Increase nurses' factual knowledge of commonly abused illegal drugs
- Highlight critical aspects of drug treatment and recovery
- Encourage nurses to engage with victims and uphold a sense of hope with empathy, sincerity, and warmth
- Support nurses to continue to learn drug culture and advance addiction recovery management

With the right attitude and skills, nurses can provide a comprehensive approach to meet the needs of these clients. Nurses as mandated reporters must follow their employers' protocols about how to report.

THE SPECTRUM OF DRUG ADDICTION IN SEX TRAFFICKING

Are you aware whether you have seen any sex-trafficked children or women in your practice? Would you suspect an addicted child or women you have seen in your practice to be a victim of trafficking? Consider the possibility that you may be the person to identify a child or woman with a drug problem who is being sexually exploited. Identifying victims is a challenge because victims of trafficking and drug abusers are virtually invisible to most of society. Some factors that increase risk are:

- Drug use at an early age, leaving home at an early age, injection frequency, and dependence on multiple types of illegal drugs
- Exposure to trauma such as being held captive, being threatened with a weapon and witnessing torture, serious injury, and death
- Drug use patterns, demographic characteristics, psychiatric comorbidity
- How sex work is conducted; for instance, being able to work longer and minimize the consequences and the distress (Cusick, McGarry, Perry, & Kilcommons, 2010; Hedden et al., 2011; Mosedale, Kouimtsidis, & Reynolds, 2009; Roxburgh, Degenhardt, Copeland, & Larance, 2008; Ulibarri et al., 2011; Wechsberg et al., 2009)

There are mutually reinforcing barriers to overcoming drug addiction. Addiction is not curable but it is treatable. Coming down from highs does not necessarily lead to detox or treatment. Drug-addicted women and children may be further inhibited by negative experiences they have had with mainstream health care services, perhaps because of feeling ashamed or unworthy, sexually objectified, or being blamed for their situation. There is a vicious cycle of knowing they need help but being afraid to ask.

WHAT DO THE NUMBERS SAY?

We know that sex trafficking victims face drug abuse and addiction. An estimated 85% of prostitutes in the United States are addicted to crack, heroin, prescription drugs, or alcohol (Delancey Street Foundation, 1997).

To describe the scope of addiction, the following information from the 2010 National Survey on Drug Use and Health (NSDUH) is presented. These results are from an annual survey sponsored by the Substance Abuse and Mental Health Services Administration (SAMHSA). This report is the primary source of information on the use of illicit drugs and alcohol in the civilian, noninstitutionalized population of the United States aged 12 years or older. The survey interviews approximately 67,500 persons each year. Unless otherwise noted, all comparisons in this report using terms such as "increased," "decreased," or "more than" are statistically significant at the .05 level. All material appearing in this report is in the public domain and may be reproduced or copied without permission from SAMHSA.

Illicit Drug use in the United States

In 2010, an estimated 22.6 million Americans aged 12 or older used an illicit drug during the month prior to the survey interview. This estimate represents 8.9% of the population aged 12 or older. The illicit drugs included: marijuana/hashish, cocaine (including crack), heroin, hallucinogens, inhalants, and prescription-type psychotherapeutics not used medically. The rate of current illicit drug use among persons aged 12 or older in 2010 (8.9%) was similar to the rate in 2009 (8.7%), but higher than the rate in 2008 (8.0%).

In 2010, there were 1.5 million current cocaine users aged 12 or older, comprising .6% of the population. These estimates were similar to the number and rate in 2009 (1.6 million or .7%).

Hallucinogens were used by 1.2 million persons (.5%) aged 12 or older in 2010, including 695,000 (.3%) who had used Ecstasy. These estimates were similar to estimates in 2009. The number of methamphetamine users decreased between 2006 and 2010, from 731,000 (.3%) to 353,000 (.1%).

Among youths aged 12 to 17, the current illicit drug use rate was similar in 2009 (10.0%) and 2010 (10.1%), but higher than the rate in 2008 (9.3%). Between 2002 and 2008, the rate declined from 11.6% to 9.3%. The rate of current Ecstasy use among youths aged 12 to 17 declined from .5% in 2002 to .3% in 2004, remained at that level through 2007, and then increased to .5% in 2009 and 2010.

The rate of illicit drug use among young adults aged 18 to 25 increased from 19.6% in 2008 to 21.2% in 2009 and 21.5% in 2010, driven largely by an increase in marijuana use (from 16.5% in 2008 to 18.1% in 2009 and 18.5% in 2010).

Among young adults aged 18 to 25, the rate of nonmedical use of prescription-type drugs in 2010 was 5.9%, similar to the rate in the years from 2002 to 2009. There were decreases from 2002 to 2010 in the use of cocaine (from 2.0% to 1.5%) and methamphetamine (from .6% to .2%).

Among persons aged 12 or older in 2009 to 2010 who used pain relievers nonmedically in the last 12 months, 55.0% got the drug they most recently used from a friend or relative for free. Another 17.3% reported they got the drug from one doctor. Only 4.4% got pain relievers from a drug dealer or other stranger, and .4% bought them on the Internet. Among those who reported getting the pain reliever from a friend or relative for free, 79.4% reported in a follow-up question that the friend or relative had obtained the drugs from just one doctor.

Among unemployed adults aged 18 or older in 2010, 17.5% were current illicit drug users, which was higher than the 8.4% of those employed full time and 11.2% of those employed part time. However, most illicit drug users were employed. Of the 20.2 million current illicit drug users aged 18 or older in 2010, 13.3 million (65.9%) were employed either full or part time.

Cocaine

In 2010, there were 637,000 persons aged 12 or older who had used cocaine for the first time within the past 12 months. This averages to approximately 1,700 initiates per day. This estimate was similar to the number in 2009 (617,000) and 2008 (722,000). The annual number of cocaine initiates declined from 1.0 million in 2002 to 637,000 in 2010.

The number of initiates to crack cocaine declined during this period from 337,000 to 83,000. Most (71.6%) of the .6 million recent cocaine initiates were 18 or older when they first used. The average age at first use among recent initiates aged 12 to 49 was 21.2 years, which was similar to the average age in 2009 and 2008 (20.0 and 19.8 years, respectively). These average age estimates have remained fairly stable since 2002.

In 2010, there were 140,000 persons aged 12 or older who had used heroin for the first time within the past 12 months. This estimate was similar to the estimate in 2009 (180,000) and to estimates during 2002 to 2008 (ranging from 91,000 to 118,000 per year). The average age at first use among recent initiates aged 12 to 49 was 21.3 years, and was significantly lower than the 2009 estimate (25.5 years).

Hallucinogens

In 2010, there were 1.2 million persons aged 12 or older who had used hallucinogens for the first time within the past 12 months. This estimate was not significantly different from the estimate in 2009 (1.3 million), but was higher than the estimates from 2003 to 2005 (ranging from 886,000 to 953,000). The number of past year initiates of lysergic acid diethylamide (LSD) aged 12 or older was 377,000 in 2010, which was similar to the number in 2009 (337,000), but higher than the estimates from 2003 to 2007 (ranging from 200,000 to 270,000). Past year initiates of phencyclidine (PCP) decreased from 123,000 in 2002 to 45,000 in 2009 and 2010.

The number of past year initiates of Ecstasy was similar in 2009 (1.1 million) and 2010 (937,000). The estimate was 1.2 million in 2002, declined to 642,000 in 2003, and increased by about 50% between 2005 (615,000) and 2010 (937,000). Most (59.2%) of the recent Ecstasy initiates in 2010 were aged 18 or older at the time they first used Ecstasy. Among past year initiates aged 12 to 49, the average age at initiation of Ecstasy in 2010 was 19.4 years, similar to the average age in 2009 (20.2 years). In 2010, among persons aged 12 or older, the number of first-time past year Ecstasy users who initiated the use prior to the age of 18 was 382,000. This estimate was significantly higher than the estimate in 2005 (209,000).

Alcohol

Slightly more than half of Americans aged 12 or older reported being current drinkers of alcohol in the 2010 survey (51.8%). This translates to an estimated 131.3 million people that was similar to the 2009 estimate of 130.6 million people (51.9%).

In 2010, nearly one-quarter (23.1%) of persons aged 12 or older participated in binge drinking. This translates to about 58.6 million people. The rate in 2010 was similar to the estimate in 2009 (23.7%). Binge drinking is defined as having five or more drinks on the same occasion on at least 1 day in the 30 days prior to the survey.

In 2010, heavy drinking was reported by 6.7% of the population aged 12 or older, or 16.9 million people. This rate was similar to the rate of heavy drinking in 2009 (6.8%). Heavy drinking is defined as binge drinking on at least 5 days in the past 30 days among young adults aged 18 to 25 in 2010, the rate of binge drinking was 40.6%, and the rate of heavy drinking was 13.6%. These rates were similar to the rates in 2009.

The rate of current alcohol use among youths aged 12 to 17 was 13.6% in 2010, which was lower than the 2009 rate (14.7%). Youth binge and heavy drinking rates in 2010 (7.8% and 1.7%) were also lower than rates in 2009 (8.8% and 2.1%). There were an estimated 10.0 million underage (aged 12–20) drinkers in 2010, including 6.5 million binge drinkers, and 2.0 million heavy drinkers. Past month and binge drinking rates among underage persons declined between 2002 and 2010. Past month use declined from 28.8% to 26.3%, while binge drinking declined from 19.3% to 17.0%.

In 2010, 55.3% of current drinkers aged 12 to 20 reported that their last use of alcohol in the past month occurred in someone else's home, and 29.9% reported that it had occurred in their own home. About one-third (30.6%) paid for the alcohol the last time they drank, including 8.8% who purchased the alcohol themselves and 21.6% who gave money to someone else to purchase it. Among those who did not pay for the alcohol they last drank, 38.9% got it from an unrelated person aged 21 or older, 16.6% from another person younger than 21 years old, and 21.6% from a parent, guardian, or other adult family member.

In 2010, an estimated 11.4% of persons aged 12 or older drove under the influence of alcohol at least once in the past year. This percentage had dropped since 2002, when it was 14.2%. The rate of driving under the influence of alcohol was highest among persons aged 21 to 25 (23.4%).

In 2010, an estimated 3.0 million persons aged 12 or older used an illicit drug for the first time within the past 12 months. This averages to about 8,100 initiates per day and was similar to the estimate for 2009 (3.1 million). A majority of these past year illicit drug initiates reported that their first drug was marijuana (61.8%). About one-quarter initiated with psychotherapeutics (26.2%, including 17.3% with pain relievers, 4.6% with tranquilizers, 2.5% with stimulants, and 1.9% with sedatives). A sizable proportion reported inhalants (9.0%) as their first illicit drug, and a small proportion used hallucinogens as their first drug (3.0%).

In 2010, the illicit drug categories with the largest number of past year initiates among persons aged 12 or older were marijuana use (2.4 million) and nonmedical use of pain relievers (2.0 million). These estimates were not significantly different from the numbers in 2009. However, the number of marijuana initiates increased between 2007 (2.1 million) and 2010 (2.4 million). In 2010, the average age of marijuana initiates among persons aged 12 to 49 was 18.4 years, significantly higher than the average age of marijuana initiates in 2002 (17.0 years).

The number of past year initiates of methamphetamine among persons aged 12 or older was 105,000 in 2010. This estimate was significantly lower than the estimate in 2007 (157,000) and only about one-third of the estimate in 2002 (299,000). The number of past year initiates of Ecstasy aged 12 or older was similar in 2009 (1.1 million) and 2010 (937,000), but these estimates were an increase from 2005 (615,000).

The number of past-year cocaine initiates aged 12 or older declined from 1.0 million in 2002 to 637,000 in 2010. The number of initiates of crack cocaine declined during this period from 337,000 to 83,000. In 2010, there were 140,000 persons aged 12 or older who used heroin for the first time within the past year, not significantly different from the estimates from 2002 to 2009. Estimates during those years ranged from 91,000 to 180,000 per year. Most (82.4%) of the 4.7 million past year alcohol initiates were younger than 21 at the time of initiation.

Deciding to increase awareness and knowledge of drug addiction can directly help identify victims of sex trafficking. The nurse may be the initial contact between a victim and the health care system. It is critical to have an understanding of the nature and origins of drug abuse. All who present with warning signs of drug addiction should be evaluated as potential victims of sex trafficking.

METHODS OF RECRUITMENT AND COPING

Although some enter prostitution as substance abusers, many are deliberately addicted by their pimps or have been forced into prostitution in exchange for drugs. There are cases when parents are drug users and will use their children to obtain money. Others pimp their children to obtain money for their own drugs or to pay household expenses. It is understandable that victims use drugs to survive the realities of frequent beatings, traumas, and repeated rapes by their pimps and johns. The progression of drug use can be slow or rapid, with the most common drugs being alcohol, cocaine, and heroin.

IMPLICATIONS FOR NURSING

Components of a routine nursing assessment include performing a physical exam, taking a complete medical history, psychiatric history, and family, social and employment history. Assessment of a person who is drug addicted is complex and many victims are not recognized as victims.

The best starting point is to identify one's own feelings and attitudes about drug use. The client also forms an impression of the nurse during the initial assessment and will notice unfavorable attitudes. Look for general physical signs of substance abuse while building trust. Avoid judgments. Be alert for unhealthy general appearance:

- Very thin or malnourished body
- Runny nose, yawning, or flu-like symptoms
- Abnormal mental status of drowsiness to unexplained agitation
- Unexplained dilated pupils or unusual smell on clothes or breath
- Impaired coordination, attention, or concentration
- Abnormal affect, withdrawn, guarded, odd behaviors
- "Track marks" at injection sites on hands, arms, legs, feet, groin, or neck, wasted muscles, swollen or damaged hands, skin complaints, and poor complexion

The first point of assessment is to evaluate the possibility of drug use. Individuals from diverse ethnic backgrounds may find the screening and assessment process intrusive, threatening, or foreign. Screening must be approached with sensitivity in a way the client can accept. How questions are asked will influence the nurse's ability to establish trust. Proceed slowly, using language appropriate to the patient, and seek feedback to verify understanding. It may be necessary to breakdown information in short sessions and repeat some material. Allow time for questions. How one presents can be as important as the actual information given and sets the tone for the relationship.

CLINICAL ASSESSMENT STRATEGIES

Understanding the extent and nature of a person's drug addiction and life situation is essential. Standardized screening and assessment instruments such as surveys, questionnaires, and interview protocols will identify some problems, but may not specifically identify sex-trafficked victims.

Structured interviews include a series of prepared questions (Rollnick et al., 2008). For instance, the general mental status exam nurses routinely perform systematically covers functioning, awareness, orientation with regard to time and place, attention span, memory, judgment, insight, thought content and processes, mood, and appearance. Formal interview questions include structured questions about the quantity and frequency of use, any adverse situations or consequences of using, and attitude toward using drugs. Laboratory drug screens identify illegal drug use, addiction disorders, infectious disease, pregnancy, and general health status.

Having a conversation that includes both health questions and questions about housing, work, school, and family is a less formal approach. Seek detailed information by asking open-ended questions such as: "Tell me about yourself." Follow the client's lead and place no constraints on what they can discuss. The nurse who takes steps to learn as much as possible about an individual such as who are they, what their life is like, and what are their complaints will learn more about the presenting symptoms. It is important to pay attention to information inconsistencies.

There are hundreds of assessment tools and screening instruments for substance abuse. Here are standard examples provided by SAMSHA (2010 NSDUH Computer-Assisted Interviewing (CAI) Instrumentation www.samhsa.gov/data/nsduh/2K10MRB/2k10Q.pdf). The 2010 NSDUH CAI instrument included questions designed to measure alcohol and illicit drug dependence and abuse in adults. These substance abuse questions were based on the criteria in the *DSM-IV* (2004).

Specifically, for marijuana, hallucinogens, inhalants, and tranquilizers, a respondent was defined as having dependence if he or she met three or more of the following six dependence criteria:

- Spending much time over a month getting, using, or getting over a substance
- Using more than intended; cannot stick to limits
- Changes in need patterns; needing more to get the same effect
- Inability to stop or cut down on use
- Continuing to use even when problems with mental or physical health develop
- Use interferes with activities

For alcohol, cocaine, heroin, pain relievers, sedatives, and stimulants, a seventh withdrawal criterion was added, defined by a respondent reporting a certain number of withdrawal symptoms that vary by substance (e.g., having trouble sleeping, cramps, and hands tremble). Respondents were considered dependent if they met three or more of seven dependence criteria.

For substances that include alcohol, marijuana, cocaine, heroin, hallucinogens, inhalants, pain relievers, tranquilizers, stimulants, and sedatives, a respondent was defined as having abused that substance if he or she met one or more of the following four abuse criteria and was determined not to be dependent on the respective substance in the past year:

EXHIBIT 14.1
Screening Tools

- Screening and assessing adolescents for substance use disorders.
  www.ncbi.nlm.nih.gov/books/NBK64364
- DAST-10 Questionnaire: A list of questions concerning information about
  potential involvement with drugs.
  www.integration.samhsa.gov
- AUDIT (Alcohol Use Disorders Identification Test)
  http://whqlibdoc.who.int/hq/2001/WHO_MSD_MSB_01.6a.pdf
- TCUDS II (The Texas Christians University Drug Screen).
  http://whqlibdoc.who.int/hq/2001/WHO_MSD_MSB_01.6a.pdf.

- Serious problems at home, for example, neglecting children, missing work,
  and losing job
- Did something to put you in physical danger
- Did something to get in trouble with the law
- Kept using if problems with family

For screening to be useful, it must be applicable to a broad range of people. For more information on screening tools, refer to the sources in Exhibit 14.1. These instruments have been designed more specifically for women and screen for alcohol consumption and some adapted for specific drugs.

RED FLAG IDENTIFIERS

Regardless of the style of assessment or screening tool used, find ways to help victims trust you. Determine the best course for gathering information by providing privacy, staying in touch with your own feelings, and let kindness and respect guide you.

The following "red flags" are considered hallmarks of the disease of addiction: denial, deception, and distortions in thinking. Know that any truthful answers to questions about their drug use or drinking would be the exception rather than the rule. Despite the value of a clinical interview, there are limits to getting accurate information. Most likely the victim will try to present in the best light and tend to avoid personal topics. They may protect themselves by providing inaccurate information. For example, they may describe a story they made up to camouflage their real-life situation. Red flags should also be noticed in the following:

Personality Assessment

Are they vague or uncomfortable talking about their future or what they want to do? Do they have a plan for what they will do or seem to have no options? Are they defensive, disrespectful, verbally and physically abusive? Do they act angry, paranoid, confused, depressed, or have mood swings? Do they seem secretive, or lie about what they have done or where they are going?

Physical Assessment of Red Flags

Are they taking care of hygiene and grooming? Why not? Are they tired, do they say they do not sleep, sleep too much, or tired all the time? Are they hungry? Do they have a loss of appetite or unplanned weight loss?

Physical Screening Methods

- Urine toxicology or hair analysis (for drugs and alcohol)
- Blood testing—Liver function tests, hepatitis B/C antibodies
- Breathalysers
- Abnormal temperature, pulse, respirations, blood pressure, or body weight

Whether you see red flags or not, the best way to get to know people is to take time to observe reactions to questions, listen to their responses, watch them observing you, and generally get a sense of who they are as well as who they are not.

Whether the interview has a formal or informal approach, be aware that you may make subjective judgments that skew the information you gathered. For example, you may rely too heavily on first impressions if you do not take time to process information. Your biases may influence the way you interpret what you hear. Victims may respond differently depending on the nurse's style; for example, they might feel less comfortable with coldness or distance and offer less information than they would to someone with a warm and supportive style.

Make a practice of monitoring your own feelings and thoughts during the interview. Having insight into your own thinking will be most helpful to make a stronger connection with the victim. A major red flag is feeling angry at victims for taking drugs, neglecting their health, or for lying.

This is only a beginning to identify and understand the complex problems of drug addiction. Proper screening, assessment, and diagnosis will lead to appropriate referrals for further evaluation in order for treatment to be meaningful. Use the sites in Exhibit 14.1 to access assessment tools and Exhibit 14.2 for additional resources.

TRUST-BUILDING INTERVIEWS

In order to obtain the most truthful responses possible, it helps victims to know that not every detail of information will be shared. A person who feels safe will offer more information. Reassessments help monitor progress and can be used to guide treatment because symptoms may change. Explain exactly what

EXHIBIT 14.2
Nursing Resources for Information

- *Substance Abuse and Mental Health Publications*: Order and download substance abuse and mental health issues-related publications.
www.samsha.gov
- *National Institute on Drug Abuse*: The mission of the National Institute on Drug Abuse (NIDA) is to lead the nation in bringing the power of science to bear on drug abuse and addiction.
www.drugabuse.gov
- *NIDA for Teens: The Science Behind Drug Abuse*: NIDA created the NIDA for Teens website to educate adolescents aged 11 through 15.
teens.drugabuse.gov
- *Drug abuse: MedlinePlus Medical Encyclopedia*: Drug abuse and illegal drugs.
www.nlm.nih.gov/.../001945.htm
- *NIDAMED: Medical & Health Professionals*: The NIDA is part of the National Institutes of Health (NIH), a component of the U.S. Department of Health and Human Services.
http://www.drugabuse.gov/medical-health-professionals
- Comorbid Drug Abuse and Mental Illness: What is comorbidity and what are its causes? When two disorders or illnesses occur simultaneously in the same person, they are called comorbid.
www.drugabuse.gov/comorbid-drug-abuse-mental-illness
- TWEAK for samples of the actual instruments in Spanish are not included in this online version. For printed copies, please contact the source listed on each fact sheet. pubs.niaaa.nih.gov
- White House Drug Policy
www.whithousedrugpolicy.gov/drugfact/cocaine/index.html
- Safety and Risk Assessment—Child Welfare Information Gateway.
www.childwelfare.gov/responding/iia/safety_risk/
- The manual "Clinical Protocols for Detoxification in Hospitals and Detoxification Facilities" has been prepared by John B. Saunders and Junie Yang and staff at:
www.health.qld.gov.au/atod/documents/24904.pdf
- *Detoxification and Substance Abuse Treatment Training Manual Treatment Improvement Protocol (TIP)*: 45 detoxification and substance for emergency rooms, hospital medical/surgical wards, and acute care clinics.
http://kap.samhsa.gov/products/trainingcurriculums/pdfs/tip45_curricu
lum.pdf

information you are obligated to share and with whom. For example, if there is a court-ordered evaluation for a judge or probation officer, information must be shared. Be clear that if there is a possibility or threat that they may injure

214 II: Clinical Perspectives

themselves or others, this information has to be shared with the doctor and clinical supervisor or appropriate staff. Finally, a victim's chaotic drug abuse lifestyle can cause them to fear legal repercussions, putting them in danger of more violence from their traffickers. Inform them about the established security standards for protecting their confidentiality.

Become familiar with privacy rules for your agency. Know the local and federal laws that limit what information can be released by health care providers. Some states have confidentiality laws where a consent release form has to be signed first, before any information is shared about such things as selling drugs, where their drugs are obtained, or names of peers. Toxicology tests on body fluids such as urine and saliva, or on hair samples is usually a routine part of the assessment, and can be done intermittently during and after treatment. Collecting samples must be done with consent of the person. Since drugs stay in the body for a limited time only, a negative toxicology report does not mean that the person does not use drugs.

Children and adolescents differ from adults emotionally and physiologically. Physical size, maturity, and cognition vary. Any drug use is an indication that the young person is struggling to deal with problems, but drug use can impair normal growth and development. Unfortunately, the younger the age, the less ability they have to recover. Even a brief assessment of a young person's mental health and risk assessment can make a difference in their lives. These are complex cases and will require a multidisciplinary team approach to provide developmentally specific care.

Brain Development Review

Cognitive ability and developmental skills take place at stages during normal growth and development. The brain develops for about 20 years and is shaped in part by environmental experiences. Drugs and alcohol can have permanent detrimental effects on the way the brain develops, works, and perceives the world.

The age range of 5 to 10 is a critical time. The brain is being molded. Most synaptic connections are established but logical pathways are not fully developed. Synapses are strengthened by the process of myelination. This dynamic process is the basis of learning and accounts for long-term memory.

Adolescence is from age 10 to 20 years when fine tuning the frontal lobes for functional proficiency occurs. The more primitive limbic system becomes more refined. Processing of information and attention span improve and emotional responses gradually become more reasoned. Some may describe a teenager as ill-tempered, grumpy, and confusing. Complicating factors are the hormonal influences on the brain during puberty. Illicit drugs and alcohol during adolescence are likely to disturb the brain and any change at this time will be permanent. Continued drug use will produce negative influences on mood, emotional responses, judgment, thinking, memory, interpersonal skills, and attention.

Risk Assessment

When assessing risk for children or adults, it is important to remember that risks are often higher when other indicators of mental illness are present. Several areas should be considered in the risk assessment: self-harm and suicide, vulnerability to assault, violence to others, risk of being abused, risk of self-neglect, and risk of relapse or nonengagement with services. Competence to consent to treatment may be required. As mandated reporters, nurses must follow their facility's protocols and report abuse to either local child protective services or police departments.

Providing the client an opportunity to talk about the benefits of using before talking about the disadvantages will help reduce defensiveness. If they feel safe enough they may open up more. The process of discussing the positives first and then a negative of drug use is called "pay off matrix." This will help the nurse to understand their concerns. The goal is to help clients make informed choices, and not react based on the crisis they are in. Focus on their needs as they state them. Detailed assessment is important, so questions exploring the age of onset of using, patterns of their use, progression, names and use of specific drugs, the places and times they use, any descriptions may be helpful. However, starting with these questions might increase clients' anxiety and distress making them less likely to be candid.

During the assessment, clients have little or no motivation to change. They do not think they have a problem or are too afraid to say so. In this case, plant a seed for thought. It will show you care and are attempting to understand them. If they want to continue using, provide them with a harm reduction tip. For example, if they are using solvents to mix drugs advise them not to use a plastic bag; use a paper bag to avoid interaction of the drug with the plastic, which can be toxic. Consider clients' level of understanding and literacy level. Document if they have attempted to decrease or stop using, if they are being forced to continue, or any other major concerns they have about using.

The basics discussed here when working with young people who abuse drugs are the same as working with any young person. It is up to the nurse to develop a safe place and a climate of caring. Be respectful and nonjudgmental.

Symptoms

The *DSM-IV* identifies seven symptoms governing the diagnosis of substance dependence, at least three of which must be met during a given 12-month period. These include:

- Tolerance, as defined either by the need for increasing amounts of the substance to obtain the desired effect or by experiencing less effect with extended use of the same amount of the substance
- Withdrawal, as exhibited either by experiencing unpleasant mental, physiological, and emotional changes when drug-taking ceases or by using the substance as a way to relieve or prevent withdrawal symptoms

- Longer duration of taking the substance or use in greater quantities than was originally intended
- Persistent desire or repeated unsuccessful efforts to stop or lessen substance use
- A relatively large amount of time spent in securing and using the substance, or in recovering from the effects of the substance
- Important work and social activities are reduced because of substance use
- Continued substance use despite negative physical and psychological effects of use

Although not explicitly listed in the *DSM-IV* criteria, "craving," or the overwhelming desire to use the substance regardless of countervailing forces, is a universally reported symptom of substance dependence. In the child and adolescent age group, the diagnostic determination of substance abuse requires at least three of the above criteria to be present such as:

- Withdrawal symptoms
- Loss of control over use
- Tolerance of the drug

Symptoms of substance abuse, as specified by *DSM-IV*, include one or more of the following occurring during a given 12-month period:

- Substance use resulting in a recurrent failure to fulfill work, school, or home obligations (work absences, substance-related school suspensions, and neglect of children)
- Substance use in physically hazardous situations such as driving or operating machinery
- Substance use resulting in legal problems such as drug-related arrests. Continued substance use despite negative social and relationship consequences of use

In addition to the *DSM-IV* symptoms, there are other physical signs of substance abuse that are related to specific drug classes:

- Signs of alcohol intoxication include slurred speech, lack of coordination, unsteady gait, memory impairment, and stupor, as well as behavior changes shortly after alcohol ingestion, including inappropriate aggressive behavior, mood volatility, and impaired functioning
- Signs of amphetamine use are rapid heartbeat, elevated or depressed blood pressure, dilated (enlarged) pupils, weight loss, as well as excessively high energy, inability to sleep, confusion, and occasional paranoid psychotic behavior
- Signs of cocaine use are rapid heart rate, elevated or depressed blood pressure, dilated pupils, weight loss, in addition to wide variations in energy level, severe mood disturbances, psychosis, and paranoia

- Signs of hallucinogen use are anxiety or depression, paranoia, and unusual behavior in response to hallucinations (imagined sights, voices, sounds, or smells that appear real). Also included are dilated pupils, rapid heart rate, tremors, lack of coordination, and sweating. Flashbacks, or the reexperiencing of a hallucination long after stopping substance use, are also a sign of hallucinogen use
- Signs of inhalant use are dizziness, spastic eye movements, lack of coordination, slurred speech, and slowed reflexes. Associated behaviors may include belligerence, tendency toward violence, apathy, and impaired judgment
- Signs of opioid drug use are slurred speech, drowsiness, impaired memory, and constricted (small) pupils. They may appear slowed in their physical movements
- Signs of use of any sedative, hypnotic, or anxiolytic drugs show slurred speech, unsteady gait, inattentiveness, and impaired memory. They may display inappropriate behavior, mood volatility, and impaired functioning

UNDERSTANDING ADDICTION

Drugs can lead to physical and psychological dependency that is as much a disorder of the brain as any other neurological or psychiatric illness. Drug addiction occurs when a person becomes dependent on a drug to the point that it is the central part of life. Drug-related disorders are caused by the use of substances that affect the central nervous system (CNS), such as cocaine, heroin, and alcohol.

Technically, the term "drug" applies to any substance other than food that alters mental functioning or changes the body. All drug misuse will lead to different kinds of abnormal functioning. Drug use causes changes in behavior, emotion, and thought such as intoxication, a temporary state. Continuous drug use can then lead to physical dependency, psychological dependency, or both. Physical dependency means that the body has become so used to the drug that physical withdrawal symptoms result if deprived of the drug. Psychological dependency means that one takes the drug to feel good, and then may feel that one cannot stop using even though not physically dependent.

The regular use of drugs can lead to longer-term patterns of maladaptive behaviors and changes in the body's response to the substance. They experience withdrawal symptoms if they suddenly stop taking the drug. The diagnosis for substance abuse requires clinically significant levels of distress or impairment.

Tolerance occurs when a person needs increasing amounts of drugs in order to keep getting the desired effect. Similarly, regular long-term use can cause withdrawal, a state of unpleasant and dangerous symptoms. Withdrawal symptoms can begin within hours of the last use, and intensify over several days before subsiding.

Detoxification, commonly called "detox," usually requires the use of medications to detox safely. Normally, benzodiazepines and other sedatives are used for treating alcohol withdrawal, while buprenorphine (Suboxone®) is given with other medications for opiate withdrawal. If complications of withdrawal are not managed appropriately, death can occur.

What Are Barriers to Treatment?

Trafficked victims encounter enormous barriers to treatment. First, there is the wide range of withdrawal symptoms that occurs whenever any chronic drug use is reduced, stopped, or ignored. Second, the violence experienced and witnessed by victims, leaves them vulnerable and compelled to survive by continuing to feed their habit. They will be compliant to the demands of traffickers in order to preserve themselves from further harm. Traffickers will stalk, harass, forcibly return, beat, emotionally punish, or kill their victims. In some cases a victim's fear of having her family threatened will be sufficient to comply with the traffickers.

Few resources are available to address victims unique situations and few nurses have been oriented to identify victims. There are treatment programs that coincide with state regulations and standards set by the Joint Commission on Accreditation of Health Care Organizations (JCAHO). However, sex trafficking victims may not know where to turn. Victims may not be allowed to participate in programs for substance abuse or receive care for psychiatric disorders. Any emergency medical problems they have would not likely be treated. Finally, medically assisted and monitored detoxification and use of anticraving drugs would not be available to trafficking victims.

PRACTICAL STREET DRUG INFORMATION

The drugs we will review fall into four categories:

1. Stimulants stimulate the CNS; examples include cocaine and amphetamines
2. Depressants depress the CNS; examples include alcohol and opioids
3. Hallucinogenic drugs cause changes in sensory perceptions
4. Polysubstance abuse can include all of the above, plus marijuana, which can have hallucinogenic, depressant, and stimulant effects

Knowledge of drug abuse can be used in a variety of settings, including hospitals, and residential environments. This section provides information about street drugs and their harmful effects.

Cocaine Abuse and Addiction

History
Cocaine has been ingested for thousands of years making it one of the oldest known psychoactive substances. Pure cocaine is a naturally occurring plant alkaloid derived from the leaf of the *Erythroxylum coca* bush. It was grown primarily in Bolivia and Peru until those countries began efforts to reduce crops. In the

1990s, Colombia became the country with the largest cultivated coco crops. The purified chemical, cocaine hydrochloride, is the main active ingredient and has been abused for 100 years or more. Elixirs and tonics were used to treat a variety of illnesses in the 1900s. Today, cocaine is considered to be one of the greatest drug threats to the world because of the violence related to trafficking and use.

Street Name
Crack, rock, and freebase. Cocaine is known also as coke, snow, flake, Charlie, blow, nose candy, big C, white, lady, and snowbirds. Cocoa puffs, gummers, or numbies are some of the names referring to the drug being rubbed in the mouth. Snow bomb is another oral method when cocaine is rolled up in rolling papers and swallowed.

What Does it Look Like?
Cocaine, when refined from leaves and sold on the street, appears as a fine powder that is crystalline. When pure, it is white; when not pure, it can be yellowish, off-white, tan, or pinkish in color. Traffickers buy wholesale cocaine from regional distributors and importers in kilograms or multikilogram amounts. This is the weight when it is shipped from Colombia and other countries.

Once it arrives in the "consuming country," it is packaged into retail quantities of either ounces or grams. During the packaging process, pure cocaine may be mixed with other products; this mixing process is referred to as "cutting." Cutting is done to increase the quantity and increase the profit potential. Drugs are processed and pass through the hands of many people before they eventually get to the street. Street dealers then usually dilute the drugs further with inert substances such as talcum powder, cornstarch, or sugar. The common types of sugars used are lactose and dextrose. Sometimes other stimulant drugs such as amphetamines are mixed (or "cut") in. Other types of drugs used to cut cocaine are local anesthetics, such as lidocaine, procaine, or benzocaine, which mimic or add to cocaine's numbing effect on mucous membranes.

Sometimes cocaine is combined with heroin to make a "speedball." It is not unusual to find substances in illegal drugs that are much more harmful than the drugs themselves. Some unfortunate drug users ingest other impurities in their cocaine, such as rodent poison.

There are two chemical methods that can be used that alter the appearance of cocaine. Both chemical manufacturing processes are known as freebasing. First, a water-soluble hydrochloride salt combines with the water-insoluble cocaine base for injecting or snorting. Second, dealers may also convert the cocaine hydrochloride into crack by simply dissolving it in a solution of water and heating it with a chemical reagent such as sodium bicarbonate (baking soda) or ammonia to free the alkaloid base from the salt. A solid substance forms after the solution is boiled and this is called "crack." The solid substance is then removed and left to dry to produce a substance that can be smoked. The term "crack" derived from the crackling sound is heard when this substance is smoked.

This form of cocaine is then cut into pieces called "rocks" that usually are the size of a raisin. A rock can weigh from one-tenth to 1 gram. The crack rocks are estimated to be 75% to 90% pure cocaine for street selling.

How Are Cocaine and Crack Abused?

Cocaine use ranges from occasional use to compulsive use or "binges." There is no safe way to use cocaine, not even orally. Oral use is uncommon because it produces a less high effect than other routes. To use orally, the drug is rubbed onto mucous tissue in the mouth. The three more commonly used routes are snorting (intranasal), injecting (into a vein), and smoking. These routes enable the drug to be absorbed into the bloodstream through the tissues or veins. The language referring to paraphernalia and practices of smoking cocaine varies greatly in different areas and in different countries. What remains constant is that all three of the more common routes can lead to a fast absorption rate that can produce overdose. Regardless of the route or frequency of use, abusers can experience acute cardiovascular or cerebral vascular emergencies such as a heart attack or stroke that may cause sudden death. Cocaine-related deaths are often the result of cardiac arrest or seizure and respiratory arrest.

"Snorting," "sniffing," or "blowing" are the terms used for this most common method of self-administration where cocaine is used intranasally. The process involves inhaling cocaine powder through the nose using a rolled up dollar bill, a hollowed-out pen, a cut straw, the pointy end of a key, a long fingernail, or even an empty tampon applicator. These makeshift devices are used to insufflate cocaine from "lines," "rails," or "bumps," which is cocaine powder laid out on a flat surface. The effect of snorting cocaine is similar to smoking crack but is less intense, because of slower absorption; the high can last 15 to 30 minutes.

Injecting or intravenous use with a needle releases the drug directly into the bloodstream. This delivery method produces the fullest effects of the drug within 5 to 10 seconds, and heightens the intensity of the effect. Injecting drugs is also referred to as "slamming," "shooting [up]," "banging," "pinning," or "jacking-up," depending on the type of drug used and the specific drug subculture environment. This more intense short high can lead to physical and psychological dependency, both developing more quickly than with other routes of drug self-administration.

Smoking crack is done in a pipe or glass tube, plastic bottle, or in foil. Smoking involves inhaling cocaine vapor into the lungs with devices called "stems," "horns," "blasters," and "straight shooters." Other methods include smoking by placing it at the end of the pipe. A flame held close to it produces vapor, which is then inhaled by the smoker. Crack smokers also sometimes smoke through a beer or soda can with small holes in the bottom, with the effect as rapid as injecting. Pure cocaine base/crack is easy to smoke because it vaporizes smoothly. The smoke produced from cocaine base is usually described as having a very distinctive and pleasant taste. If not done correctly, cocaine hydrochloride does not vaporize until heated to a high temperature that destroys some of the cocaine, and produces a foul-tasting smoke. Compulsive cocaine use may develop more quickly if the substance is smoked rather than snorted. The high from smoking may last only 5 to 10 minutes. In order to stay high the drug is used repeatedly and frequently at increasingly higher doses, which is why it is abused in binges.

What Does Using Feel Like?

Using cocaine makes you feel on top of the world, with a feeling of wellness and confidence, of being very alert and awake, with increased energy, and feeling ready to take risks. The person becomes euphoric, talkative, and hypersensitive to sights, sounds, and touch. When the effects diminish, users may experience irritability and confusion. Strong cravings occur to use more especially during the crash period that sometimes can linger for days afterward. Although a psychological dependence can easily cause lows and depression, it is the physical withdrawal symptoms that cause the user to want and need more.

How Do Nurses Make a Diagnosis?

A physical examination and a clinical history are required. Stimulant use can be confirmed by urinalysis and/or oral fluid swab. Physical assessment, a good history, and urine and blood tests to screen for drugs can confirm opiate use. The definition of cocaine opioid dependence is a maladaptive pattern of opioid use leading to clinically significant impairment or distress, as manifested by three (or more) of the following, occurring at any time in the same 12-month period (American Psychiatric Association, 2000; *DSM-IV*, 2004):

* Tolerance—either of the following:
  a. Need increasing amounts for effect
  b. Weaker effect with same amount
* Withdrawal—either of the following:
  a. The characteristic syndrome for that substance
  b. Taking the same or closely related substance relieves withdrawal
* The substance is taken in larger amounts or over a longer period
* Persistent desire but unsuccessful efforts to cut down or control substance use
* Much time spent in obtaining, using the substance, or recovering from effects
* Substance use replaces important activities or responsibilities
* Use is continued despite knowledge of having a persistent or recurrent physical or psychological problem likely to have been caused by the substance

In short, opioid dependence is not just physical dependence on opioids, but also continuing use despite consequences.

What Are the Effects on the Body?

Cocaine produces its effects by working on three neurotransmitters: dopamine, serotonin, and adrenalin. Cocaine's primary acute effect on brain chemistry is to raise the amount of dopamine and serotonin in the nucleus acumens—the pleasure center in the brain. Cocaine acts by preventing dopamine from being recycled causing it to build up in excessive amounts. The receiving and transmitting neurons get amplified messages causing cocaine's euphoric effects. Long-term use changes the brain's reward system; tolerance to a "cocaine high" develops. This explains the feelings of depression as a "crash" after the initial high.

- **Small-to-moderate amounts cause:** increased heart rate and arrhythmias, rapid respirations, elevated blood pressure from constricted blood vessels, dilated pupils, sweating, excessive body movements, talkativeness, and behavioral changes such as nervousness, agitation, and irritability.
- **Binge pattern causes:** mood instability, anxiety, restlessness, and irritability, musculoskeletal problems include muscle spasms, tremor, twitches, sleep disturbance, grandiose thinking, and more risk-taking behaviors.
- **Larger amounts cause:** chest pain, palpitations, cardiac arrest, dizziness, blurred vision, headaches, abdominal pain, nausea, impaired coordination, seizures, panic, and a temporary state of paranoid psychosis in which the person loses touch with reality and experiences hallucinations and delusions, leading to bizarre, erratic, and violent behavior.
- **Mixing drugs** is highly dangerous. For example a mixture of cocaine and heroin called a speedball increases the risks from each drug making it more likely for the user to have harmful effects.
- **Overdose:** The risk of overdose increases if crack is used in combination with other drugs or alcohol. Since cocaine is also highly pyrogenic (stimulation and increased muscular activity cause greater heat production), the person will have a high temperature. Cocaine-induced hyperthermia can cause muscle cell destruction resulting in renal failure from myloglobinuria. Other symptoms can include coma, convulsions, and hallucinations.

Most deaths due to cocaine are accidental. Immediate medical treatment is needed. Emergency treatment consists of administering a sedative agent to decrease the elevated heart rate and blood pressure. The body temperature must be lowered with medication such as acetaminophen, or by physical cooling such as hypothermia blanket, ice, cold blankets, and so on. There is no Federal Drug Administration (FDA)-approved antidote for cocaine overdose.

What Are the Complications of Using?

A different method of using cocaine produces different adverse effects. Polydrug use increases the risk of serious side effects. The combination is dangerous because the body produces coca-ethylene, a toxic chemical in the liver. Researchers believe coca-ethylene can increase the euphoric effects of cocaine and has a greater risk of sudden death than if cocaine were used alone (Harris et al., 2003). Specific complications are as follows:

- **Snorting** can cause ulcerated nasal mucosa, perforation as the result of necrosis, infection or ischemia, loss of the sense of smell, nosebleeds, chronic runny nose, acute and chronic sinusitis may occur along with bone destruction problems, difficulty in swallowing, and voice hoarseness. Over time snorting damages the cartilage in the nose and heavy users can end up with just one big nostril or misshapen nose as the cartilage is damaged.
- **Injecting** leaves track marks on the arms, legs, or trunk. Ulcers and gangrene or clots and abscesses can result from the collapse of veins. Sharing needles can spread HIV/AIDS and viral hepatitis C infection.
- **Smoking** can cause lung damage such as asthma that might be acute, severe, and occasionally fatal, bleeding (hemoptysis), shortness of breath, chronic cough or chest pain, or pulmonary infections such as pneumonitis. Crack keratitis can occur due to the local anesthetic effect, causing the user to rub eyes excessively. Tooth enamel erodes. Hands will show burns consistent with holding cocaine pipes and cracked calluses on the fingers from the repeated use of a lighter.

What Is Physical Withdrawal Like?
Symptoms can be mild to moderate and differ for each victim, from flu-like symptoms to physiological changes that include vivid and unpleasant dreams, insomnia or hypersomnia, hostility, agitation, or psychomotor retardation. Crack users often use alcohol to ease cocaine withdrawal (or to enhance the effects of the drug) and this combination results in possibly the highest number of drug-related deaths (Burnett, 2010).

Long-Term Effects
Cocaine decreases the appetite to the point of significant weight loss. Crack is also associated with furring coronary arteries with fatty deposits leading to hypertension, chest pain, shortness of breath, or ventricular fibrillation.

What Treatment Options Exist?
The best treatment is to combine medical with comprehensive mental health services including behavior therapy. The FDA currently has not approved medications for cocaine treatment. Research is being done to develop medications to alleviate the severe cravings. Several compounds that would seize cocaine in the blood and prevent it from reaching the brain are under investigation.

There are many effective behavioral treatment programs for outpatient and residential settings. Community-based recovery groups such as Cocaine Anonymous that use a 12-step program like Alcoholics Anonymous (AA) can help sustain abstinence. Cognitive behavioral therapy (CBT) is a learning process that can help reduce drug use by avoiding the triggers that produce craving for the drug.

What Are the Nursing Implications?

Be alert to possible victims of sex trafficking. Explain there are drug treatment services with trained nurses with required skills and knowledge. Even the memory of using cocaine can trigger cravings and relapse. The risk of relapse is high even following periods of abstinence, especially when new stressors occur.

Heroin Abuse and Addiction

History

Heroin is a semisynthetic opiate and analgesic. It is a drug made from morphine, which is the substance derived from the resin of the Asian opium poppy, an annual herb called *Papaver somniferum*. This is the key ingredient for all narcotics. When morphine is made into heroin to be used as medicine, it is called diamorphine and it is stronger than morphine or opium. Many drugs made from opium are called opiates, and heroin is the most rapid acting.

The opium poppy was documented a very long time ago in 3400 BC. Opium did not have legal restrictions until the early 1900s. Today, opium is cultivated and converted into heroin in many countries. Opium production occurs primarily in the countries of southeast/southwest Asia and Latin America, enough to generate significant worldwide problems. There are many long-established trafficking and distribution networks. For example, Mexico primarily supplies the United States heroin market.

Heroin is broken down into alkaloid constituents when imported. It was not widely used in medicine until the beginning of the 20th century when it was first made from morphine. It was marketed as a cough suppressant. Today drug abusers smoke, ingest, or inject heroin and can overdose using any route.

What Are the Street Names?

Heroin, an illegal opiate drug, is known on the street as "dope," "smack," "junk," "horse," "brown sugar," "skunk," and a variety of other names in drug subcultures. "Mud," "black tar," and "big H" are some additional common street names.

What Does it Look Like?

Heroin has different appearances. It is a powder that can vary in color from white if pure, to dark brown or black with impurities from the manufacturing process. Black tar heroin is black like coal but with the consistency of roofing tar that is sticky and black. It can be manufactured in remote laboratories using simple equipment that presses the powder into bricks for bulk shipment. An uncut bag of heroin contains approximately 100 mg of powder. It takes approximately 10 kg of opium to make a kilogram of heroin. Heroin can be sold on the street in its tar-like state or in "bags," which is a slang term for single dosage units. Heroin usually is cut with sugar, starch, powdered milk, quinine, or paracetamol for added weight and to increase quantity for more profit. Users cannot be sure if the heroin they are given has been "cut" with nutmeg or a more dangerous substance such as brick dust or ground-up gravel.

How Is Heroin Used?

Heroin is most frequently dissolved, diluted, and injected. The onset of heroin's effect depends upon the route of administration. The fastest route of injection is intravenous, followed by smoking, snorting, and ingestion.

Injection

A typical heroin user will inject up to 4 times a day obtaining a high in less than 10 seconds. To inject heroin, it is mixed in a spoon with water and citric acid or lemon juice and heated until it becomes a solution. The hydrochloride salt form of heroin commonly found in the United States requires just water to dissolve. Homemade filters such as cigarette filters, or cotton bud tips are used to remove any large particles (not bacteria) from the solution. The solution with filter material is now ready to inject and the onset of the rush can occur in a few seconds.

Injection is known as "slamming," "banging," "shooting up," or "mainlining" and begins in easily accessible arm veins that eventually collapse or get damaged over time from the acid. The user will then use any veins they can find. Intramuscular injection effects are slower with the onset of euphoria in 5 to 8 minutes.

Snorting/Insufflation

Heroin can be inhaled by placing it in aluminum foil and then heating it from the bottom so that the vapors rise up to inhale the resulting smoke. This method is also known as "Chinese blowing," "chine sing," or "chasing the dragon." It can also be smoked in glass pipes made from Pyrex tubes or light bulbs.

Another popular route to use heroin is snorting the crushed powder spread out in lines like cocaine. It is sharply inhaled usually with a straw or a rolled up dollar bill where it is absorbed in the mucous membrane of the sinus cavity and straight into the bloodstream. Heroin sniffed or smoked has peak effects within 10 to 15 minutes. This method is preferred by users who do not want to prepare and administer heroin for injection or smoking but still experience a fast onset with a rush.

Oral Ingestion

Oral use of heroin is less common than other methods of administration, mainly because there is little to no "rush," and the effects are less potent. The oral route of administration requires approximately half an hour before the high begins.

What Does Using Feel Like?

"Using" the first time may cause dizziness and vomiting. Heroin is a pain killer. In small doses, heroin gives a sense of well-being, and a feeling of warm flushing of the skin, heavy feeling in the extremities, and dry mouth. Larger doses can make you feel very relaxed, mentally cloudy, and sleepy, or severely itchy and nauseated. The effects last for hours.

Heroin is highly addictive. Using on a regular basis produces "tolerance" that increases so that a higher dose is needed to get the same high, but then the higher dose is needed to feel "normal." In time, more drug is needed to avoid unpleasant withdrawal symptoms. High levels of use produce ataxia, confusion, agitation, or delusions and hallucination.

How Do Nurses Make a Diagnosis?

Physical assessment, good history, and urine and blood tests to screen for drugs can confirm opiate use.

How Do You Diagnose Opium-Related Disorders?

Opioid dependence leads to clinically significant impairment or distress, as manifested by three or more of the following conditions in the same 12-month period (American Psychiatric Association, 2000):

- Tolerance—either of the following:
  a. Need increasing amounts for effect
  b. Weaker effect with same amount
- Withdrawal—either of the following:
  a. The characteristic syndrome for that substance
  b. Taking the same or closely related substance relieves withdrawal
- The substance is taken in larger amounts or over a longer period
- Persistent desire but unsuccessful efforts to cut down or control substance use
- Much time spent in obtaining, using the substance, or recovering from effects
- Substance use replaces important activities or responsibilities
- Use is continued despite knowledge of having a persistent or recurrent physical or psychological problem likely to have been caused by the substance

What Are the Effects on the Body?

Opiates act on many parts of the brain and nervous system. Heroin is converted into morphine and binds rapidly to opioid receptors. This is what causes the "rush" or surge of pleasure sensation. There are mu-opioid receptors (MORs) in the brain. MORs have a high affinity for heroin because heroin crosses the blood–brain barrier rapidly. Both natural and synthetic opioid derivatives affect MORs increasing addictiveness (Yu, 1996). Overdose is common if the person is using heroin with other drugs and even alcohol. Overdose can lead to coma and death usually from respiratory failure. Since it is impossible to know how pure heroin is, it is easy to overdose. The risk of sedation can occur to the point that there is no cough reflex and aspiration can occur if vomiting while unconscious. There is also a considerable risk of respiratory depression that can develop quickly with prolonged use or during withdrawal. It is difficult to determine whether a heroin overdose was an accident, suicide, or homicide.

What Are the Complications of Using?

Tolerance develops with frequent use of heroin and drops rapidly, creating risk of an overdose from taking too much the next time.

Immune reactions to contaminates used to cut heroin can cause arthritis and other rheumatological problems. Chronic use has been shown to cause liver and kidney disease because of hypernatremia as a result of excess vasopressin secretion. Some of the most detrimental effects result from chemical and molecular changes in the brain.

- **Snorting** can cause lightheadedness, dizziness, pupil constriction, nausea, and drowsiness as a result of stimulation of the opioid receptors in the cerebrum.
- **Injecting IV** can lead to infections or gangrene—usually a finger, toe, or limb. Using and sharing needles and equipment increases risk of hepatitis B, hepatitis C, and HIV/AIDS. Positive HIV can lead to lung abscesses or empyema from aspiration. Also found are tuberculosis (TB) or community-acquired pneumonia, pleural or mediastinal infection, septic emboli, and endocarditis.
- **Smoking** may cause bronchiectasis or bronchitis. Substances inhaled like talc can lodge in the pulmonary vasculature causing a foreign body reaction that can lead to fibrosis.
- **Ingestion** can cause gastrointestinal or gastrourinary effects such as urethral spasms and urinary retention due to CNS stimulation of sympathetic pathways.

What Is Physical Withdrawal Like?

Opioid withdrawal reactions are not life threatening, but they are very uncomfortable. Symptoms usually start within 12 hours of the last heroin use, and within 30 hours of the last methadone dose. Early symptoms of withdrawal include restlessness, agitation, anxiety, muscle and bone pain, increased tearing, runny nose, sweating, yawning, vomiting, diarrhea, and insomnia. Later symptoms of withdrawal are dilated pupils, goose pumps, cold flashes, abdominal cramping, nausea, vomiting, diarrhea, and uncomfortable leg movements. Major withdrawal peaks between 24 and 48 hours after the last use and can last for a week to several months with persistent withdrawal symptoms. Withdrawal is not fatal in healthy children or women, but it can cause death to a fetus (National Institute on Drug Abuse, 2009).

What Are the Treatments for Heroin Addiction?

Sex trafficking victims are not usually able to access effective treatment for heroin addiction. Nurses need to be informed that treatment can be successful if supportive care, counseling, and medications are provided. Interventions are aimed at achieving humane withdrawal by minimizing medical complications and relieving withdrawal symptoms. The chronic disease of addiction is a medical condition and, it cannot be cured but it can be managed. Nurses are in a position to identify addictive patterns and help people understand the issues that trap them.

A person has to take heroin to feel "normal" because of their level of tolerance and dependence. The cravings are strong and the fear of withdrawal is great. Medications are often the best choice for treating heroin addiction. The three most commonly used medications are methadone, buprenorphine, and naltrexone. Methadone is a synthetic opiate medication that binds to the same receptors as heroin and is only available through specialized opiate treatment programs. Buprenorphine produces less risk for overdose and withdrawal effects. It can only be dispensed by authorized physicians and can give opiate-addicted victims more medical options. Naltrexone is not as widely used due to the nature of poor compliance. This medication prevents an addicted individual from feeling the effects of the drug. Naltrexone is used in medical detoxification residential settings to prevent withdrawal symptoms. Individuals must be opiate-free for several days and medically detoxified before taking naltrexone (National Institute on Drug Abuse, 2009).

Careful assessment is required to identify the best medication for the client. The person taking the medication has to be able to follow the directions carefully because taking the medication improperly can lead to overdose and death. It is critical to avoid illegal drugs that interact with the medication. People can take the medication safely as long as needed. Nurses can refer, support, and encourage clients through the recovery process.

What Support Groups Are Available?

Methadone Anonymous www.methadoneanonymous.info
Rational Recovery www.rationalrecovery.org
Dual Recovery Anonymous www.draonline.org
Life Ring www.unhooked.com
National Alliance of Methadone Advocates www.methadone.org
National Alliance of Advocates for Buprenorphine www.naabt.org

Check with each organization for details. This is not a complete list. If you are unable to find a community support group in your area, another option is to contact a local chapter of AA. Meetings are sometimes open to people in recovery from substances other than alcohol.

What Are the Nursing Implications?

Like any chronic disease, heroin addiction can be treated. Recovery is a long process, starting with physical detoxification, learning to cope with the withdrawal symptoms, and learning to live without heroin.

Alcohol Abuse and Addiction

Alcohol is often not thought of as a drug and yet is the oldest and most widely used drug in the world. Beer might have been a staple of diet in ancient times and there is documentation that alcoholic drinks were made from berries or honey. Wine was documented in Egypt around 4000 BC (Blum, 1969; Lucia, 1963; Patrick, 1952). Alcohol is associated with fun and sociability, but abusing alcohol has life-threatening consequences.

According to the World Health Organization (WHO) Global Status Report on Alcohol (2004), alcohol consumption in Europe, Africa, and the Americas peaked in the early 1980s. Europe and the Americas show the highest levels of consumption, followed by Africa and the Western Pacific regions, while the southeast Asian and eastern Mediterranean regions show the lowest level of consumption. While alcohol consumption has increased steadily in the southeast Asian and Western Pacific regions, it is stable or falling in the other regions.

In the United States during 1970 to 1975 the minimum drinking age was lowered in 29 states from 21 to 18 and 19 or 20 following the enactment of the 26th Amendment to the U.S. Constitution, which lowered the legal voting age to 18. The younger the age at first drink, the more likely the person will have a problem with alcohol. Nearly half of all Americans over the age of 12 are consumers of alcohol (WHO) Global Status Report on Alcohol (2004). The extent and frequency with which people drink influences the severity of health and behavioral issues. Continued use despite harmful effects can lead to alcohol addiction, a serious and sometimes life-threatening disease.

What Is Alcohol?

Alcohol is an organic compound composed of carbon, oxygen, and hydrogen; its chemical formula is C_2H_5OH. It is a clear volatile liquid that burns (oxidizes) easily. It has a slight characteristic odor and is highly soluble in water. Alcohol is the liquid form of ethanol, or ethyl alcohol. It is a powerful and addictive CNS depressant.

How Is Alcohol Made?

An alcoholic beverage is produced by the action of yeast on carbohydrates when distilling various fruits, vegetables, or grains. Fermentation is a process that uses bacteria or yeast to convert the sugars into alcohol. Alcohol in different forms can be classified as a sedative, antiseptic, or cleaner.

What Are the Street Names for Alcohol?

Beer, wine, and hard liquor are the most commonly used, also known as drunk, drink, booze, brew, and hooch. The word "moonshine" is generally assumed to mean whiskey, a widely abused psychoactive drug.

How Is it Used?

A drink can come in many forms. It can be a shot of hard liquor or a mixed drink containing vodka, rum, tequila, gin, scotch, or some other liquor. It can also be wine, a wine cooler, beer, or malt liquor. There are three basic types of alcoholic drinks that are ingested. Beer is made from fermented grains. Wine is made from fermented fruits and has more alcohol content. Liquor is made by distilling a fermented product that usually contains the highest percentage of alcohol such as 40-proof or 80-proof (percent alcohol). Some people think beer and wine is safer than liquor, but any form of alcohol can cause problems. One 12-ounce bottle of beer or a 5-ounce glass of wine (about a half cup) has as much alcohol as a 1.5-ounce shot of liquor.

There are three main patterns of drinking alcohol:

- Binge drinking
  For women, four or more drinks during a single occasion.
  For men, five or more drinks during a single occasion.
- Heavy drinking
  For women, more than one drink per day on average.
  For men, more than two drinks per day on average.
- Excessive drinking includes heavy drinking, binge drinking, or both. Drinkers who experience blackouts consume large quantities of alcohol too much and too quickly, which causes their blood alcohol levels to rapidly rise.

How Does Alcohol Affect You?

Within moments of ingestion, alcohol reaches the brain. Alcohol initially serves as a stimulant, and then induces feelings of relaxation and reduced anxiety. Consumption of two or three drinks in an hour can impair judgment, lower inhibitions, and induce mild euphoria. Then alcohol depresses and sedates producing calmness and tranquility, can induce a hypnotic state and sleep, to the point of anesthetizing.

The properties of alcohol that affect the CNS are directly proportional to the concentration of alcohol in the blood. Alcohol moves from the bloodstream into every part of the body that contains water, including major organs such as the brain, lungs, kidneys, and heart, and distributes itself equally both inside and outside of cells. How alcohol affects a person depends on how much alcohol is consumed, the time period in which it is consumed, how much food is in the stomach, and body weight.

What Are the Signs of Intoxication?

Physical symptoms of the state of being drunk are the smell of alcohol on the breath or skin, bloodshot or glazed eyes, and flushed skin. The person can become passive or argumentative. Cognitively, there is a decreased attention span and memory loss. Deterioration in the person's appearance or hygiene is common.

How Do Nurses Make a Diagnosis?

There is no one test that is definitive for alcohol disorder. Therefore, health care practitioners diagnose these disorders by gathering comprehensive medical, family, and mental health information. *DSM-IV* criteria for alcohol abuse are:

- Tolerance—either of the following:
  a. Need increasing amounts for effect
  b. Weaker effect with same amount
- Withdrawal—either of the following:
  a. The characteristic syndrome for that substance
  b. Taking the same or closely related substance relieves withdrawal
- The substance is taken in larger amounts or over a longer period
- Persistent desire but unsuccessful efforts to cut down or control substance use
- Much time spent in obtaining, using the substance, or recovering from effects
- Failure to fulfill major role obligations at work, school, or home (e.g., repeated absences or poor work performance related to substance use, substance-related absences, suspensions or expulsions from school, or neglect of children or household)
- Recurrent alcohol use in physically hazardous situations (e.g., driving an automobile or operating a machine)
- Recurrent alcohol-related legal problems (e.g., arrests for alcohol-related disorderly conduct)
- Continued alcohol use despite persistent or recurrent social or interpersonal problems caused or exacerbated by the effects of the alcohol (e.g., arguments with spouse about consequences of intoxication or physical fights)

What Are the Effects on the Body?

Hangover is a withdrawal state a person experiences after drinking where there is a combination of physical symptoms: headache when blood vessels in the head dilate and stretch as they return to their normal state, upset stomach as alcohol irritates the gastric lining, and a state of dehydration as alcohol acts as a diuretic by stimulating the kidneys to process and pass more water than is ingested.

Tolerance to alcohol is the lessening of the effectiveness of alcohol after a period of prolonged or heavy use. With tolerance the blood alcohol concentration level remains high. Prolonged and heavy use of alcohol can lead to addiction. If there is a sudden interruption in the long-term heavy use of alcohol, withdrawal symptoms may occur. These are severe anxiety, tremors, hallucinations, and convulsions.

What Is Physical Withdrawal Like?

According to the *DSM-IV* (2004), alcohol withdrawal occurs following cessation or reduction of intake. Simple withdrawal symptoms are perspiration, tachycardia, hypertension, increased respirations, low-grade temperature, poor motor coordination, slurred or incoherent speech, tremor, nausea, vomiting, malaise, poor concentration, impaired judgment, impulsivity, agitation, irritability, mood instability, anxiety, depressed mood, sedation, insomnia, and blackouts.

Complicated withdrawal symptoms are hyperactivity, tremors, agitation, clouding of consciousness, disorientation, hallucination, paranoid ideation, delusions stupor and coma, grand mal seizures, and delirium tremens. Signs and symptoms of alcohol withdrawal, experienced by both alcoholics and problem drinkers are tremors, agitation, anxiety and panic attacks, paranoia, delusions, hallucinations (usually visual), nausea and vomiting, increased body temperature, elevated blood pressure and heart rate, convulsions, and seizures.

What Is Alcoholism?
Dependence is the most severe end of the spectrum of substance misuse. Alcoholism is a syndrome that develops after repeated use over months or years. Alcohol addiction is characterized by increased tolerance, causing the abuser to drink greater amounts to achieve the same desired effect. When alcoholics stop drinking, they experience withdrawal because large doses of alcohol invade the body's fluids and interfere with cell metabolism.

What Are the Dangers of Alcohol Abuse?
In addition to risk of injury or death as a result of accident or violence, alcohol abuse poses a broad range of physiological and psychological dangers such as:

- Alcohol does not relieve depression—it makes it worse
- Miscarriage and stillbirth, or a combination of physical and mental birth defects for children of pregnant women
- Alcohol poisoning is a medical emergency from the CNS depression that can cause loss of consciousness, low blood pressure, coma, and respiratory depression
- Neurological problems including blackouts, hallucinations, dementia, impaired motor coordination, seizures, stroke, neuropathy, brain cell deterioration, and atrophy
- Cardiovascular problems, including hypertension, myocardial infarction, atrial fibrillation cardiomyopathy, and heart failure
- Irreversible liver damage occurs in three irreversible stages: fatty liver; alcoholic hepatitis when liver cells swell, become inflamed, and die; and cirrhosis, when fibrous scar tissue forms in place of healthy cells. A diseased liver will not convert stored glycogen into glucose (producing hypoglycemia), manufacture bile for fat digestion, prothrombin for blood clotting, albumin for maintaining healthy cells, or change the production of digestive enzymes (preventing the absorption of the vitamins A, D, E, and K)
- Hepatic encephalopathy can cause changes in sleep patterns, mood, and personality, psychiatric conditions such as anxiety and depression, severe cognitive effects such as shortened attention span, and problems with coordination such as a flapping or shaking of the hands (asterixis)

- Alcohol can inflame the mouth, esophagus, and stomach, possibly causing cancer in these locations. The stomach's digestive enzymes irritate the stomach wall, producing heartburn, nausea, gastric ulcers, sluggish digestion, vomiting, or inflame the small and large intestines (American Council for Drug Education, n.d.)

How Does Alcohol or Drugs Affect Pregnancy?

Alcohol is an especially dangerous drug for pregnant women. Drinking during pregnancy raises the risk of low birth weight babies and intrauterine growth retardation, increasing the danger of infection, feeding difficulties, small head circumference, heart defects, behavior issues, and long-term developmental problems. Heavy drinking during the early months of pregnancy can result in the birth of babies with fetal alcohol syndrome, a common cause of mental retardation (Mayo Clinic, n.d.).

How Do Nurses Screen for Alcoholism?

Tools used in the diagnosis of any substance abuse include screening questionnaires and patient histories, physical examination, and laboratory tests. There are short and long screening tests—all with advantages and disadvantages. Some are more sensitive than others. Much information on screening tests and other useful clinical guides for medical professionals can be found on the website of the National Institute on Alcohol Abuse and Alcoholism (NIAAA) (www.niaaa.nih.gov/publications/clinical-guides-and-manuals).

What Are the Treatments for Alcohol Addiction?

According to the NIAAA, substance abuse can involve any of the following classes of substances:

- Alcohol
- Amphetamines including "crystal meth"
- Cannabis including marijuana and hashish
- Cocaine including "crack"
- Hallucinogens (including LSD, mescaline, and 3,4-methylenedioxymethamphetamine (MDMA) "Ecstasy"
- Inhalants including compounds found in gasoline, glue, and paint thinners
- Opioids including morphine, heroin, codeine, methadone, and oxycodone
- Phencyclidine including PCP, angel dust, and ketamine.

What Treatments Are Available?

According to the American Psychiatric Association, there are three goals for the treatment of people with substance use disorders:

- Reduce the use and effects of the substance
- Reduce the frequency and severity of relapses
- Develop the skills necessary to recovery functioning

Treatment itself consists of three parts. The first step in treatment is assessment followed by a comprehensive medical and psychiatric evaluation, and formulation of a treatment plan and psychiatric management.

Treatment begins with detoxification. Stopping suddenly or "cold turkey" is potentially life threatening and requires medical intervention. There are many multidimensional treatments for alcohol acute and chronic disease. The following sources are particularly helpful:

- WHO; www.who.int/substance
- International Center for Alcohol Policies (ICAP); www.icap.org
- NIAAA; www.nih.gov
- Clinical protocols for detoxification in hospitals and detoxification facilities prepared by John B. Saunders and Junie Yang and staff; www.health.qld.gov.au/atod/documents/24904.pdf
- Detoxification and substance abuse treatment training manual treatment improvement protocol (TIP) and 45 detoxification and substance for emergency rooms, hospitals, medical, surgical units, and acute care clinics; http://kap.samhsa.gov/products/trainingcurriculums/pdfs/tip45_curriculum.pdf.

What Support Groups Are Available?

AA has been intensively studied, and a 1996 meta-analysis noted that long-term sobriety appears to be positively related to AA involvement (official site of the AA World Services Inc. www.aa.org). Other resources are:

- Alcohol research and health and additional resources can be downloaded from NIAAA's website; www.niaaa.gov
- Programs for young children; www.soberrecovery.com/
- Al-Anon logo and Alateen; www.al-anon.alateen.org

In the emergency department (ED), a red flag of chronic drug abuse pattern is found on physical exam. The nurse understands what type of street drugs are commonly used, identifies a range of issues associated with their use, recognizes

CASE STUDY: SHERRY

Sherry is a 17-year-old African American girl who entered the life at the age of 12 when her mother said she should just go to the street. Sherry was found by neighbors outside an abandoned building on a cold winter day. She was unresponsive, barely breathing, partially dressed, and very thin. An ambulance was called and began treatment maintaining her airway, starting an IV, and then transporting her to the ED 5 minutes away. The paramedics report possible intoxication/acute influence of a substance. They perceive this to be "a typical drug addict."

the signs and symptoms, and is familiar with treatment approaches for a drug use problem.

Since SUD often coexist with mental disorders, Sherry receives a psychiatric consultation. Sherry is assessed upon admission for alcohol and drug use history. Seizure and delirium tremens (DT) precautions are initiated and symptom-triggered doses of medication such as lorazepam are recommended. Emergency intubation equipment is ready to assist maintaining airway because her CNS is depressed.

Desired Patient Outcomes:

- Sherry will experience minimal discomfort and complications related to withdrawal syndrome and detoxification
- Sherry will experience the promotion of dignity and psychiatric stabilization
- Sherry will experience stable medical and obstetrical status

Clinical Assessment and Care:

- Monitor neurological status
- Vital signs (temperature, pulse, respiratory rate, and blood pressure)
- Monitor intake and output
- Maintain patient safety
- Provide interdisciplinary treatment planning

Sherry's mental status changes in the ED from unresponsive to awake, screaming and thrashing, and trying to get up and leave. Her aggression and violent behavior is directed at the nursing staff. Sherry experiences hallucinations that can affect one or all of her five senses. Drug users are likely to suffer from tactile hallucinations and alcoholics from visual hallucinations. The nurse monitors and treats Sherry's medical and cardiac instability, maintains her safety in the ED while showing kindness, compassion, and patience.

Sherry has no family or friends to call. She looks terrified and weak. Her judgment is impaired and the nurse notes suicidal and homicidal ideation. Vital signs are unstable, blood pressure is low, and pulse is rapid and irregular. Cardiac monitoring shows sinus tachycardia with occasional premature ventricular contractions. Chest x-ray is normal. Exam and blood tests are done showing multiple drugs in her system. Pregnancy test is positive. The nurse now must also consider the stage of pregnancy and the possibility of miscarriage, premature labor, or damage to the fetus. Detoxification and withdrawal protocols are reviewed by the nurse who will be taking over Sherry's care as she is transferred to the intensive care unit (ICU).

In the ICU Sherry's mental status improves and she is less hostile and agitated. She refuses to talk with the staff. The nurse is careful to deescalate each episode and continues showing respect. Sherry tells that nurse she fears the police are after her and fears the legal consequences for using drugs, but is really terrified her pimp will find her and kill her. Sherry continues to be observed for the complex physical and psychological disturbances that can occur upon withdrawal of addicting agents. Severity of the autonomic and psychomotor disturbances varies with the agent, length of addiction, and size of dosage she has been using. Consultation with an obstetrician is made and active monitoring of the effects of withdrawal from cocaine, heroin, and alcohol continues. Testing is done to assess for possible TB, hepatitis B and C, and sexually transmitted infections such as chlamydia, gonorrhea, and HIV.

Effective treatment must attend to her multiple needs and not just her polysubstance drug use. Sherry's circumstances are discussed in team meetings and social service is consulted for discharge planning. Discharge is scheduled in 3 weeks. Sherry receives medical care to improve her overall health and seems to be working with the doctor to adjust medication and doses as needed as she stabilizes and is moved out of ICU.

Sherry is transferred to a step-down unit and taught about what the drugs have done to her body. On this unit she tells the nurse about a girl she knew who died of an overdose. Sherry also learns about preventing accidental overdoses for herself. Sherry's stress as a trafficking victim is constant and threat is always present. The nurse continues to be nonjudgmental, warm, and supportive. She helps Sherry see her self-worth and her strength as a survivor.

Once discharged medically, Sherry is admitted to a psychiatric unit where she can begin to learn new life skills. The staff must allow time for a therapeutic alliance to build. Sherry may identify any person as a potential abuser. Therefore, it is important for the nurses to be aware of their own internal and external reactions, vulnerabilities, and unresolved conflicts.

One of the most difficult issues to understand is that many people in treatment will relapse one or more times before getting better and remaining drug free. Sherry is discharged but relapses. Each of Sherry's relapses is a setback but not a failure. She has strong cravings to use; however, she continues with treatment and hopefully will achieve full recovery. Many drug-dependent persons are ambivalent about starting treatment and stopping their drug use. They may not find treatment services that are responsive to their individual needs.

WHAT ARE CO-OCCURRING DISORDER TREATMENTS?

Treatment of co-occurring disorders (COD) is a relatively new field. Services that offer a wide range of treatment options and support programs increase motivation and empower victims. As in Sherry's case, care and treatment can be conducted in different settings (hospital, residential treatment, partial hospitalization, or outpatient treatment). Substance use disorders are considered a chronic condition requiring long-term care, and therefore these plans need to be flexible but based on the individual's needs and strengths. Individuals vary in their readiness to change. The stages of change model are useful to understanding of the nature and cycle of change (Prochaska & DiClemente, 1983). Some minimize or deny their problems (precontemplation stage), some recognize their problem but are not ready (contemplation stage), while some are ready to change and make changes (action stage). Relapse is a normal part of change.

Patients typically undergo psychosocial therapy and pharmacologic treatment. Pharmacologic treatment may include medications that ease withdrawal symptoms, reduce craving, interact negatively with substances of abuse to discourage drug-taking, or treat associated psychiatric disorders. Psychosocial therapeutic modalities include cognitive-behavioral therapy, behavioral therapy and individual psychodynamic, interpersonal therapy, group therapy, and self-help groups.

SUMMARY

Recovery from substance use is notoriously difficult, even with exceptional treatment resources. When drug users are also victims of sex trafficking, treatment is complicated by cultural and social factors beyond the control of the person who struggles to overcome the medical issues as well as the control by traffickers. When the patient is younger than 18, the resources for child abuse intervention are available, but when over 18, the person likely has few resources to help. The role of the nurse as a compassionate and nonjudgmental professional is critical to success.

REFERENCES

American Council on Drug Education. (n.d.). Basic facts about drugs: Alcohol. Author. Retrieved July 8, 2012, from http://www.acde.org/common/alcohol.htm

American Psychiatric Association. (2000).

Blum, R. H. (1969). *Society and drugs*. San Francisco, CA: Jossey Bass.

Burnett, L. (2010). Cocaine toxicity in emergency medicine. Retrieved July 8, from http://emedicine.medscape.com/article/813959-overview.

Clancy, C., Coyne, P., & Wright, S. (1997). *Substance use: Guidelines on good clinical practice for specialist nurses working with alcohol and drug users*. London: Association of Nurses in Substance abuse (ANSA). Retrieved March 31, 2012, from http://ansauk.org/downlouds/resource/ansabooklets/ansa alcolol.pdf

Clawson, H., Small, K., Go, E., & Myles, B. (2003). *Needs assessments for service providers and trafficking victims*. Fairfax, VA: National Criminal Justice Reference Service. Retrieved April 22, 2012, from http://www.ncjrs.gov/pdffiles1/nij/grants/202469.pdf

Cusick, L., McGarry, K., Perry, G., & Kilcommons, S. (2010). Drug services for sex workers: Approaches in England and Ireland. *Safer Communities, 9*(4), 32–39.

Delancey Street Foundation, San Francisco, Sarah McNaught, Working for the man, *The Boston Phoenix*, 23–30, October 1997.

Diagnosis and Statistical Manual of Mental Disorders (DSM-IV). (2004). Washington, DC: Author. American Psychiatric Association.

Harris, D. S., Everhart, E. T., Mendelson, J., & Jones, R. (2003). The pharmacology of cocaethylene in humans following cocaine and ethanol administration. *Drug and Alcohol Dependency, 72*(2), 169–182.

Hedden, S., Hulbert, A., Cavanaugh, C., Parry, C., Moleko, G., & Latimer, W. (2011). Alcohol, drug, and sexual risk behavior correlates of recent transactional sex among female black South African drug users. *Journal of Substance Use, 16*(1), 57–67.

Lucia, S. P. (1963). The antiquity of alcohol in diet and medicine. In: S. P. Lucia (Ed.) *Alcohol and civilization* (pp. 151–166). New York: McGraw-Hill.

Mayo Clinic. (n.d.). Fetal alcohol syndrome. Retrieved July 7, 2012, from http://www. mayoclinic.com/health/fetal-alcohol-syndrome/ds00184/dsection=symptoms.

Mosedale, B., Kouimtsidis, C., & Reynolds, M. (2009). Sex work, substance misuse and service provision: The experiences of female sex workers in south London. *Drugs: Education, Prevention and Policy, 16*(4), 355–363.

National Institute for Alcoholism and Alcohol Abuse. (n.d.). Retrieved July 7, 2012, from http://www.niaaa.nih.gov/publications/clinical-guides-and-manuals.

National Institute on Drug Abuse. (2009). *InfoFacts: Heroin*. Rockville, MD: US Department of Health and Human Services. Retrieved from http://www.nida.nih.gov/info facts/heroin.html

National Survey on Drug Abuse. (2010). Retrieved from http://www.oas.samhsa.gov/ NSDUH/2k10NSDUH/2k10Results.pdf

NSDUH CAI Instrumentation. (2010). Retrieved from http://www.samhsa.gov/data/ nsduh/2K10MRB/2k10Q.pdf

Patrick, C. H. (1952). *Alcohol, culture, and society*. Durham, NC: Duke University Press, Reprint edition by AMS Press, New York, 1970.

Prochaska, J., & DiClemente, C. (1983). Stages and processes of self-change of smoking: Toward an integrative model of change. *Journal of Consulting and Clinical Psychology, 51*(3), 390–395.

Rollnick, W., Miller, S., & Butler, C. (2008). *Motivational interviewing in health care: Helping patient change behavior*. New York: The Guilford Press.

Roxburgh, A., Degenhardt, L., Copeland, J., & Larance, B. (2008). Drug dependence and associated risks among female street based sex workers in the greater Sydney area, Australia. *Substance Use & Misuse, 43*, 1202–1217.

Ulibarri, M., Strathdee, S., Ulloa, E., Lozada, R., Fraga, M., Magis-Rodriguez, De La Torre, A., Amaro, H., O'Campo, P., & Patterson, T. (2011). Injection drug use as a mediator between client-perpetrated abuse and HIV status among female sex workers in two Mexico-US border cities. *AIDS Behavior, 15*, 179–185.

Wechsberg, W., Wu, L., Zule, W., Parry, C., Browne, F., Luseno, W. et al., (2009). Substance abuse, treatment needs and access among female sex workers and non-sex workers in Pretoria, South Africa. *Substance Abuse Treatment, Prevention, and Policy, 4*(11). Retrieved from http://www.substanceabusepolicy.com/content/4/1/11

WHO Global Status Report on Alcohol. (2004). Retrieved July 2, 2012, from http://www. who.int/substance_abuse/publications/global_status_report_2004_overview.pdf.

Yu, L. (1996). The mu opioid receptor: From molecular coning to functional studies. *Addiction Biology, 1*(1), 19–30.

CHAPTER 15

Sexually Transmitted Infections

GLORIA TAYLOR AND BARBARA BLAKE

Sexually transmitted infections (STIs) are caused by more than 30 bacteria, viruses, and parasites, and are primarily transmitted from one person to another through sexual activity (vaginal, anal, and oral). The most common STIs are syphilis, gonorrhea, chlamydia, and trichomoniasis. According to recent estimates, approximately 448 million curable STIs (syphilis, gonorrhea, chlamydia, and trichomoniasis) occur worldwide each year. Persons 15 to 49 years of age and women are predominately affected. STIs and their complications represent the top five disease categories for which adults seek health care. Some persons infected with STIs are asymptomatic, which can lead to chronic health problems and infertility. Any inflammatory genital disease increases the risk of acquiring an STI (Centers for Disease Control and Prevention [CDC], 2010a; World Health Organization [WHO], 2008a, 2011a).

Individuals who are sexually exploited are unable to insist on condom use or negotiate for safer sex practices. Generally, safer sex practices prevent contact with genital sores and the exchange of body fluids, such as semen, blood, and vaginal secretions. Because of the inability to negotiate for safer sex, the probability of sexually exploited victims acquiring STIs increases. Unfortunately, these victims also have fewer opportunities to access STI prevention and treatment services and are usually less knowledgeable about STI transmission. In addition, adolescent women are biologically more vulnerable because their cervical and vaginal tissues are less mature, fragile, and more susceptible to transmission of STIs. In this chapter, the authors present an overview of major STIs, including symptoms, treatment, complications, and prevention.

BEST PRACTICES: COMMON SEXUALLY TRANSMITTED INFECTIONS

Trichomoniasis

Trichomoniasis or "trich" is caused by the protozoan parasite, *Trichomonas vaginalis*. Trichomoniasis infections are more common in women than in men and older women are more likely to be infected than younger women (CDC, 2011a). Worldwide, approximately 174 million people are infected each year (Chang, 2008). Symptoms of trichomoniasis vary from person to person, but only about 30% of people infected develop symptoms.

Trichomoniasis is more difficult to diagnose in men than women. Men who are infected may feel itching or irritation inside the penis, burning after urination or ejaculation, or have a penile discharge. Some men may develop prostatitis or epididymitis from the infection. Women may notice itching, burning, redness, or soreness of the genitals, discomfort with urination, or develop a foul smelling, thin discharge that can be clear, white, yellow, or green in color. Pregnant women infected with trichomoniasis are more likely to have a preterm delivery or low birth weight baby (<5.5 lbs). In both men and women, sexual intercourse can be painful when the infection is present. Because trichomoniasis causes inflammation of the genitals, infected persons are more susceptible to other STIs (CDC, 2010a, 2011a).

Culture remains the gold standard for diagnosing trichomoniasis, but a presumptive diagnosis can be made based on evaluating symptoms, visualizing the protozoan parasite by microscopy (wet mount), or by using an antigen detection diagnostic test. Results of point-of-care antigen detection testing are available in 10 minutes. This type of testing is particularly beneficial in areas where microscopes are not available. Treatment for trichomoniasis is a single dose of an antibiotic, metronidazole or tinidazole. Drinking alcohol within 48 hours of taking the medication can cause severe nausea, abdominal pain, and vomiting (CDC, 2011a; Schwebke, 2012; Schwebke & Burgess, 2004).

Gonorrhea

Gonorrhea is caused by the bacterium *Neisseria gonorrhoeae*. Both men and women are affected by gonorrhea and the bacterium can infect the cervix, urethra, rectum, eyes, mouth, and throat. Gonorrhea is sometimes called the "clap" or "drip." Worldwide, approximately 62 million new cases occur each year, with more women being infected than men. Gonorrhea is primarily spread through contact with the penis, vagina, mouth, or rectum. However, mother-to-child transmission can occur during delivery. Symptoms of gonorrhea most often appear 1 to 14 days after exposure; however, it is possible to become infected and have no symptoms (CDC, 2011b, 2011c; National Center for Biotechnology Information [NCBI], 2011; WHO, 2012).

If women develop symptoms, they are usually mild and sometimes confused with a bladder or other vaginal infections. Symptoms include pain or burning when urinating, increased vaginal discharge, painful intercourse, or vaginal bleeding between menstrual cycles. A complication that women can experience from gonorrhea is pelvic inflammatory disease (PID), which can lead to an ectopic pregnancy or infertility. If a pregnant woman is infected during delivery, the baby can be born with a gonoccocal eye infection, which must be treated with antibiotics to prevent blindness. Symptoms of gonorrhea infection in men include a burning sensation when urinating, a white, yellow, or green discharge from the penis, and painful or swollen testicles. Gonorrhea can cause scarring of the urethra, making it more difficult for men to urinate (CDC, 2010a, 2011b; NCBI, 2011; WHO, 2012).

Symptoms of rectal infection in both men and women include discharge, anal itching, soreness, bleeding, or painful bowel movements. Infections in the mouth or throat may cause inflammation and pain. However, it is important to remember that like cervical or urethral infections, there may be no symptoms with rectal or oral gonorrhea. Complications from undiagnosed and untreated gonorrhea can occur in both men and women; they include, joint infections, heart valve infections, and meningitis (CDC, 2011b; NCBI, 2011; WHO, 2012).

When diagnosing gonorrhea, a sample from the part of the body that is likely to be infected (cervix, rectum, urethra, or throat) is obtained and sent for analysis. Gram staining or culture of the specimen is performed to confirm diagnosis. A Gram stain provides visualization of the bacteria by microscopy shortly after the specimen is collected, while culture results can take 1 to 3 days. Nonculture testing is available to detect gonorrhea infections. This nonculture technology, nucleic acid amplification tests (NAATs), amplifies and detects *N. gonorrhoeae* DNA or RNA sequences in endocervical specimens from women, urethral specimens from men, and urine from both men and women. Testing of rectal and oropharyngeal specimens with NAATs is not currently recommended. Point-of-care testing for gonorrhea using a urine specimen eliminates the need for more invasive procedures, such as a pelvic exam, and facilitates the opportunity for screening in nontraditional health care settings (CDC, 2010a, 2011b; Zenilman, 2012).

Individuals infected with *N. gonorrhoeae* are frequently coinfected with *Chlamydia trachomatis*, so it is recommended that when treating someone for gonorrhea, a regimen that is effective in treating uncomplicated chlamydia should also be administered. Antibiotics (a cephalosporin with either azithromycin or doxycycline) are successful treatment options. However, drug-resistant strains of gonorrhea are emerging in many parts of the world. Medications used in treating gonorrhea can stop the infection, but cannot repair permanent damage, infertility, ectopic pregnancy, and chronic pelvic pain, which might have been caused by the disease (CDC, 2010a, 2011b, WHO, 2012).

Hepatitis B

The most common types of hepatitis viruses are A, B, and C. These viruses are of concern because of the burden of illness and death they cause and the potential for epidemic spread. Hepatitis A, B, and C viruses can be transmitted sexually. However, the transmission of hepatitis A is more likely to occur through the ingestion of contaminated food or poor sanitation, and hepatitis C is transmitted primarily through percutaneous exposure to blood (such as sharing needles during intravenous drug use) (CDC, 2011d; National Institute of Allergy and Infectious Diseases [NIAID], 2009). For these reasons, only hepatitis B (HBV) will be discussed in this chapter because it is primarily transmitted through sexual activity.

Worldwide, an estimated 2 billion people have been infected with HBV and more than 350 million have chronic long-term infections. An estimated 600,000 people die each year from the disease. HBV is endemic in China and other parts of Asia. High rates of chronic infection are found in the Amazon and southern parts of eastern and central Europe. However, less than 1% of the population in Western Europe and North America is chronically infected (Sharapov & Hu, 2010; WHO, 2008b).

HBV can be transmitted through contact with infected blood or other body fluids (i.e., semen, vaginal fluids, and saliva). Modes of transmission include having penetrative sex (vaginal or anal) with an infected partner, sharing contaminated needles, syringes, or other drug paraphernalia, acquiring needle sticks or sharp instrument exposures, sharing items such as razors or toothbrushes with an infected person, and vertical transmission from mother to baby at birth. It is not transmitted through casual contact. It is estimated that HBV is 50 to 100 times more infectious than human immunodeficiency virus (HIV) (CDC, 2011d; NIAID, 2009).

HBV can cause both acute and chronic disease. Symptoms of acute HBV include jaundice, dark urine, fatigue, nausea, vomiting, and abdominal pain. People can take several months to a year to recover. The likelihood that HBV infection will become chronic depends upon the age at which a person becomes infected; young children are the most likely to develop a chronic infection. About 90% of healthy individuals infected with HBV will spontaneously recover within 6 months. Complications of chronic HBV infection include cirrhosis of the liver and liver cancer (CDC, 2011d; NIAID, 2009; Sharapov & Hu, 2010).

To diagnose HBV and determine the phase of infection (acute versus chronic), blood testing is required. For acute HBV infections there are no medications; treatment is supportive and based on symptoms. Persons with chronic HBV infection require long-term follow-up to assess progression of the disease and can be treated with medications that include interferon and antiviral drugs (CDC, 2011d; NIAID, 2009; Sharapov & Hu, 2010).

Hepatitis B vaccine is the backbone of HBV prevention. The vaccine can prevent the disease and consequences associated with becoming infected. As of 2007, HBV vaccine has been introduced into 171 countries and an estimated 65% of the world's population has been vaccinated. Coverage is highest in the Americas (88%) and lowest in southeast Asia (30%) (Te & Jensen, 2010; WHO, 2008b).

Syphilis

Syphilis is a systemic disease caused by the bacterium *Treponema pallidum*. It is a spirochete that is primarily transmitted through vaginal, anal, or oral sexual contact. Despite the existence of effective prevention measures and relatively inexpensive treatment options, syphilis remains a global problem. It is estimated that 12 million people become infected each year. Because of the enormous variation in the disease's symptoms, syphilis is sometimes called the "Great Imitator" (CDC, 2010a, 2010b; Sherman, 2007; WHO, 2011a).

Depending on the stage of the disease, syphilis can be characterized as primary, secondary, or tertiary (late). In the primary stage, a painless, spontaneously resolving sore (chancre) occurs. The chancre develops at the site where syphilis enters the body. The development of a rash on one or more parts of the body characterizes the secondary stage. The rash usually does not cause itching, may be so faint that it is not noticed, and often involves the palms of the hands and/or soles of the feet. Other signs and symptoms of secondary syphilis can include fever, swollen lymph glands, sore throat, patchy hair loss, headaches, weight loss, muscle aches, and fatigue. The symptoms of secondary syphilis will also resolve without treatment. Tertiary syphilis begins after the primary and secondary symptoms of syphilis disappear. Complications during this stage occur in 15% to 40% of persons and can appear years after the infection was first acquired. These complications can damage the brain, nervous system, blood vessels, liver, bones, and joints. Signs and symptoms of late-stage syphilis include difficulty in coordinating muscle movements, paralysis, numbness, gradual blindness, and dementia (CDC, 2010b; NIAID, 2010).

Syphilis can be diagnosed by examining the material from a chancre using dark-field microscopy or through blood testing. Since primary syphilis presents with a chancre or open sore, individuals with a lesion in the genital area are more susceptible to acquiring HIV if exposed. Therefore, when someone tests positive for syphilis, they should also be tested for HIV as well as other STIs. Penicillin G, administered parenterally, is the most commonly used antibiotic to treat all stages of syphilis. Dosage and length of treatment is dependent on stage and clinical manifestations of the disease. For people who are allergic to penicillin, other antibiotics, doxycycline, and tetracycline, are used for treating the disease (CDC, 2010a, 2010b).

Human Immunodeficiency Virus/Acquired Immunodeficiency Syndrome

HIV is a retrovirus that infects CD4+ T-cells of the immune system, destroying or impairing their function. As HIV infection progresses, there is ongoing damage to the immune system and the body is less able to fight-off infection. This damage results in severe immunodeficiency, opportunistic infections, certain types of cancers, and possibly death. A person is said to have acquired immunodeficiency syndrome (AIDS) as opposed to simply being HIV positive when the number of CD4+ T cells in their immune system drops below a certain level (<200 cells/μL or CD4+ T-cell percentage of total lymphocytes $<15\%$), acquires an opportunistic infection (e.g., *Pneumocystis jiroveci* pneumonia, *Mycobacterium avium* complex), or develops a certain cancer (e.g., invasive cervical cancer, Burkitt's lymphoma) (CDC, 2008; Williams, Daniels, Gedela, Briggs, & Pryce, 2011).

In 2010, approximately 34 million people around the world were living with HIV. The proportion of women was 50%. Women most affected by the disease were living in sub-Saharan Africa and the Caribbean. Globally, HIV is primarily transmitted through unprotected sexual intercourse (anal or vaginal), contaminated blood, and the sharing of contaminated injecting drug equipment (UNAIDS, 2011; WHO, 2011b). However, in resource-poor countries, mother-to-child transmission is still a major contributor to the epidemic because these countries lack access to HIV medications that can decrease transmission of the virus during pregnancy and breast feeding (Mepham, Bland, & Newell, 2011).

Recent studies have found that sex trafficking is becoming more prominent in fueling the HIV epidemic. There are several reasons why this is occurring. First, trafficked persons are forced to have unprotected sex with multiple partners and if violent sex acts occur, tearing of genital tissue is more likely, making HIV transmission easier. Second, there has been an increased demand for young girls and boys and consumers are willing to pay more for these youth. There is the assumption that younger individuals are less likely to be HIV infected and so the consumer is "safe" from the disease. Last, in some parts of the world, there is a belief that having sex with a virgin girl can "cure" AIDS. Unfortunately, because of the secrecy associated with trafficking, HIV and STI testing are almost nonexistent and ongoing transmission of these diseases continues, especially when the trafficked individual is asymptomatic, which is very common with HIV infection (Falb et al., 2011; Kamazima, Ezekiel, Kazaura, & Fimbo, 2012; Kloer, 2010; Silverman et al., 2008).

In recent years, HIV antibody testing has become quicker and less invasive. Rapid testing allows patients the opportunity to receive results on the day of their medical visit, which is important in urgent situations and settings where patients do not return for test results. These antibody tests use oral fluid, urine, and fingerstick blood samples versus the collection of blood by venipuncture. However, the initial positive rapid HIV test result must be followed up with a confirmatory test, such as a Western blot or immunofluorescence assay (CDC, 2009; U.S. Department of Health Resources and Services Administration [HRSA] HIV/AID Bureau, 2011).

Unfortunately, rapid tests are often not conclusive when someone presents with acute primary HIV infection because it takes approximately 4 weeks for the body to develop antibodies. During the acute phase of infection, two-thirds of people present with mononucleosis or flu-like symptoms that include fever, rash, fatigue, arthralgia, generalized lymphadenopathy, headache, anorexia, and urticaria. Primary HIV infection is often overlooked and difficult to diagnose, but early identification and linkage to care can decrease future HIV transmission by persons who are particularly infectious during the early phase of the disease. Unfortunately, once this stage passes, persons can remain asymptomatic for many years and continue to transmit the virus because they do not know their HIV serostatus and participate in unsafe sex practices (HRSA HIV/AIDS Bureau, 2011).

Prior to 1996, about 50% of people diagnosed with HIV progressed to AIDS within 10 years. This time varied greatly from person to person and depended on many factors, including a person's health status and health-related behaviors. Since 1996, the introduction of powerful antiretroviral (ART) medications has dramatically changed the progression of HIV infection to AIDS, and has transitioned AIDS from a death sentence to a chronic illness (UNAIDS, 2011). More than 30 medications are currently available for treatment; however, not all counties have access to these drugs. In addition, there are medical treatments that can prevent or cure some of the illnesses associated with HIV/AIDS, although these treatments do not cure AIDS. As with other diseases, early detection allows for more treatment options and preventive health care measures (Boyd, 2011; CDC, 2011e).

Bacterial Vaginosis

Bacterial vaginosis (BV) is the most common vaginal infection in women of child-bearing age. The cause of BV is not fully understood. BV is thought to be associated with an imbalance in the harmful and good bacteria normally found in a woman's vagina. With BV, there is an increase in the harmful bacteria and a decrease in the good bacteria (CDC, 2010c; U.S. Department of Health and Human Services [DHHS] Office of Women's Health, 2008).

There are activities or behaviors that can disrupt the normal balance of bacteria in the vagina; they include having a new or multiple sex partners, douching, and not using a condom. Women do not get BV from toilet seats, bedding, swimming pools, or touching objects around them. Sexually active women are more likely to get BV, but women who are not sexually active can also develop the disease (CDC, 2010c; DHHS Office of Women's Health, 2008).

Not all women with BV have symptoms. Symptoms associated with BV include an abnormal vaginal discharge with an unpleasant odor. Some women report a strong fish-like odor, especially after sexual intercourse. If a discharge is present, it is usually gray or white in color and can be foamy or watery. Other symptoms include burning during urination and itching around the vagina (CDC, 2010c; DHHS Office of Women's Health, 2008).

To diagnose BV, a health care professional must examine the vagina and perform laboratory tests on a sample of vaginal fluid. Although BV may resolve without treatment, all women with symptoms of BV should be treated to avoid further health problems, such as PID and increased susceptibility to other STIs. The antibiotics used to treat BV include metronidazole, clindamycin, and tinidazole. Depending on the antibiotic prescribed, it can be taken by mouth or used vaginally. Treatment is especially important for pregnant women to prevent premature labor and low birth weight infants. Basic prevention steps can be used to reduce the risk of disrupting the natural balance of bacteria in the vagina and developing BV; they include abstinence, limiting the number of sex partners, using latex condoms, not douching, and completing medicine prescribed for BV, even if symptoms resolve (CDC, 2010c; DHHS Office of Women's Health, 2008).

Human Papillomavirus

Human papillomavirus (HPV) represents more than 40 types. Current estimates indicate 20 million Americans are infected and 6 million new infections occur each year. It is estimated that 50% of sexually active men and women will become infected during their life times. These viruses can infect the genitals, mouth, and throat. The vast majority of persons who become infected (~90%), clear the virus within 2 years without treatment. However, if the virus is not cleared, affected persons can develop genital warts, certain cancers (cervical, vulva, vagina, penis, anus, and oropharynx), and recurrent respiratory papillomatois (a rare disorder). The HPV that causes cancer does not cause genital warts (CDC, 2010e).

The major risk factors for HPV are unprotected intercourse (vaginal and anal) at an early age and multiple sex partners. In the United States, recent studies indicate that HPV infection is lowest among women 14 to 19 years of age and highest among women 20 to 29 years of age. The four common types, HPV 16 and 18 (cervical cancers) and HPV 6 and 11 (genital warts) are responsible for most of the disease. Cervical cancers are highest among women aged 20 to 24 and genital warts are more prevalent among women 14 to 19 years of age (Dunne et al., 2011; Hariri et al., 2011). Vaccines for HPV have only been in existence since 2010. Currently, there are two quadrivalent vaccines available, Gradasil (administered to women and men, aged 9–26) and Cervarix (administered to women 9–25 years of age). However, these vaccines are most effective among persons who are naive to HPV types and protect against most, but not all, cervical cancers (McCormack & Joura, 2011). Unfortunately, about 12,000 women develop cervical cancer each year and the majority is related to HPV infection. There are many women at risk (HPV) for whom the vaccine is not appropriate because of previous sexual activity and age. Therefore, these affected women need to adhere to the American Cancer Society recommendations for cervical cancer screening to identify cervical cancers early, when treatment is most effective.

Genital warts typically appear as tumor/bump-type lesions in the genital and/or anal areas. The lesions can be singular or clustered. These lesions can also be found on the mucous membrane areas of the vagina, cervix, and rectum, and sometimes in the mouth or on the lips. Lesions can appear within weeks or months after sexual contact with an infected person. Warts can be removed by chemicals (podophyllin resin or podofilox lotion), surgical excision, cryotherapy, laser therapy, or electrocautery. In some instances, genital warts will resolve without treatment and will not become cancerous (CDC, 2010e; Edwards, 2008).

Chlamydia

Chlamydia is caused by the bacterium *Chlamydia trachomatis*. It is frequently diagnosed in the United States, especially among persons younger than 25 years of age. In 2010, 1,307,893 cases were reported; however, these numbers are probably underrepresented because many individuals are not aware of their infection. According to a recent study, asymptomatic infections worldwide are estimated to be as high as 50% to 70%. Therefore, chlamydia is known as the "silent disease" because 75% of infected women and 50% of infected men have no symptoms. Symptoms vary by gender. Women who have symptoms may have abnormal vaginal discharge, burning with urination, lower abdominal pain, nausea, fever, pain during intercourse, and bleeding between menstrual cycles. Men can experience penile discharge, burning with urination, burning and itching around the opening of the penis, and testicular pain and swelling (CDC, 2010a, 2011c, 2012).

When an individual has no symptoms the person is more likely to pass the infection to others. Also, asymptomatic women are more at risk for other gynecological conditions, such as salpingitis and PID, which can cause chronic pelvic pain and culminate in tubal occlusion and infertility. Untreated chlamydia can also cause proctitis and Reiter's syndrome (a form of arthritis characterized by inflammation of the joints). In pregnant women, a chlamydia infection can lead to premature delivery and transmission of the infection to the newborn (eye infection, which can lead to blindness if left untreated and/or pneumonia). Early diagnosis and treatment are important to prevent transmitting the infection to others and avoiding other health problems in women (CDC, 2010a, 2012; DHHS Office of Women's Health, 2011; Godinjak & Hkic, 2012).

Chlamydia is diagnosed by culture or NAATs (endocervical or intraureteral swab specimen). Both are helpful in identifying the organism. However, culture is more precise. NAATs are advantageous because they allow health care providers to make a diagnosis based on signs and symptoms and test results for immediate treatment. The medication of choice is azithromycin or doxycycline (CDC, 2002, 2010a).

Genital Herpes

Genital herpes is caused by the herpes simplex viruses type 1 (HSV-1) and type 2 (HSV-2). However, the majority of genital herpes is caused by the HSV-2 strain. HSV-1 is more commonly seen on the mouth but can be transferred to the genital area during oral sex, especially if there is an open lesion on the mouth. Open lesions are the primary source of viral shedding, contributing to person-to-person transmission. However, the virus can be passed through intact skin. The majority of persons infected are asymptomatic and sometimes not aware of their infection until there is a primary outbreak of lesions, which can be a few weeks to several years after the initial infection. Therefore, the current sex partner may not be the source of the infection, which can be important in contact follow-up and partner notification (CDC, 2010a, 2010d).

Transmission is more likely to occur from men to women. In the United States, the highest prevalence is among persons 20 to 29 years of age and 90% of these individuals are not aware of their infection. The infection is more common among women between the ages of 14 and 49. Herpes infection is treatable, not curable. It is a lifelong chronic infection characterized by periodic recurrences following the initial outbreak (CDC, 2010e; Gilbert, Levandowski, & Roberts, 2010; Nath & Thappa, 2009; Nicum & Mahida, 2010).

Most persons infected with HSV-2 do not have lesions or have very mild symptoms. Sometimes lesions associated with mild symptoms can be mistaken for another skin condition. In general, infected persons can experience malaise, fever, pain (lower back, buttocks, and legs), swelling of regional lymph nodes, and the appearance of a few to multiple vesicular lesions. Women can have lesions on the labia, vagina, cervix, anus, thighs, and buttocks. In men, the lesions can appear on the penis, scrotum, anus, thighs, and buttocks. Both women and men usually have difficult and painful urination and women may have a vaginal discharge. This array of signs and symptoms will vary from individual to individual and the largest number of lesions is usually associated with the initial outbreak. Typically, lesions and the intensity of signs and symptoms will decrease with each recurring episode. The presence of herpes infection should be confirmed by viral culture (CDC, 2010a, 2010e; Nath & Thappa, 2009; Nicum & Mahida, 2010).

Herpes infections are treated with antiviral acyclovir, valacyclovir, or famciclovir. Of these, acyclovir is the least expensive. These medications are used to minimize symptoms and improve healing of lesions, decrease the number of recurrences and their duration, and as suppressive therapy (treatment for 6–12 months) to prevent recurrences. Suppressive therapy can limit outbreak frequency, but does not guarantee that outbreaks will be eliminated. In addition, suppressive therapy helps reduce the transmission of the virus to others (Nath & Thappa, 2009; Nicum & Mahida, 2010).

Genital herpes in pregnant women is a special situation that requires close monitoring. This is because the virus can be transferred to the neonate during birth, which is associated with high morbidity and mortality. Therefore, antiviral therapy can benefit this population. Moreover, caesarean section should be considered for pregnant women who present with genital herpes at term or within 6 weeks of the expected delivery (Nicum & Mahida, 2010).

Pelvic Inflammatory Disease

PID is an infection of the female reproductive system and considered a complication of STIs. The causative agent is usually *N. gonorrhoeae* or *C. trachomatis*. More than 1 million women are affected each year. If there is a delay in recognition of this disease, scarring of the fallopian tubes can occur that leads to infertility (annual rates of 10%–15%). However, ectopic pregnancy and chronic pelvic pain are also consequences of undiagnosed PID. The majority of women affected are under 25 years of age. Young women are at greatest risk because the cervix is not fully mature. PID is usually considered a delayed or undertreated STI; therefore, it is usually treated with two or three antibiotics (ceftriaxone, doxycycline, and metronidazole) (Abatangelo et al., 2010; American College of Obstetricians and Gynecologists, 2011; CDC, 2011f).

Pubic Lice

Pubic lice are caused by the parasitic organism *Pethirus pubis* and are commonly known as "crab lice" or "crabs." This organism is primarily transmitted through sexual contact and lives and reproduces in the pubic and rectal regions of the body and other hairy areas (axilla, eyelashes, scalp, beard, and mustache). However, in rare instances, pubic lice can be transferred from one individual to another by sharing clothing, towels, or bed linens of the infected person. Infestations are typically found in sexually active young adults and teens. Young children can be affected; however, pubic lice in young children may suggest sexual exposure or abuse (Burkhart, Gunning, & Burkhart, 2000; CDC, 2010a, 2010f).

Symptoms of pubic lice infestation include intense itching in the affected area, predominately at night, and visible louse eggs (gray-white oval nits) on the hair shaft. These eggs (<1 mm) are not easily seen without the use of a strong magnifying glass. In addition, due to intense itching, secondary infections are common from bites and scratching (CDC, 2010f). The preferred treatment is a permethrin-based shampoo or lotion (over-the-counter or prescription). However, piperonyl butoxide has also been found helpful. The presence of pubic lice is a strong indicator for the need to screen for other STIs (CDC, 2010f).

BEST PRACTICES: WORKING WITH PERSONS WHO HAVE AN STI

According to the CDC (2010a), the prevention and control of STIs are based on five major strategies; they are:

- Education and counseling of persons at risk on ways to avoid STIs through changes in sexual behavior and use of recommended prevention services
- Identification of asymptomatically infected persons and of symptomatic persons unlikely to seek diagnostic and treatment services
- Effective diagnosis, treatment, and counseling of infected persons
- Evaluation, treatment, and counseling of sex partners of persons who are infected with STIs
- Preexposure vaccination of persons at risk for vaccine-preventable diseases (p. 2)

Overall, these prevention and control measures focus primarily on physical health issues and are not necessarily realistic for individuals who are being trafficked. When nurses identify and interact with trafficked individuals, they not only need to consider someone's physical health, but also personal, and psychological needs.

Effective Interviewing

Sexual History Taking

Taking an accurate health history is essential in providing comprehensive care. The information obtained will help the provider obtain a correct assessment of the person's health. An important component of this process is obtaining a thorough sexual health history. In many health care settings this is often overlooked or the history is inadequate. Sexual health questions should be routinely integrated into the health history so that sexual behaviors are not singled out or viewed by the patient in a judgmental manner. This approach allows sexual health to be perceived on the same level as other health concerns. Sexual health inquiries allow the provider to identify problems and intervene to maximize health outcomes (Nusbaum & Hamilton, 2002).

In working with patients, a general approach should include being sensitive and putting the patient at ease. This is accomplished by asking questions in a matter-of-fact manner. In addition, the provider should reassure the patient of confidentiality and inform the person that the questions being asked are routinely asked of all patients. Emphasis is placed on the importance of the questions to overall health. Providers should avoid euphemisms and ask open-ended questions, which are the most helpful. The exchange between the provider and patient should be an opportunity to teach. This approach is especially important when working with adolescents (CDC, n.d.; Nusbaum & Hamilton, 2002).

When working with adolescents, providers should create an opportunity to talk with the patient without a parent or guardian. This need for privacy should be explained during the initial encounter. Adolescents are more likely to confide in the provider if they know their conversation will be kept private. The following approach may be helpful: Explain to the teen and parent the structure of the visit and its confidential nature, and that you, the provider, is interested in speaking with both parent and adolescent after the exam. At this juncture, the parent can be directed to the waiting area (STD/HIV Prevention Training Center of New England, (n.d.)).

Areas that should be openly discussed during a sexual history are based on the 5 Ps: *Partners, Practices, Protection from STIs, Past history of STIs, and Prevention of pregnancy.* In discussing *partners*, appropriate questions include: "Are you sexually active?" "Have you had more than one sex partner in the last year?" Avoid using language that can make assumptions about a patient's sexual orientation or behavior—girlfriend, boyfriend, husband, or wife. Use of the general term "partner" allows the patient to clearly identify the relationship. *Practices* refer to the type of sexual activity the patient engages in (vaginal, oral, and anal). To assess this area, the provider might ask: "What kind of sexual practices have you had?" *Protection from STIs* can be assessed by asking questions related to condom use and personal perception of STI risk. *Past history of STIs* is important because it helps the health care provider identify conditions and behaviors that put a patient at greater risk now. This may be assessed by asking: "Have you ever been diagnosed with an STI? When?" "How were you treated?" *Prevention of pregnancy* may be assessed by asking: "Are you using contraception or practicing any form of birth control?" (CDC, n.d.; Nusbaum & Hamilton, 2002; STD/HIV Prevention Training Center of New England, n.d.).

A good sexual health history has the potential to help health care providers identify victims of trafficking. Within a clinical situation, if trafficking becomes apparent, the health care provider can be supportive because assistance is available for victims under federal law. Victims who are 18 years of age and older, if certified by the U.S. Department of Health and Human Services, are entitled to the same benefits as refugees. Child victims are immediately eligible for benefits such as housing, food, income assistance, English language training, health care assistance, and mental health services, for the protection of their lives (Administration for Children and Families, 2011).

Partner Notification and Treatment

Notification of sexual contact partners is an important aspect of reducing the spread of STIs and provides an opportunity for persons who do not know they have been infected to receive prompt treatment to reduce the morbidity associated with some STIs. The current public health system has inadequate partner notification services and partner notification is almost nonexistent in private practice. However, there are federal guidelines that specifically address partner notification for STIs such as HIV and syphilis (Hogben, 2007).

Currently, partner notification is predominately the responsibility of the person who is diagnosed with an STI. Research indicates patient referral seems to be the most effective when the index case accepts responsibility for notifying contacts instead of the health care provider (Gursahaney, Jeong, Dixon, & Wiesenfeld, 2011; Wilson et al., 2009). While partner notification is very important, achieving this goal among persons who are sex trafficked is not realistic, as a large percentage of their contacts are anonymous. Also, trafficked individuals may be reluctant to disclose the names of their partners if known.

Prevention Education and Counseling

Few good strategies exist for preventing the spread of STIs and most require male cooperation. Despite the limitation in STI prevention, all sexually active individuals should be counseled about strategies that can reduce the risk for STI transmission. Risk reduction actions include abstinence, condom use, limiting the number of sex partners, modifying sexual practices, and vaccination. Counseling someone about risk reduction is most effective when it is provided in a nonjudgmental manner that is congruent with the person's culture, language, gender, sexual orientation, age, and developmental level (CDC, 2010a). Individuals who are involved in sex trafficking often do not have the freedom to negotiate risk reduction actions, but if an opportunity arises, the counseling they receive could allow them to protect their physical health. Therefore, it is imperative for nurses to provide appropriate STI prevention education and behavioral counseling to all sexually active individuals, especially those who have a current STI or are at risk of an STI.

For STIs that are vaccine preventable, counseling about pre-exposure vaccination is one of the most effective methods for preventing transmission. As previously discussed, two HPV vaccines (Gardasil and Cervarix) are available. The nurse should also remember to question persons seeking STI services about their hepatitis vaccination history. Hepatitis B vaccine is recommended for all individuals who are unvaccinated. In addition, hepatitis A and B vaccines are strongly recommended for men who have sex with men and injection drug users (CDC, 2010a).

When counseling, it is important to discuss the two primary ways that STIs are transmitted, though infected genital (vaginal or urethral) secretions and skin-to-skin or mucosal surface contact. HIV, gonorrhea, chlamydia, and trichomoniasis are examples of STIs that are transmitted through genital secretions. Genital ulcer diseases (syphilis, genital herpes, and HPV) are STIs that can be transmitted through contact with infected skin or mucosal surfaces. Individuals need to be reminded that the best way for someone to avoid contracting or transmitting an STI is abstinence from oral, vaginal, and anal sex or having sexual activity exclusively within a long-standing monogamous relationship with an uninfected partner. It is also important to stress the fact that individuals who are infected with an STI may not have any symptoms or the initial symptoms may resolve without treatment (CDC, 2010a, 2011g).

When abstinence or monogamy is not an option, male latex condoms when used consistently and correctly, are found to be highly effective in reducing transmission of STIs. However, condoms provide a greater level of protection against STIs that are transmitted through genital secretions versus diseases that are transmitted through genital ulcers. That is because genital ulcer disease can occur in areas not covered by condoms and therefore skin or mucosal surface exposure to the disease occurs (CDC, 2010a, 2011g).

In the United States, there are two types of male condoms available that are not made of latex—polyurethane and natural membrane condoms. Polyurethane condoms protect against STIs and pregnancy equal to that of latex condoms and are recommended for persons who have a latex allergy. However, polyurethane condoms do have a higher slippage and breakage rate when compared to latex condoms and are more costly. Natural membrane condoms (mistakenly called "lambskin") are made from lamb cecum and do not allow the passage of sperm, but are not recommended for the prevention of STIs (CDC, 2010a, 2011g).

Some individuals blame the condom for breaking as their excuse for putting themselves at risk for exposure to an STI. However, condoms are regulated medical devices and are subject to random sampling and testing by the U.S. Food and Drug Administration. Rates of condom breakage during sexual intercourse and withdrawal are approximately two condoms per 100. In most cases, failure of a condom to protect from STIs is usually the result of inconsistent or improper use, not breakage (CDC, 2010a).

To help ensure that male condoms are used correctly, patients should be advised of the following recommendations:

- Use a new condom with each sex act (i.e., oral, vaginal, or anal)
- Carefully handle the condom to avoid damaging it with fingernails, teeth, or other sharp objects
- Put the condom on after the penis is erect and before any genital, oral, or anal contact with partner

- Use only water-based lubricants with latex condoms. Oil-based lubricants can weaken latex and should not be used
- Ensure adequate lubrication during vaginal and oral sex. This might require the use of water-based exogenous lubricants
- To prevent the condom from slipping off, hold the condom firmly against the base of the penis during withdrawal and withdraw while the penis is still erect (CDC, 2010a, p. 5)

The female condom is a thin sheath or pouch made of nitrile that is worn by women during sex. The sheath lines the vaginal wall and helps to prevent pregnancy and STIs, but it is not thought to be as effective as the male condom. Oil-based as well as water-based lubricants can be used with female condoms. If a female's partner refuses to use a male condom, the female condom is a good alternative and can be inserted prior to intercourse. Some women do not like female condoms because they are uncomfortable and the outer ring or frame of the condom is visible outside the vagina, making them feel self-conscious. In addition, because the female condom does not fit snugly against the vaginal wall, complaints of "noise" during intercourse have been reported. It is important to note that some individuals are using female condoms during anal sex. However, this use has not been officially approved or recommended to prevent the transmission of STIs during anal sex (AVERT, n.d.; Beksinska, Smit, Joanis, Usher-Patel, & Potter, 2011; CDC, 2010a).

Only a few studies have examined the relationship between trafficking and condom negotiation (Decker, McCauley, Phuengsamran, Janyam, & Silverman, 2011; Sarkar et al., 2008). Most of the current literature on condom negotiation is focused on sexually active adolescents and sex workers. Findings in this literature indicate that the ability to negotiate condom use is related to both personal and environmental attributes. Personal attributes include self-efficacy, feelings of empowerment, and knowledge about STI prevention. Environmental factors include violence, access to condoms, substance use, and financial benefit (East, Jackson, O'Brien, & Peters, 2010; Shannon et al., 2009; Urada, Morisky, Hernandez, & Strathdee, 2012).

Finally, women need to be counseled about the ineffectiveness of birth control methods, such as diaphragms, sponges, cervical caps, and spermicides, in reducing or preventing the transmission of STIs. Research has found that using spermicides containing nonoxynol-9 can cause irritation of the vaginal lining and anal wall, thus creating a more conducive environment for the transmission of STIs. Douching should also be discouraged because it alters the vaginal flora and predisposes women to BV and other STIs. Unfortunately current studies using topical microbicides for the prevention of STIs have demonstrated that these products are also ineffective in preventing STI transmission. However, there is hope they will be available in the future. Effective microbicides would provide women with an STI prevention method that would not require male cooperation or permission (CDC, 2010a; Cottrell, 2010).

CASE STUDIES

The following cases illustrate key aspects of assessment and treatment of selected STIs. The answers provided should be viewed as tentative since all data/variables relative to the situation are not provided. Readers are referred to other chapters in this book for more detailed information on how to approach patients if trafficking is suspected.

CASE STUDY 1

A 14-year-old female adolescent comes into a walk-in primary care clinic accompanied by a gentleman who identifies himself as her "uncle and legal guardian." The young girl is complaining of painful urination for the past 2 weeks. When the "uncle" is asked to leave the exam, he protests. However, the nurse examiner explains the need for privacy and he begrudgingly retreats to the waiting area. Prior to starting the exam, the nurse practitioner explains to the young girl the need for a thorough health history. The nurse integrates questions consistent with a detailed sexual history and explains to the young girl that she asks all patients the same questions.

The results of the health history were: general health history within normal limits, menarche age 12 with a regular 5-day menstrual cycle. The patient denies any sexual activity. The nurse practitioner explains the need for a physical examine that includes the perineal area. As the nurse practitioner prepares the patient for examination, she reflects on the fact that the teen has made very little eye contact during the interview and used close-ended responses to the nurse practitioner's open-ended questions. In addition, the young teen appeared to be on the verge of tears several times.

The nurse practitioner proceeds with the exam being mindful of her observations. The nurse observed: inflammation throughout the perineal area (redness and swelling), perineum was sensitive to touch, and a milky white, and odorous discharge near the vaginal opening. When the nurse asks about the discharge, the young patient openly cries and discloses that she had intercourse with several men in the past 2 weeks and three sexual encounters prior to arriving at the clinic today.

Questions

What Should the Nurse Practitioner Do Next?
Continue with the exam in a reassuring manner to collect the appropriate specimens for diagnosis. Inquire about the patient's relationship with the parent or

guardian. Is the person who accompanied her to the visit a relative or sex trafficker?

What About the "Uncle/Legal Guardian"?
Inform the uncle/guardian in the waiting area that the exam is taking longer than anticipated. This is a ploy to keep the uncle/guardian in the waiting area until authorities arrive.

What Specimens or Tests Should be Conducted?
Syphilis screening, chlamydia, and gonorrhea screening—point of care, HIV screening—rapid HIV screening, hepatitis B screen (if no previous immunization), and pregnancy test.

What Is the Probable Diagnosis?
Probable gonorrhea and trauma to the perineal area due to recent frequent sexual encounters.

Is any Treatment Necessary? If Yes or No, Provide a Rationale
Perineal irritation and odorous milky vaginal discharge is an indicator of possible gonorrhea based on the patient's history of sexual activity. Yes. Gonorrhea is typically treated based on signs and symptoms.

Is HIV Counseling Necessary? If Yes or No, Provide a Rationale
Yes, the patient needs to understand that a primary risk factor for HIV is unprotected sex with multiple partners.

What About Notification of Authorities?
On the basis of the patient's disclosure regarding recent multiple sex partners, this is considered suspected child abuse; therefore, a notification of children and youth services is necessary. Also, the current situation needs to be explained to the local law enforcement authorities. When doing so, the nurse should be very specific about her assessment findings and concerns.

CASE STUDY 2

An 18-year-old female adolescent presents at the emergency department (ED) with a history of a faint rash covering her body for the past 5 days. She is accompanied by a female "friend."

A detailed health history with integrated questions related to sexual history and activity is taken by the nurse. The health history is negative,

(continued)

except for the current rash and a genital sore that occurred about 4 months ago. The sore resolved spontaneously and did not cause any pain or discomfort. The woman believed that the sore was related to "American detergents." However, the woman admits to having unprotected intercourse with multiple male partners over the last few months. She also informs the nurse that she came to the United States 6 months ago as a prospective mail-order-bride from Croatia and her female "friend" is from the sponsoring agency. The client's English is limited, but she is able to communicate effectively. Upon physical exam, the nurse observes a symmetrical, reddish-pink nonitchy rash on the woman's trunk and extremities, including the palmer and planter surfaces. The vaginal exam was within normal limits.

Questions

What Is the Probable Diagnosis?
Secondary syphilis

Is Any Treatment Necessary? Provide a Rationale for Your Response
Yes. The patient should be treated for secondary syphilis and a pregnancy test.

How Should the Patient be Counseled Regarding Multiple Sex Partners?
Explain the probable diagnosis. Teach prevention regarding use of condoms. Emphasize the likelihood of acquiring a sexually transmitted infection via unprotected intercourse with multiple partners. The patient should be counseled regarding modes of transmission. Explore with the patient regarding her involvement with multiple sex partners.

Is it Within the Realm of Nursing Practice for the Nurse to Initiate a Discussion Regarding the Relationship Between the Patient and Her Friend? Provide a Rationale for Your Response
Further discussion regarding the relationship between the patient and friend is needed. Is this a same-gender relationship or does the friend have "power" over the patient? If the patient is also having same-gender intimate encounters, some STIs can be passed female to female. For example, use of sex toys, oral sex, and so on.

CASE STUDY 3

An 18-year-old Asian man presents to the health department for a HIV test because he recently attended a health education class about HIV infection. The young man was concerned because he recently had a sexual encounter

(continued)

with a man 20 years his senior, who convinced him there was no need to use a condom since they were both HIV negative. They had unprotected anal intercourse, the young man being the receptive partner.

The nurse learns that the young man entered the United States 2 years ago with his parents under the pretext of finishing school and securing a job in the garment industry. However, soon after arriving he learned that his work environment promoted involvement in anonymous sexual encounters with potential clients of the company. He feared losing his job and having his family deported to their country of origin if he did not participate. The young man's rapid HIV tests result was positive.

Questions

How Should the Nurse Handle This Preliminary Positive Result?

Engage the patient in further discussion about the meaning of the HIV rapid test. What is the patient's knowledge level regarding HIV? Explain to the patient that a confirmatory test, a Western blot, needs to be done to verify the results of the rapid test. However, it will be several weeks before the outcome will be known; therefore, this patient is considered a presumptive positive and should abstain from sexual activity or use a condom with each sexual encounter.

In Addition to Dealing With the Positive HIV Test, What Other Medical and Social Needs Will This Young Man Need?

If there is truly a chance that the patient will lose his employment, referral to appropriate agencies may be necessary. Until the outcome of the Western blot is known, the patient may benefit from mental health counseling. Also, the patient can be advised regarding immigration and naturalization services.

What Responsibility Does the Nurse Have Regarding the Young Man's Employer?

With the patient's permission the nurse can advocate on behalf of the patient and notify the local law enforcement about the employer. However, considering the circumstances, there may be little if anything that can be done if the patient is terminated by his employer.

SUMMARY

STIs continue to be a major public health problem worldwide and are a leading cause of morbidity, especially among individuals who have asymptomatic infections. Unfortunately, there are only a limited number of strategies available that reduce the transmission of STIs among sexually active individuals and cooperation between partners is needed to initiate them. For individuals who are trafficked for sex, STI prevention and treatment are almost nonexistent, which contributes to ongoing transmission. Therefore, nurses must be vigilant in obtaining an accurate sexual history, providing appropriate education and counseling about STIs to all persons who are sexually active, and act as an advocate for victims of sex trafficking. This chapter highlighted the major STIs and the impact these infections can have on someone's health.

REFERENCES

Abatangelo, L., Okereke, L., Parham-Foster, C., Parrish, C., Scaglione, L., Zotte, D. et al. (2010). If pelvic inflammatory disease is suspected empiric treatment should be initiated. *Journal of the American Academy of Nurse Practitioners*, *22*(2), 117–122. doi:10.1111/j.1745-7599.2009.00478.x

Administration for Children and Families. (2011). *Fact sheet: Victim assistance.* Retrieved from http://www.acf.hhs.gov/trafficking/about/victim_assist.html

American College of Obstetricians and Gynecologists. (2011). *Pelvic inflammatory disease.* Retrieved from http://www.acog.org/~/media/For%20Patients/faq077.pdf?dmc=1&ts=20120329T1542383624

AVERT. (n.d.). *The female condom.* Retrieved from http://www.avert.org/female-condom.htm

Beksinska, M., Smit, J., Joanis, C., Usher-Patel, M., & Potter, W. (2011). Female condom technology: New products and regulatory issues. *Contraception*, *83*(4), 316–321. doi:10.1016/j.contraception.2010.07.022

Boyd, S. D. (2011). Management of HIV infection in treatment-naïve patients: A review of the most current recommendations. *American Journal of Health-System Pharmacy*, *68*, 991–1001. doi: 10.2146/ajhp100156

Burkhart, C. N., Gunning, W., & Burkhart, C. G. (2000). Scanning electron microscopic examination of the egg of the pubic louse (Anoplura: *Pthirus pubis*). *International Journal of Dermatology*, *39*, 201–202. doi: 10.1046/j.1365-4362.2000.00901.x

Centers for Disease Control and Prevention. (n.d.). *A guide to taking a sexual history.* Retrieved from http://www.cdc.gov/std/treatment/SexualHistory.pdf

Centers for Disease Control and Prevention. (2002). Screening tests to detect *Chlamydia trachomatis* and *Neisseria gonorrhoeae* infections. *Morbidity and Mortality Weekly Report*, *51*(RR-15), 1–46. Retrieved from http://www.cdc.gov/mmwr/pdf/rr/rr5115.pdf

Centers for Disease Control and Prevention. (2008). Revised surveillance case definitions for HIV infection among adults, adolescents, and children aged <18 months and for HIV infection and AIDS among children aged 18 months to <13 years—United States. *Morbidity and Mortality Weekly*, *57*, 1–12. Retrieved from http://www.cdc.gov/mmwr/pdf/rr/rr5710.pdf

Centers for Disease Control and Prevention. (2009). *HIV testing.* Retrieved from http://www.cdc.gov/hiv/topics/testing/index.htm

Centers for Disease Control and Prevention. (2010a). Sexually transmitted diseases treatment guidelines, 2010. *Morbidity and Mortality Weekly Report*, *59*, 1–110. Retrieved from http://www.cdc.gov/std/treatment/2010/STD-Treatment-2010-RR5912.pdf

Centers for Disease Control and Prevention. (2010b). *Syphilis.* Retrieved from http://www.cdc.gov/std/syphilis/STDFact-Syphilis.htm

Centers for Disease Control and Prevention. (2010c). *Bacterial vaginosis—CDC fact sheet.* Retrieved from http://www.cdc.gov/std/bv/stdfact-bacterial-vaginosis.htm

Centers for Disease Control and Prevention. (2010d). *Human papillomavirus (HPV).* Retrieved from http://www.cdc.gov/hpv/

Centers for Disease Control and Prevention. (2010e). *Genital herpes CDC—Fact sheet.* Retrieved from http://www.cdc.gov/std/herpes/stdfact-herpes.htm

Centers for Disease Control and Prevention. (2010f). *Pubic "crab" lice.* Retrieved from http://www.cdc.gov/parasites/lice/pubic/

Centers for Disease Control and Prevention. (2011a). *Trichomoniasis—CDC fact sheet.* Retrieved from http://www.cdc.gov/std/trichomonas/STDFact-Trichomoniasis.htm

Centers for Disease Control and Prevention. (2011b). *Gonorrhea—CDC fact sheet.* Retrieved from http://www.cdc.gov/std/Gonorrhea/STDFact-gonorrhea.htm

Centers for Disease Control and Prevention. (2011c). *STD trends in the United States: 2010 National data for gonorrhea, chlamydia, and syphilis.* Retrieved from http://www.cdc.gov/std/stats10/trends.htm

Centers for Disease Control and Prevention. (2011d). *Viral hepatitis.* Retrieved from http://www.cdc.gov/hepatitis/

Centers for Disease Control and Prevention. (2011e). *Basic information about HIV and AIDS.* Retrieved from http://www.cdc.gov/hiv/topics/basic/index.htm

Centers for Disease Control and Prevention. (2011f). *Pelvic inflammatory disease (PID).* Retrieved from http://www.cdc.gov/std/pid/stdfact-pid.htm

Centers for Disease Control and Prevention. (2011g). *Condoms and STDs. Fact sheet for public health personnel.* Retrieved from http://www.cdc.gov/condomeffectiveness/latex.htm

Centers for Disease Control and Prevention. (2012). *Chlamydia—CDC fact sheet.* Retrieved from http://www.cdc.gov/std/Chlamydia/STDFact-Chlamydia.htm

Chang, A. K. (2008). *Trichomoniasis.* Retrieved from http://www.emedicinehealth.com/trichomoniasis/article_em.htm

Cottrell, B. H. (2010). An updated review of evidence to discourage douching. *The American Journal of Maternal Child Nursing [MCN]*, 35(2), 102–107. Retrieved from http://www.nursingcenter.com/pdf.asp?AID=984319

Decker, M. R., McCauley, H. L., Phuengsamran, D., Janyam, S., & Silverman, J. G. (2011). Sex trafficking, sexual risk, sexually transmitted infection and reproductive health among female sex workers in Thailand. *Journal of Epidemiology and Community Health*, 65(4), 334–339. doi:10.1136/jech.2009.096834

Dunne, E. F., Sternberg, M., Markowitz, L. E., McQuillan, G., Swan, D. C., Patel, S. et al. (2011). Human papillomavirus (HPV) 6, 11, 16 and 18 prevalence among females in the United States—National Health and Nutrition Examination Survey, 2003–2006: Opportunity to measure HPV vaccine impact? *Journal of Infectious Diseases*, 204, 562–565. doi:10.1093/infdis/jir342

East, L., Jackson, D., O'Brien, L., & Peters, K. (2010). Condom negotiation: Experiences of sexually active young women. *Journal of Advanced Nursing*, 67(1), 77–85. doi: 10.1111/j.1365-2648.2010.05451.x

Edwards, M. (2008). Genital warts and genital herpes: A public health perspective. *Practice Nurse*, 36(10), 20–23. Retrieved from http://www.accessmylibrary.com/article-1G1-213230963/genital-warts-and-genital.html

Falb, K. L., McCauley, H. L., Decker, M. R., Sabarwal, S., Gupta, J., & Silverman, J. G. (2011). Trafficking mechanisms and HIV status among sex-trafficking survivors in Calcutta, India. *International Journal of Gynecology & Obstetrics, 113*(1), 86–87. doi: 10.1016/j.ijgo.201.11.009

Gilbert, L. K., Levandowski, B. A., & Roberts, C. M. (2010). Characteristics associated with genital herpes testing among young adults: Assessing factors from two national data sets. *Journal of American College Health, 59*(3), 143–150. doi:10.1080/07448481. 2010.497522.

Godinjak, A., & Hkic, M. (2012). *Chlamydia trachomatis* and female infertility. *Health Medical Journal, 6*(2), 690–693. Retrieved from http://www.healthmedjournal. com/index.htm

Gursahaney, P. R., Jeong, K., Dixon, B. W., & Wiesenfeld, H. C. (2011). Partner notification of sexually transmitted diseases: Practices and preferences. *Sexually Transmitted Diseases, 38*, 821–827. doi: 10.1097/OLQ.0b013e31821c390b

Hariri, S., Unger, E. R., Sternberg, M., Dunne, E. F., Swan, D., Patel, S. et al. (2011). Prevalence of genital HPV among females in the United States, the National Health and Nutrition Examination Survey, 2003–2006. *Journal of Infectious Diseases, 204*, 566–573. doi:10.1093/infdis/jir341

Hogben, M. (2007). Partner notification for sexually transmitted diseases. *Clinical Infectious Diseases, 44*, 160–174 doi:10.1086/511429.

Kamazima, S. R., Ezekiel, M. J., Kazaura, M. R., & Fimbo, B. (2012). Understanding the link between trafficking in persons and HIV and AIDS risk in Tanzania. *Tanzania Journal of Health Research, 14*(1), 1–12. Retrieved from http://www.ajol.info/index.php/ thrb/article/viewFile/70053/62135

Kloer, A. (2010). Sex trafficking and HIV/AIDS: A deadly junction for human. *Human Rights, 37*(2), 8–25. Retrieved from http://www.americanbar.org/publications/ human_rights_magazine_home/human_rights_vol37_2010/spring2010/sex_traf ficking_and_hiv_aids_a_deadly_junction_for_women_and_girls.html

McCormack, P. L., & Joura, E. A. (2011). Spotlight on quadrivalent human papillomavirus (Types 6, 11, 16, 18) recombinant vaccine (Gardasil) in the prevention of premalignant genital lesions, genital cancer, and genital warts. *BioDrugs, 29*, 339–343. doi:10.2165/11205060-000000000-00000

Mepham, S. O., Bland, R. M., & Newell, M. L. (2011). Prevention of mother-to-child transmission of HIV in resource-rich and -poor settings. *BJOG. An International Journal of Obstetrics and Gynaecology, 11*, 118, 202–218. doi: 10.1111/j.0528.2010.02733.x

Nath, A. K., & Thappa, D. M. (2009). Newer trends in the management of genital herpes. *Indian Journal of Dermatology, Venereology, and Leprology, 75*, 566–574. doi: 10.4103/0378-6323.57716

National Center for Biotechnology Information. (2011). *Gonorrhea*. Retrieved from http://www.ncbi.nlm.nih.gov/pubmedhealth/PMH0004526/

National Institute of Allergy and Infectious Diseases. (2009). *Hepatitis B*. Retrieved from http://www.niaid.nih.gov/topics/hepatitis/hepatitisb/Pages/Default.aspx

National Institute of Allergy and Infectious Diseases. (2010). *Syphilis*. Retrieved from http://www.niaid.nih.gov/topics/syphilis/Pages/default.aspx

Nicum, S., & Mahida, N. (2010). The presentation and management of genital herpes. *InnovAiT, 3*(3), 124–127. doi: 10.1093/innovait/inp259

Nusbaum, M. R. H., & Hamilton, C. D. (2002). The proactive sexual history. *American Family Physician, 66,* 1705–1713. Retrieved from http://www.aafp.org/afp/2002/1101/p1705.pdf

Sarkar, K., Bal, B., Mukherjee, R., Chakraborty, S., Saha, S., Ghosh, A. et al. (2008). Sex-trafficking, violence, negotiating skill, and HIV infection in brother-based sex workers of eastern India, adjoining Nepal, Bhutan, and Bangladesh. *Journal of Health, Population, and Nutrition, 26*(2), 223–231. Retrieved from http://www.bioline.org.br/request?hn08024

Schwebke, J. R. (2012). Vaginitis. In J. M. Zenilman, & M. Shahmanesh (Eds.). *Sexually transmitted infections* (pp. 57–65). Sudbury, MA: Jones & Bartlett Learning.

Schwebke, J. R., & Burgess, D. (2004). Trichomoniasis. *Clinical Microbiology Reviews, 17*(4), 794–803. doi: 10.1128/CMR.17.4.794-803.2004

Sharapov, U. M., & Hu, D. J. (2010). Viral hepatitis A, B, C: Grown-up issues. *Adolescent Medicine: State of the Art Reviews, 21*(2), 265–286.

Shannon, K., Strathdee, S. A., Shoveller, J., Rusch, M., Kerr, T., & Tyndall, M. W. (2009). Structural and environmental barriers to condom use negotiation with clients among female sex workers: Implications for HIV strategies and policy. *American Journal of Public Health, 99*(4), 659–665. doi: 10.2105/AJPH.2007.129858.

Sherman, I. W. (2007). *Twelve diseases that changed our world.* Washington, D C: American Society of Microbiology Press.

Silverman, J. G., Decker, M. R., Gupta, J., Dharmadhikari, A., Seage, G. R., III, & Raj, A. (2008). Sexually transmitted co-infections among HIV-infected sex-trafficked women and girls, Nepal. *Emerging Infectious Diseases [serial on the Internet].* 2008 Jun [date cited]. Available from http://wwwnc.cdc.gov/eid/article/14/6/08-0090_article.htm

STD/HIV Prevention Training Center of New England. (n.d.). *Asking the right questions.* Retrieved from http://www.hawaii.edu/hivandaids/Self%20Study%20Module%20I%20%20%20Asking%20the%20Right%20Questions.pdf

Te, H. S., & Jensen, D. M. (2010). Epidemiology of Hepatitis B and C: A global overview. *Clinics in Liver Disease, 14*(1), 1–21. doi: 10.1016/j.cld2—9.11.009

UNAIDS. (2011). *UNAIDS World AIDS Day Report: 2011.* Retrieved from http://www.unaids.org/en/media/unaids/contentassets/documents/unaidspublication/2011/JC2216_WorldAIDSday_report_2011_en.pdf

U.S. Department of Health and Human Resources and Services Administration HIV AIDS Bureau. (2011). *Guide for HIV/AIDS clinical care.* Retrieved from http://www.aidsetc.org/aidsetc?page=cg-00-00

U.S. Department of Health and Human Services Office of Women's Health. (2008). *Bacterial vaginosis fact sheet.* Retrieved from http://womenshealth.gov/publications/our-publications/fact-sheet/bacterial-vaginosis.cfm

U.S. Department of Health and Human Services Office of Women's Health. (2011). *Chlamydia.* Retrieved from http://www.womenshealth.gov/publications/our-publications/fact-sheet/chlamydia.cfm

Urada, L. A., Morisky, D. E., Hernandez, L. I., & Strathdee, S. A. (2012). Social and structural factors associated with consistent condom use among female entertainment workers trading sex in Philippines. *AIDS and Behavior.* Advanced online publication. doi. 10.1007/s10461-011-0113-x

Williams, I., Daniels, D., Gedela, K., Briggs, A., & Pryce, A. (2011). HIV. In K. E. Ragstad (Ed.) *ABC of sexually transmitted diseases* (pp. 95–109). West Sussex, UK: Blackwell Publishing Ltd.

Wilson, T. E., Hogben, M., Malka, E. S., Liddon, N., McCormack, W. M., Rubin, S. R. et al. (2009). A randomized controlled trial for reducing risks for sexually transmitted infections through enhanced patient-based partner notification. *American Journal of Public Health, 99*, pS104–pS110. doi:10.2105/AJPH.2007.112128

World Health Organization. (2008a). *10 facts on sexually transmitted infections.* Retrieved from http://www.who.int/features/factfiles/sexually_transmitted_diseases/en/index.html

World Health Organization. (2008b). *Hepatitis B.* Retrieved from http://www.who.int/mediacentre/factsheets/fs204/en/index.html

World Health Organization. (2011a). *Sexually transmitted infections.* Retrieved from http://www.who.int/mediacentre/factsheets/fs110/en/index.html

World Health Organization. (2011b). *Global HIV/AIDS response. Epidemic update and health care sector progress towards universal access.* Progress Report 2011. Retrieved from http://whqlibdoc.who.int/publications/2011/9789241502986_eng.pdf

World Health Organization. (2012). *Sexually transmitted diseases: Gonorrhoea.* Retrieved from http://www.who.int/vaccine_research/diseases/soa_std/en/index2.html

Zenilman, G. M. (2012). Gonorrhea and chlamydia. In J. M. Zenilman, & M. Shahmanesh (Eds.). *Sexually transmitted infections* (pp. 31–42). Sudbury, MA: Jones & Bartlett Learning.

CHAPTER 16

Physical Trauma

MARY DE CHESNAY AND JORDAN GREENBAUM

*P*rostituted women and children suffer the same types of physical trauma that victims of rape, intimate partner violence, and accidents suffer, but their experiences are recurrent and in many cases, more severe. Although victims of intimate partner violence also experience long-term abuse, they usually have more control over their lives and more resources than sex-trafficked victims, who might be kept in locked rooms and deprived of food and sleep. Pimps or traffickers do not allow the girls to obtain health care for minor injuries or illnesses because time is money and they are indifferent to the suffering of their victims. To allow frequent visits with health care professionals increases the risk of escape attempts. When victims do present, they are likely to have major problems or comorbid conditions such as substance abuse that complicate the presenting condition.

In this chapter the authors will present examples of how nurses and physicians who are in a position to recognize the commercially sexually exploited children (CSEC) might address the special circumstances presented by these patients. The case study treatment strategies might be performed by physicians, sexual assault nurse examiners (SANEs), or nurse practitioners. Examples of acute problems are set in the emergency department (ED) because that is a common place for health care providers to encounter trafficking victims, although patients may present in a variety of settings including a community-based clinic, health department, private clinic, or school nurse's office. The chapter on policy and procedures for the ED provides further direction on how to engage law enforcement and social services.

APPROACHING PATIENTS

It is critical to assume a nonjudgmental attitude that is kind and respectful without being overly sympathetic. Paradoxically, saying things like, "You poor dear" and "What an awful time you have had" can reinforce shame and embarrassment when the intention is to develop rapport. The patient is likely to be less cooperative and may even leave without treatment if she feels that staff members are going to invade her privacy. CSEC children have no control over most of their lives and what little control they have, they exert. Information is power and they may lie about their ages, how they sustained their injuries, and their living arrangements to maintain some control over their situations.

Health care settings may have their own systems for how to interview patients with suspected intimate partner violence or child abuse, but may not know how to approach patients who have been trafficked. Several chapters in this book present ideas for screening, but agencies should hold meetings to orient the staff about the unique features of trafficking, especially when CSEC is suspected. Tables 16.1 and 16.2 present a place to start.

EXAMPLES OF HOW PATIENTS MIGHT PRESENT

The literature contains many examples of health and mental health issues that CSEC patients experience. In this chapter, we present some scenarios of common presenting problems and how to adapt traditional best-practice treatment for CSEC. Since it is most likely that nurses will meet CSEC victims in settings where physicians and surgeons are accessible, the examples will focus on these types of agencies, but nurses in any setting might be in a position to identify and refer CSEC victims. For any CSEC patient who presents for a health care condition, it should be assumed that one should screen for sexually transmitted infections (STIs). We have not made a point in this chapter of discussing STI screening but readers are referred to the chapter by Taylor and Blake that contains detailed information on STIs.

In the chapter on ED policies and procedures, suggestions are given for how managers might develop protocols that could be standardized for sex trafficking, much similar to the protocols in place for child abuse and intimate partner violence. Some of the same special considerations apply to CSEC: treating

TABLE 16.1   Questions Regarding Reproductive History

a. Any current or recent genitourinary signs/symptoms?

b. Are you sexually active? How long have you been active?

c. How many partners?

d. Ever had an STI? Was it treated?

e. Ever been pregnant or had an abortion/miscarriage?

f. Do you use any form of birth control?

g. Any prior trauma/injuries associated with sexual activity?

h. Any menstrual problems?

TABLE 16.2 Potential Questions Regarding Prior Trauma, Substance Abuse, and Mental Health Injuries/Abuse

Questions Regarding Prior Trauma	Substance Abuse	Mental Health Screen
1. Any prior history of being hit, kicked, slapped, choked, and so on by a parent/caregiver? By anyone else (dating violence, peer violence, and CSEC violence)? 2. Did this ever result in injury? Was medical treatment sought? 3. Have you ever had any broken bones, loss of consciousness, significant lacerations, or other wounds? Inquire about circumstances. 4. What happens when you get in trouble at home? 5. Any prior history of sexual abuse? 6. Ever had to exchange sex for money, food, shelter, and so on? Ever had sex when you did not want to?	1. Obtain details of types of drugs/alcohol used, frequency, patterns of use, withdrawal symptoms, and use while driving. 2. Were you ever forced to use drugs/alcohol? 3. What kinds of things did you do to help you relax, or "chill"? 4. Did you ever take any drugs or use alcohol to help you get through the night? 5. Has anyone ever given you drugs when you did not know about it?	*Inquire of any recent or current problems with*: 1. Nightmares? 2. Difficulty in sleeping? 3. Repetitive thoughts or images in your mind that will not go away? 4. Times when you feel very anxious? 5. Panic attacks? 6. Times when you feel like a part of you "goes somewhere else"—is not part of what your body is experiencing? 7. Periods of feeling sad and/or hopeless? 8. Thoughts of hurting yourself or others? 9. Have you attempted to hurt yourself or others? Ask about circumstances, method used, and so on.

the patient with careful respect, avoiding confrontational questions, explaining procedures, careful observation of old injuries, matching the story with the injury, and careful screening interviews.

CASE STUDY: CARLA

Carla is a 14-year-old female adolescent who presents to the ED of an American suburban community hospital with a chief complaint of intermittent vaginal bleeding and pelvic pain of 2 days' duration. She is accompanied by her female "aunt," who says she is the child's guardian. Carla is quiet

(continued)

and withdrawn while the aunt provides information to the medical staff and answers questions. As you try to obtain information about the child's symptoms, you notice the aunt interrupts the child and tends to minimize the severity of the situation. The patient will not look at you and defers to the aunt. However, she does say that she is not bleeding now and has not had significant bleeding today. The aunt is very reluctant to leave the room so you can speak with the child alone and refuses to do so until you explain that it is hospital practice to interview adolescents alone whenever possible and that she will need to wait in the family waiting room.

Once the child is alone you begin to build rapport, asking about school, recreational activities, and friends. You observe her demeanor and body language. Eventually you move on to explain that you will be asking her some personal questions that will help you determine what she may need, and how you can best treat her; you explain the limits of confidentiality and ask her if she understands. You say that sometimes when you ask adolescents these questions, they may feel anxious, embarrassed, or feel some other way. This is okay and you would like her to tell you if she has any of these feelings so that you can address them. You do not want to make her feel uncomfortable. Then you begin asking questions about her vaginal bleeding and abdominal/pelvic pain. She says this began after having sex with her boyfriend, that he stuck something plastic inside her, and it had a sharp edge. She does not know what it was but she felt a lot of pain. The bleeding was brisk initially (soaked much of a small towel), but stopped after a few hours and has returned intermittently since then. Each time the blood soaks 1 to 2 sanitary pads, but the volume has decreased considerably today. The pelvic pain is constant, dull, and midline, without radiation. You take a detailed gynecologic history, including questions listed in Table 16.1. You find out she has had gonorrhea in the past, and has been sexually active since age 11. She has a boyfriend who is about 30 years old. You ask about prior injuries to her anogenital region, and injuries involving other areas of the body. All the time you are talking to her, you monitor her behavior and facial expressions, looking for signs that the conversation is causing significant stress. As you obtain history related to current/prior injuries and abuse, substance use/misuse, and mental health screening (Table 16.2), you note that some of her answers contradict others and she is reluctant to talk about certain topics, especially those involving her home life and her "boyfriend."

When you begin your exam you immediately notice a tattoo of the letter "D" below the child's right axilla. You ask her about this and she mutters something unintelligible and becomes quiet. You also notice a cluster of ~1 cm round contusions on the left upper arm, a healed burn

(continued)

on the flexor aspect of the right forearm, and amorphous red–blue bruising in a 5 cm area on the medial right thigh. You document the location, size, shape, color, and tenderness of each injury. You ask the patient about the injuries in a nonthreatening manner ("There's an old scar here on your arm—do you remember how you got this?"). She gives you vague answers about accidental trauma. You document her general nutritional status, cleanliness, and assess for untreated medical conditions. As you proceed through your exam you ask a few more questions, such as "Have you ever broken a bone, or had trouble bearing weight for an extended time?" (as you examine her extremities). You ask whether she gets treatment when she has an injury or when she is sick, and if so, where she is taken and by whom.

You explain the process of your anogenital exam (need for exam, the process itself, the sexual assault evidence kit, STI testing, and prophylaxis) before proceeding and then begin a detailed examination of the vulvar structures. You note some bruising of the left labia majora and clitoral hood with mild swelling, an unremarkable vaginal vestibule, an estrogenized hymen with a complete transection at 6:00 in the supine position (indicative of prior blunt force penetrating trauma), bruising of the perineum, and a blood clot noted within the vagina. The anus has a normal configuration and is without evidence of acute trauma, scarring, or focal lesions. You contact the surgery service and collect swabs and trace evidence for the sexual assault kit as best as you can.

An abdominal/pelvic computer tomography (CT) scan shows no free air or fluid. The surgeon performs an exam under anesthesia, and notes a 3 cm laceration of the posterior vaginal wall that is ~5 mm deep and does not extend to the serosa. There is oozing upon dislodgement of the clot; the laceration is closed with sutures. There is bruising of the cervix, but no active bleeding. No apparent anorectal involvement.

Genital Injuries

Genital injury may be classified in a scoring system ranked from I to V and progressing from isolated injuries distal to the hymen, to those including the hymen, those including the vagina, to hymenal vaginal injury with partial tear of the anorectum, and vaginal injury with complete tear of the anorectum (Onen et al., 2005). Injuries may range from small abrasions, contusions, redness, and swelling, to deep lacerations of the perineum, and/or penetration of the vaginal wall. There is evidence to suggest that sexual assault with a foreign object is associated with a greater risk of injury than is assault involving penile penetration (Sturgiss, Tyson, & Parekh, 2010). The extent of the injury may be greater than is suggested by the external appearance of the genitalia. Careful evaluation is critical in identifying internal injuries (vagina and anorectum). This may entail exam under anesthesia, CT of the abdomen/pelvis, exploratory laparoscopy, or laparotomy.

Vulvar Hematomas/Abrasions/Lacerations

Hematomas from blunt force trauma may be small and cause only mild pain and swelling, or may be large and painful and may interfere with urine outflow and cause local tissue necrosis, especially of overlying skin. Mild injuries may be treated conservatively, with ice packs and bed rest. Contusions involving the vulva, including the hymen, may disappear within several days to a few weeks, and are not associated with residual scarring (McCann, Miyamoto, Boyle, & Rogers, 2007). Large hematomas that distort genital anatomy and interfere with bladder emptying may be treated with urinary catheterization, and in some cases, evacuation of the blood clot and resection of devascularized tissue (Merritt, 2009). Hematomas in this region may track along fascial planes and may take days to weeks to resolve completely.

Abrasions and superficial lacerations of the external genitalia tend to heal quickly and completely, often within a few days. Size and location help determine healing time. The time to resolution for moderate-to-deep lacerations depends on their depth and severity, ranging from a few days for superficial lacerations of the hymen or vestibule, to 3 weeks or longer for some deep perineal lacerations. The deep nonhymenal injuries may cause scarring, although this is not typically associated with transections of the hymen (McCann, Miyamoto, Boyle, & Rogers, 2007). Superficial lacerations of the vulva may be treated with oxidized cellulose to stop bleeding, or with steri-strips, while deep lacerations require sutures (Lentz, 2012).

Vaginal Laceration and Perforation

Laceration or perforation of the vaginal wall may result from blunt force trauma, either from forceful penile penetration, or penetration with another object. Risk factors for coital vaginal injury include "rough" or nonconsensual coitus, hurried coitus (insufficient time for lubrication to occur as part of sexual response), and disproportion between vaginal vault size and penetrating object (Hoffman & Ganta, 2001). The posterior fornix is a common site of injury for laceration (Habek & Kulas, 2007), as are the lateral walls of the vaginal vault. Patients with vaginal trauma may present with abdominal pain and vaginal bleeding; some may present in hemorrhagic shock (Hoffman & Ganta, 2001). Substantial bleeding may occur secondary to injury to the descending branches of the uterine artery or vein, or the ascending branches of the internal pudendal artery and vein, which travel along the lateral vaginal walls. Bleeding may be external or concealed within various nearby spaces, including the paravesical and pararectal spaces, and the retroperitonum of the broad ligaments (Townsend, 2012).

Deep lacerations and perforations require sutural repair. Potential complications of perforation include peritonitis from introduction of vaginal flora, sepsis, severe hemorrhage, prolapse of intraabdominal contents, and fistula formation.

Vaginal Fistula

One unusual and potentially very serious condition affecting some victims of sex trafficking is obstetric or traumatic fistula caused by early childbirth or repeated rape. Vesicovaginal fistula is simply an abnormal duct between the vaginal wall and bladder or urethra. Rectal–vaginal fistula occurs between the rectum and vagina. In the United States and other developed countries, fistulas usually occur after pelvic surgery or as a normal risk of hysterectomy (Miklos, 1999). However, they can also occur due to repeated vaginal or anal rape. Early childbirth among child brides and violent rape with foreign objects are common in some developing countries where children are married as young as 5 years old and where militia routinely use rape as a form of control over tribal villages.

In sub-Saharan Africa and India, girls are often married at early ages to older men, who usually break their promises to families to abstain from sex until the child is mature and consequently force their child brides to bear children at young ages (Alio et al., 2011). The result is pregnancy among children whose vaginal length is short and who have difficult childbirth, with labor often lasting several days. Long labor with no medical intervention makes it difficult to give birth to live babies. If a young bride produces a stillborn and has the complication of a recto-vaginal fistula, she is likely to be rejected by the husband and family due to the smell of fecal incontinence. She lives in shame and embarrassment. In rural areas, girls are often forced to live in their own huts apart from other people. If rejected by their husbands and families they may resort to prostitution to survive or may be prostituted by their husbands. It is estimated that approximately 3.5 million women suffer from vaginal fistula and about 2 million of these are untreated (Rai, 2011). These women live primarily in sub-Saharan Africa, Arab region, and southeast Asia and it is estimated that between 50,000 and 100,000 new cases will appear each year (Semere & Nour, 2008).

In developing countries, particularly when child brides give birth at young ages, these fistulas are a common and heartbreaking disability leading to urinary and fecal incontinence (Ijaiya et al., 2010; Narcisi, Tieneber, Andriani, & McKinney, 2010). They are categorized as simple or complicated depending partly on vaginal length (related to age of the person) and size of fistula as under or over 3 cm (Kohli & Miklos, 2003). Fistulas produce intense shame and self-consciousness among the women who suffer from them and sometimes require several surgeries to treat. In places like the Congo where rape by the militia is the norm, girls who are successfully treated but who remain in the Congo are likely to be raped again (Longombe et al., 2008). Interviews with 82 Eritrean women who had undergone obstetric vaginal fistula surgery revealed that although they described improvements in their conditions, many had continued problems with incontinence and sexual health, and lacked specific information about their conditions and how they might cope (Turan, Johnson, & Polan, 2007).

In the United States vaginal fistula would be treated surgically often by laparoscopy at a cost of $7,000 to 8,000. Affluent women who can afford medical tourism can obtain specialized surgical treatment fistula repair in India at a cost under $400 for the surgery plus the added travel expenses. One Indian clinic reported the results of a retrospective study of 558 women with high success rates for fistulas under 4 cm (Khumar et al., 2009). Obviously, adequate surgical intervention is out of reach of victims who have not been rescued since traffickers are not concerned with caring for their victims.

CASE STUDY: IFE

Ife is a 12-year-old Nigerian girl (whose name means "love") who presents in the ED of a large American hospital with a fractured right ulna and numerous contusions and abrasions. She is accompanied by an older man who says he is her uncle and he will translate since she does not speak English. As a nurse working in a city that has many Nigerian immigrants, you have made a point of learning a little about Nigeria and know that the official language is English, though many rural people speak only one or two of their tribal languages. Therefore, you are skeptical of the man's claim and find a way to distract him while you examine the girl. You explain that you will accompany her to the rest room to obtain a urine sample while he provides information to the intake clerk. When the two of you are alone and you begin the exam, you see that her panties are stained and there is evidence of urinary and fecal incontinence. As you conduct the assessment, you discover that she has been pregnant and 1 year ago she delivered a stillborn child in Nigeria after 3 days of labor. Given her age and demographic data, you suggest the resident look for a vaginal fistula. He finds a 4 cm fistula on the vaginal wall near the urethra. Finally, Ife admits that the man is her husband and that she had been sold to him at age 6 by her parents, who were led believe he would take care of her and give her a better life than they could. He brought her to America where she is treated as a domestic slave in her husband's house.

Treatment Best Practices for Ife

Appropriate nursing and medical care would include the following:

- Clean the abrasions
- Set the broken arm
- Recognize the shame and embarrassment she feels at being incontinent. Communicate that the fistula is not her fault and that she is not alone in having this condition
- Refer for surgical repair of the fistula
- Review postsurgical care
- Teach her about available diapers for women—must be done with great sensitivity due to the embarrassment

Special considerations:

- She may be legally married to him in Nigeria but the marriage would likely not be recognized as legal in the United States
- She is at risk for abandonment for the incontinence—the typical response of men who force early pregnancy on child brides
- While the fistulas can be treated surgically, whether she can receive help is unclear since her status is unclear, there would be a cost to the surgery that she cannot afford, and there would be immigration issues until her status is clarified

Rectal Fistula/Perforation

On occasion, CSEC patients may present with anal trauma from rape with foreign objects and/or fisting. Fisting literally refers to the practice of placing one's fist into the rectum of another. In a case report, Delacroix et al. (2011) described rectal perforation occurring as the result of rape and fisting of a woman 16 years old. The following case illustrates the clinical issues for a CSEC victim.

CASE STUDY: TASHA

Tasha is a 15-year-old African American girl who presents in the ED with shivering, multiple abrasions, rectal bleeding, and fecal incontinence. She is withdrawn and frightened. After careful, nonjudgmental interviewing, she reports that she was fisted by a violent male customer who inserted his entire forearm into her rectum. She lay in severe pain in the fetal position for several hours and finally managed to make it to the ED. An IV was inserted for hydration and blood was drawn for drugs and STIs testing. Her condition deteriorated with increasing nausea and diffuse abdominal pain. Colposcopic examination and tomography revealed a two-inch laceration in the posterior aspect of the anus and free air and fluid in the abdominal cavity. Under general anesthesia, a sigmoidoscopy and exploratory laparoscopy were done and the tear repaired. A proximal sigmoid colostomy was used for temporary fecal diversion and successfully reversed within a year. She received follow-up treatment for STIs and was referred for counseling.

A 4-year-old girl presented to a sexual abuse clinic with severe penetrating trauma of vagina and rectum resulting in a recto-vaginal fistula, caused by her father roughly placing his penis and fingers into her mouth, vagina, and rectum. She was examined 2 months later where colposcopy revealed erythema to both labia, some hymenal tissue, thickened tissue along the perineum, and confluence between the vaginal and rectal orifices. The child was placed in protective custody and surgery delayed until legalities were finalized and her medical condition stabilized. A sigmoid colostomy was performed for fecal diversion and perineal structures were repaired. The surgery and outcomes were considered successful, though reversal of the colostomy was delayed until the anal sphincter became functional (Parra & Kellogg, 1995).

Injuries Resulting From Beatings and Torture by Traffickers

Beatings appear to occur so frequently that the effects are often considered minor injuries and not worthy of medical treatment. Some victims report that they treated fractured fingers, toes, cuts and abrasions themselves with over-the-counter (OTC) medications, or folk remedies (Anonymous, personal communication, 2011). Table 16.3 is a chart showing some substances that people might use in various cultures to treat the conditions for which they cannot obtain medical attention.

CSEC patients might present with multiple injuries from repeated beatings by exploiters. The medical and nursing care of patients with the following injuries is the same for CSEC patients as for any other patient, but follow-up would require comprehensive services specific to CSEC victims as described in other chapters in this book. After safety is ensured, mental health evaluation and therapy along with other social services and a long-term plan for vocational training would be important.

- Facial fractures: Might need surgery
- Other fractures: Casting or other immobilization, analgesics, antibiotics (if open fractures), teaching cast care, elevation, and ice for swelling
- Cuts and abrasions: Cleanse, bandage, provide antibiotics, teach follow-up care, and possible sutures
- Sprains and bruises: Protection of site, rest, ice, compression, and elevation
- Burns from hot water or cigarette or chemical burns: Determine if first, second, or third degree (may need to refer to a burn center). First-degree burns are red, with swelling, and pain. Second-degree burns are characterized by blisters, extreme redness, and intense pain and swelling. Third-degree burns cover an area over 3 inches or affect the hands, feet, buttocks, or are over a joint and appear charred-black or white and dry. If minor burn, cleanse with cool water (but not ice) and cover loosely with sterile dressing. Different products are used after cleansing, such as silver sulfadiazine cream. Do not apply egg-whites, butter, or oils that may cause infection. Elevate and administer tetanus shot. Minor burns usually heal without extensive treatment. If major burn, check airway, breathing, and circulation (ABCs) immediately as there may have been smoke inhalation (American Burn Association, n.d.; Mayo Clinic, n.d.; Ryssel et al., 2010).

TABLE 16.3 Herbal Treatment Chart

Health Issue	Herbal Treatment	How Used	Side Effects/Cautions
Anxiety	Omega 3 fatty acids (fish oil)	Oral supplement 3000 mg/day (FDA does not recommend higher doses)	Use cautiously if diabetic, pregnant, or taking blood thinners
	Chamomile	Oral supplements and teas	Allergic reactions have been noted in people with allergies to plants in the daisy family
	Lavender	Aromatherapy or essential oil applied to skin	Do not take by mouth May cause irritation
Dental Overall health, plaque	Probiotics	Oral ingestion in the form of dairy products	Generally safe; if on oral antibiotics take 2 hours apart
	Cranberry	Beverages or oral supplements	Generally safe
GI Indigestion, vomiting, and diarrhea	Turmeric	Oral ingestion in supplements or powder	Generally safe
	Cranberry	See above	Generally safe
	goldenseal	Teas and oral supplements	Safe for short-term use May interact with other medicines Not used in pregnancy or infants and children

(continued)

TABLE 16.3 Herbal Treatment Chart *(continued)*

Health Issue	Herbal Treatment	How Used	Side Effects/Cautions
Nausea	Ginger	Capsule, liquid, and topical	Safe in small doses
	Peppermint oil		Safe in small doses
Headaches	Riboflavin	Oral supplement (400mg/day) Prevents migraines	Generally safe
	Coenzyme Q 10	Oral supplements	Generally safe
	Feverfew	Oral supplements	Do not use if pregnant Allergic reactions seen in those with allergies to plants in the daisy family
	Butterbur	Oral supplements	Only use products that have pyrrolizidine alkaloids removed
Infections			
Bacterial	Tea tree oil	Topical application	Dilute to avoid skin irritation, do not swallow
Eye	Goldenseal	Oral tablet, teas, and extracts	Generally safe, undergoing research
			See above
Fungal	Tea tree oil	Topical application	See above
Upper respiratory	Echinacea	Oral	No side effects if taken orally, may cause allergic reaction in those with allergies to plants in daisy family

Condition	Herb	Form	Safety
Urinary tract	Cranberry	See above	
Vaginitis	Goldenseal	See above	
Inflammation	Turmeric	Oral supplement	Generally safe
Pregnancy (Nausea)	Ginger	Tablets, fresh teas and extracts	
Physical abuse/trauma			
Pain	Ginger	Tablets, fresh teas	Safe in small doses
Cigarette burns	Aloe vera	Gel	Safe for topical use
Rashes, and itching	Evening primrose oil	Capsule	Well tolerated in most
	Tea tree oil		
Sores/skin lesions	Aloe	Topical application	
Abrasions/wounds		Gel skin paste	
	Turmeric		Generally safe
Insomnia	Valerian	Oral supplements and teas	Generally safe in short-term use
	Melatonin	Oral supplements	

Adapted by Katrina Embrey, MSN, and RN from the following sources: U.S. Department of Health and Human Services, National Institutes of Health, National Center for Complementary and Alternative Medicine. (2010). *Herbs at a glance: A quick guide to herbal supplements* (NIH Publication NO. 10–6248). Retrieved from http://nccam.nih.gov/.

CASE STUDY: KARA

Kara is a 20-year-old woman who comes to your community-based clinic for pain medication and treatment for her right forearm, which is swollen, deformed, and painful. She says she was hit by a car but cannot describe the setting and says the car drove away but as you take her to x-ray, she says, "He didn't mean to do it." When you ask her who did not mean to do what, she becomes agitated, and wants to leave without treatment. You calmly explain that you do not wish to complicate her life but it will help the physician to know exactly what happened to her. She confides that she went home the previous night without enough money to make her quota and her pimp beat her, twisting her arm, throwing her across the room, kicking her, and standing on her arm while he burned her with cigarettes and berated her, calling her worthless, and threatening to kill her.

X-ray reveals fractures of the right ulna and radius and the physician explains that this kind of fracture almost always requires surgery in adults and she tells Kara she will refer for surgery. Kara strongly resists, saying that her pimp will kill her if she cannot work. Because she is over 18, she has the right to refuse protection as well as treatment. She begs the physician to cast her arm and the physician agrees when she realizes Kara is ready to leave without any treatment. Her anxiety level is high and she is in much pain. You cleanse and treat the burns and abrasions, administer pain medication, explain what she can do at home to relieve the pain, and try to get her to agree to stay and talk through the treatment options, but she tearfully thanks you and leaves. Afterward, you and the physician talk about how difficult it was to treat Kara, knowing there was not much you could do for her and how tempting it would have been to judge her as wanting the life she had. You resisted this impulse, though, and told her that the door was open for her to return to the clinic and that you would do what you could to help her if she did choose to return.

One of the most difficult things to understand about trafficking victims their resistance to rescue. Unless they are in a stage of change that enable them to take action, they are likely to sabotage efforts to help them. The rightly understand the risk of retaliation from their controllers who may hav threatened their families and certainly have threatened them. In this situatio the brutality of Kara's pimp is clearly demonstrated by her injuries; yet she not ready to make the break. Respecting her decision is to respect her and wh little control she has over her life. Leaving the door open may be all you can d

Incised/Stab Wounds

Victims of commercial sexual exploitation may be assaulted by the trafficker, buyer, or another person, and some assaults involve sharp force injury. Woun from sharp instruments (knives, scissors, and ragged glass, for example) may be described as "incised wounds" if they are longer than they are deep. If the wound depth is greater than the skin length, it is described as a "stab wound" (Saukko & Knight, 2004). Sharp force injuries differ in appearance from those resulting from blunt force trauma, the latter resulting from tearing (laceration) of the tissues, rather than cutting. An incised or stab wound typically has clean, nonabraded edges, and no bruising (unless the skin is impacted by the hilt of the knife). The ends may be blunt or tapered. Lacerations, on the other hand, have abraded, and often bruised edges. They may have a linear or irregular shape, and they are identifiable by the presence of tissue "bridging" within the wound. Because the tissues are torn irregularly, bits of fascia, vessels, and other tissues may remain intact, leaving tiny strands that cross from one side of the wound to the other. In contrast, the clean cut of a sharp object leaves no intact and bridging fragments. In reality, the difference between lacerations and sharp force injuries may be difficult to discern as objects may have both blunt and sharp characteristics. Thus, there is a spectrum of appearances from classic blunt to classic sharp force injury.

A detailed description of sharp force injuries is important to investigators, especially in as much as you are able to differentiate trauma from blunt versus sharp weapons. Measuring the location of the injury (centimeter from top of head, and from midline) is helpful, as is measurement of the wound itself. The latter is best done by gently reapproximating the edges of the wound before measuring, as tension from underlying muscle or Langers' lines may cause gaping and artificial shortening of the wound. Photographs of the wound are important, if feasible. If one can determine the direction and depth of the wound track, this should be documented. It is important to keep in mind that the depth of the track does not necessarily correspond to the length of the knife blade, as the full length of the blade may not have been inserted, and compression of tissue (e.g., the abdominal wall) may cause the length of the wound track to exceed the length of the blade. The appearance of the wound is influenced by movement of the body or blade during the assault, and by the depth of penetration of a tapered blade, and multiple wounds from the same weapon can look remarkably different. At times, the wound may be v-shaped, for example, if the blade has been twisted while entering/exiting the body.

Sharp force injuries may need surgical exploration and repair, depending on depth, and tissues involved. Superficial incised wounds without involvement of major vessels and nerves may be treated with simple suturing.

Gunshots

Victims of commercial sexual exploitation may experience a plethora of violent injuries, including gunshot wounds. When a victim presents with a penetrating injury from a firearm it is important to document characteristics of the wounds that will aid law enforcement in their investigation. If feasible in an emergent situation, the medical provider should note whether a penetrating injury appears to be an entrance versus exit wound (Table 16.4), and describe the characteristics of an entrance wound that help discern the range of discharge. Injuries from tight contact of the muzzle with the body have a different appearance than those resulting from a gun fired at close or distant range. With tight contact, the contents of the discharge are propelled into the tissues and very little, if any, leaks out to appear on the surrounding skin. There may be reddening of underlying tissue from the deposited carbon monoxide and soot within the soft tissues. If the wound involves skin overlying the bone, the tremendous gas expansion may split the skin of the entrance wound, leading to a cruciate appearance. In wounds resulting from a pistol shot at close range, soot and unburnt propellant flakes may be deposited on the skin, and burnt propellant may cause punctuate burns (tattooing) of the skin around the entrance wound. As the distance between pistol muzzle and skin increases, the appearance of soot diminishes (soot travels approximately 6–8 inches), and gradually tattooing disappears (propellant may travel approximately 12–18 inches). Wounds from firing distances greater than 16 to 24 inches typically lack soot, burning of the skin, and powder tattooing (Saukko & Knight, 2004).

Besides documenting the appearance of the entrance and exit wounds, medical staff should obtain photographs if at all possible. If there is unburnt powder around the entrance wound, a swab moistened with water may be rubbed on the skin to retrieve a sample; this helps investigators identify ammunition in the event that there is no retrievable bullet. In addition, it is important to provide information regarding wound location and wound track. Obtaining an exact measurement of the location of the wound relative to the top of the head and the midline allows estimation of the wound path (e.g., an entrance wound

TABLE 16.4   Characteristics of Entrance Versus Exit Wounds From Rifled Weapons

Entrance Wound	Exit Wound
Always present	May or may not be present (perforating versus penetrating injury); may be multiple "exit wounds" if bullet fragments or bone bits exit the body
Abrasion collar and frayed keratin ring around edge of wound	Usually no abrasion ring (unless skin supported by object such as belt)
Circular hole (unless tight contact overlying the bone, or distant discharge with tumbling bullet)	Varied shape (circular, slit-like, and irregular); often with everted edges
± Soot, tattooing, and unburnt propellant, depending on the range of discharge	No soot, tattooing, and unburnt propellant

50 cm below the top of the head, 8 cm right of midline on the anterior aspect of the body, compared to an exit wound 60 cm below the top of the head, and 4 cm left of midline on the posterior aspect of the body indicates a front to back, right to left, and downward direction of the bullet). It is important to note that this direction applies to the body in an anatomical position and does *not* necessarily indicate the position of the victim and assailant at the time the shot was fired. A downward trajectory may result from an assailant shooting downward at the victim, or from him/her shooting horizontally, with the victim bent over. In addition, if the bullet ricochets off the bone during its course through the body, the exit wound may not correspond to the original bullet path.

During surgical exploration, a note should be made of the tissues damaged, the size of the wound cavity, and the severity of injury. Any bullets retrieved should be handled with plastic instruments rather than metal ones, to avoid scratching the bullet and complicating future analysis. The bullet should be stored in a labeled container and submitted to law enforcement, maintaining the chain of custody. Clothing worn by the victim should also be made available to investigators.

SUMMARY

In this chapter the authors have presented common injuries that might appear in CSEC patients as they present for health care. Many of the interventions discussed are the responsibility of physicians rather than nurses, especially in the ED, but we maintain that nurses need to be knowledgeable about how to identify CSEC, collaborate with other staff in the ED, advise team members about best ways to interact with victims, and assist with appropriate referrals. The chapter on ED policies and procedures will elaborate on the roles of nurses in the ED, but all health professionals are encouraged to educate themselves about human trafficking and devise protocols for their own professions and settings.

REFERENCES

Alio, A. P., Merrell, L., Roxburgh, K., Clayton, H. B., Marty, P. J., Bomboka, L. et al. (2011). The psychosocial impact of vesico-vaginal fistula in Niger. *Archives of Gynecology and Obstetrics, 284,* 371–378.

American Burn Association. (n.d.). Retrieved July 7, 2012, from http://www.ameriburn. org/Preven/ScaldInjuryEducator'sGuide.pdf.

Delacroix, J., Brown, J., Kadenhe-Chiweshe, A., Bodenstein, L., Stimell-Rauch, M., & Lowe, T. (2011). Rectal perforation secondary to rape and fisting in a female adolescent. *Pediatric Emergency Care, 27*(2), 116–119.

Habek, D., & Kulas, T. (2007). Nonobstetrics vulvovaginal injuries: Mechanism and outcome. *Archives of Gynecology and Obstetrics, 275,* 95–97.

Hoffman, R. J., & Ganta, S. (2001). Vaginal laceration and perforation resulting from first coitus. *Pediatric Emergency Care, 17*(2), 113–114.

Ijaiya, M., Rahman, A., Aboyeji, A., Olatinwo, A., Esuga, S., Ogah, O. et al. (2010). Vesicovaginal fistula: A review of Nigerian experience. *West African Journal of Medicine, 29*(5), 293–298.

Khumar, A., Goyal, N., Das, S., Trivedi, S., Dwivedi, U., & Singh, P. (2009). Our experience with genitourinary fistula. *Urologia Internationalis, 82*(4), 404–410.

Kohli, N., & Miklos, J. (2003). Meeting the challenge of vesicovaginal fistula repair: Conservative and surgical measures. *OBG Management, 15*(8), 16–27.

Lentz, G. M. (2012). Pediatric and adolescent gynecology. *Comprehensive gynecology* (6th ed.) Philadelphia: Mosby.

Longombe, A. O., Claude, K. M., & Ruminjo, J. (2008). Fistula and traumatic genital injury from sexual violence in a conflict setting in Eastern Congo: Case studies. *Reproductive Health Matters, 16*(31), 132–141.

Mayo Clinic, Burns: First Aid. Retrieved June 20, 2012, from http://www.mayoclinic.com/health/first-aid-burns/FA00022.

McCann, J., Miyamoto, S., Boyle, C., & Rogers, K. (2007). Healing of hymenal injuries in prepubertal and adolescent girls: A descriptive study. *Pediatrics, 119,* e1094.

Merritt, D. F. (2009). Genital trauma in the pediatric and adolescent female. *Obstetrics and Gynecology Clinics of North America, 36*(1), 85–98.

Miklos, J. (1999). Laparascopic treatment of vesicouterine fistula. *The Journal of the American Association of Gynecologic Laparoscopists, 6*(3), 339–341.

Narcisi, L., Tieneber, A., Andriani, L., & McKinney, T. (2010). The fistula crisis in sub-Saharan Africa: An ongoing struggle in education and awareness. *Urologic Nursing, 30*(6), 341–346.

Onen, A., Ozturk, H., Yayla, M. et al. (2005). Genital trauma in children: Classification and management. *Urology, 65*(5), 987.

Parra, J., & Kellogg, N. (1995). Repair of a recto-vaginal fistula as a result of sexual assault. *Seminars in Perioperative Nursing, 4*(2), 140–145.

Rai, D. (2011). Women living with obstetric fistula and nurse's role in preventive measures. *International Journal of Nursing and Midwifery, 3*(9), 150–153.

Ryssel, H., Gazyakan, E., Germann, G., Hellmich, S., Riedel, K., Reichenberger, M. A. et al. (2010). Antiseptic therapy with a polylactic acid-acetic acid matrix in burns. *Wound Repair & Regeneration, 18*(5), 439–444.

Saukko, P., & Knight, B. (2004). *Knight's forensic pathology* (3rd ed.). New York: Oxford University Press.

Semere, L., & Nour, N. (2008). Obstetric fistula: Living with incontinence and shame. *Review of Obstetrics and Gynecology, 1*(4), 193–197.

Sturgiss, E. A., Tyson, A., & Parekh, V. (2010). Characteristics of sexual assaults in which adult victims report penetration by a foreign object. *Journal of Forensic Legal Medicine, 17*(3), 140–142.

Townsend, C. (2012). Gynecologic surgery. *Sabiston textbook of surgery* (19th ed., Chapter 71). Amsterdam: Saunders, An Imprint of Elsevier.

Turan, J., Johnson, K., & Polan, M. (2007). Experiences of women seeking medical care for obstetric fistula in Eritrea: Implications for prevention, treatment, and social reintegration. *Global Public Health, 2*(1), 64–77.

CHAPTER 17

Pediculosis, Scabies, and Tuberculosis: Effects of Overcrowding in Trafficked Children

REBECCA L. SHABO

*I*n addition to the sexual, physical, and emotional abuse that trafficked children may endure, they are also at risk for diseases due to housing situations. Trafficked children are often housed in dirty and crowded living conditions depriving them of living in a restful, clean environment (Farr, 2005; O'Connell Davidson, 2005). These living conditions, combined with poor nutrition, can precipitate the development of health conditions such as scabies, lice infestation, tuberculosis (TB), and other communicable diseases. Frontline health providers play an important role in identifying and treating these conditions but also in realizing that these conditions could be a warning sign of a child that is trafficked. Also, health providers should assess for these conditions in a child that is known to have been trafficked.

PEDICULOSIS

Head lice (*Pediculus humanus capitis*) are one of the most common types of human ectoparasites in children. Lice are wingless, 2 to 3 mm long, six-legged tan to grayish-white insects that crawl but cannot fly or jump (Frankowksi & Bocchini, 2010). Lice are quick crawlers, moving up to 23 cm/min (Ko & Elston, 2004). The life cycle of the head louse is approximately 25 to 26 days. A mature female louse can lay up to 10 eggs/day. The egg encasement (nit) attaches firmly to the human hair shaft near the scalp with a glue-like substance produced by the louse. The nymph hatches after a 7- to 10-day incubation period with the use of the host's body heat. Lice feed by sucking tiny amounts of blood from the human scalp every few hours. Head lice usually survive for less than 48 hours if away from the scalp (Meinking et al., 2010).

Pediculosis capitus (head lice infestation) does not pose a serious health threat but often causes significant discomfort due to severe itching and sensation of lice movement (Chosidow, 2000; Ko & Elston, 2004). This discomfort can interfere with rest, sleep, and learning. The infested child may not feel the effects of the lice for up to 6 weeks when sensitivity to the lice saliva develops (Downs, Harvey, & Kennedy, 1999; Meinking et al., 2002a). Secondary bacterial infections are also a possibility due to subsequent scratching and excoriation in response to these symptoms. On rare occasions, impetigo can develop and then local adenopathy could be present (Chunge, Scott, Underwood, & Zaverella, 1991).

Pediculosis is common in children aged 3 to 12 years of age, particularly if the children are in situations where they are in close contact. Girls are more likely to be affected than boys possibly due to their tendency toward sharing personal articles and having closer physical contact. Homeless children, children in shelters, or in overcrowded situations are at high risk for infestation (Estrada, 2003; Orion, Marcos, Davidovici, & Wolf, 2006). Head lice are most often transmitted by close contact with infested individuals and less often by indirect contact via hats, pillow, combs, or toys (Ko & Elston, 2004; Flinders & De Schweinitz, 2004; Frankowski & Bocchini, 2010).

Diagnosis

Diagnosis is made by visualizing a live louse in the hair or identifying nits. Using a louse comb may make it quicker and easier to locate a live louse due to their speed (Mumcuoglu, Friger, Ioffe-Uspensky, Ben-Ishai, & Miller, 2001). A microscope or magnifying glass is often helpful in diagnosis. Nits typically fluoresce white under Wood's light, which may aid in identification as well. Nits are often confused with dandruff, loose scabs, lint, or hair product residue. Nits, however, are difficult to remove from the shaft and typically are found 1 cm from the scalp. The nape of the neck and behind ears are common areas where nits adhere to hair. Bright light or sunlight may make it easier to visualize nits but live lice tend to crawl away from light. Scratch marks and inflammatory papules caused by secondary infection may be found on the scalp as well (Frankowski & Bocchini, 2010).

Treatment

Before modern insecticides were developed petroleum products and inorganic poisons were used to treat head lice infestation (Jones & English, 2003). Today available pediculosis capitus treatment includes prescription medications as well as over-the-counter (OTC) medications. Treatment should not be initiated unless there is a clear diagnosis of head lice. Improper use of these medications has been known to cause serious toxicity complications (Meinking, Taplin, Kalter, & Egerle, 1986). Another issue is the growing problem of resistance, which may be related to improper use of products, using the products in higher amounts or more frequently than recommended, and/or using the products when pediculosis is not present (Burkhart, 2004; Frankowski & Weiner, 2002; Hansen, 2000; Koch, Brown, Selim, & Isam, 2000; Magee, 1996). Unsafe uses of medications and home remedies have also been reported including the use of kerosene, insecticides, and other harmful products (Koch et al., 2000; Magee, 1996).

Manual removal of nits after treatment is recommended by some because none of the medications kill all of the eggs (Plastow et al., 2001). Removal of nits can be time consuming and tedious (Vander Stichele et al., 2002). Special lice combs that are fine toothed tend to make the procedure easier (Flinders & De Schweinitz, 2004; Plastow et al., 2001). One study suggested that pediculicides use alone is just as effective as when combined with manual removal (Meinking et al., 2002a).

Pediculocide Medications

Lindane (1%)

Lindane is an organochloride prescription shampoo available in a 1% concentration (Kwell) and is available only by prescription. Originally introduced in 1951, the U.S. Food and Drug Administration (FDA) recommends that lindane 1% only be used when other nonprescriptions options have been unsuccessful. Lindane has the potential of causing neurotoxicity and several cases of seizures have been reported with use (Frankowski & Bocchini, 2010). The FDA has warned that it should not be used in neonates and should be used with caution with any child, particularly those at risk for seizures or those with HIV infection (Burkhart, 2004). Also, lindane has developed a poor efficacy in the United States and some other areas due to resistance (Hansen, 2000; Meinking et al., 1986). When using the product it should be applied to the scalp, being careful to avoid the eyes and mucous membranes. It is left on for 4 min only and then rinsed thoroughly. A second application should not be applied (Frankowksi & Bocchini, 2010).

Malathion (0.5%)

Malathion, a prescription organophosphate (cholinesterase inhibitor), is marketed in a 0.5% concentration (Ovide). Malathion has high ovicidal activity (Meinking et al., 1986) and typically one application is effective. It is pediculicidal and partial ovicidal. Limited side effects reported for malathion include conjunctivitis and mild scalp irritation (Dodd, 2001; Jones & English, 2003) A concern of malathion is the high alcohol content (78% isopropyl alcohol) making it flammable. It also has the potential to cause respiratory depression if ingested. Caregivers must be cautioned to not smoke or use electrical heat sources such as hair dryers while using the hair product or while the hair is still wet with the product (Flinders & De Schweinitz, 2004). The product is contraindicated in children younger than 24 months and safety has not been established in children less than 6 years of age.

Benzyl Alcohol (5%)
Benzyl alcohol (5%) lotion (Ulesfia) is approved by the FDA for the treatment of head lice in children over 6 months of age by prescription only. Benzyl alcohol (5%) works by asphyxiation of head lice and is applied topically for 10 min and then rinsed thoroughly (Barker & Altman, 2010). It is a pediculicide but not an ovicide; therefore, a second treatment is recommended 7 to 10 days after the first treatment. Benzyl alcohol (5%) is not neurotoxic (Meinking et al., 2010). Common adverse reactions are minimal and include pruritus, erythema, and ocular irritation (Dodd, 2001; Jones & English 2003; Meinking et al., 2010).

Pyrethrins Plus Piperonyl Butoxide
Pyrethrins are naturally occurring pyrethroid extracts from the chrysanthemum plant and are combined with piperonyl butoxide for an OTC pediculocide treatment (Rid, Pronto). Pyrethrins are neurotoxic to lice but have not been found to be neurotoxic to humans. Allergic reactions are a concern for people who are allergic to chrysanthemums. The product is left on for 10 min and then rinsed thoroughly. Pyrethrins typically kill only 70% to 80% of eggs and therefore require a second treatment in 7 to 10 days. The effectiveness of pyrethrins have decreased since initially used in the 1980s due to resistance (Burkhart, 2004).

Permethrins 1%
Initially introduced as a prescription medication in 1986, permethrin 1% (Nix), a synthetic pyrethroid, was approved for over-the-counter use in 1990. Potential adverse effects are erythema, edema, and pruritis. Permethrin 1% lotion is applied to damp hair, left on for 10 minutes, and then rinsed thoroughly. A non-conditioning shampoo should be used before the treatment. Permethrin is a pediculocide but not an ovicide. It will continue to kill newly hatched lice for several days after treatment; however, silicone-based additives and conditioning agents in many hair products can interfere with effectiveness, thus requiring a second application if live lice are noticed in 7 to 10 days (Hansen, 2000; Meinking et al., 2002b). Owing to limited side effects, over-the-counter availability and low toxicity, many recommend permethrin 1% as a drug of choice for head lice in children over 2 months of age (Frankowski & Bocchini, 2010; Frankowski, & Weiner, 2002; Jones & English 2003).

Environmental Measures
When a child is diagnosed with head lice, all household members should be assessed as well and treated if the condition is present. Items that have been in contact with the child's affected head within the last 48 hr before treatment should be cleaned even though there is only a small risk for transmission. Head lice rarely live past 48 hours once detached from the warm scalp and blood supply (Orion et al., 2006). Clothing, bedding, and cloth toys can be washed in hot water (>130°F) and heat dried. Cloth items that cannot be washed can be placed in plastic bags for 2 weeks since any nymphs would

have died without a food source. Combs, brushes, and hair clips should be soaked in hot water for a minimum of 10 minutes. Furniture, carpets, and car seats can be vacuumed but pediculocide sprays are not recommended due to the potential toxic effects to children and/or pets (Flinders & De Schweinitz, 2004; Frankowksi & Bocchini, 2010).

SCABIES

Scabies is caused by infestation of the ectoparasite mite *Sarcoptes scabiei*. The life expectancy of a female mite is about 30 days. The mite is oval shaped and white with four pairs of legs. It is too small to be seen without magnification (Orion, Marcos, Davidovici, & Wolf, 2006). The mite burrows into the stratum corneum and deposits feces and lays eggs that hatch into larvae in 3 to 4 days. The mite sucks human tissue fluids for nourishment. Maturation to the adult larvae stage occurs in about 14 to 17 days (Flinders & De Schweinitz, 2004). Mites can only live about 3 days without a live host (Fawcett, 2003). The host's body begins to respond to the secretions of the mite, which are highly antigenic, within about 3 weeks of infestation. Factors including lack of hygiene, overcrowding, poor sanitary conditions, and geographical regions with high humidity and temperature can all play a role in increasing the risk of scabies infection.

Skin-to-skin contact with an infected person is the prominent route of transmission but scabies can be acquired through indirect infestation as well, such as shared clothes or linen. Clinical symptoms include pruritis, a papular rash that might include pustules, vesicles, nodules, and crusting. Excoriated crusted lesions are more common in immunocompromised children. The axillae, hands, feet, popliteal folds, inguinal area, wrists, elbows, and interdigital spaces are common sites in children (Flinders & De Schweinitz, 2004). The scalp is not a common site except in the case of immunocompromised patients or infants.

Diagnosis

Diagnosis is based on classic symptoms such as nocturnal pruritus, and location and appearance of rash or possibly the classic linear burrows of feces sometimes visible near lesions. The burrow appears as a small linear, grayish brown, threadlike line with a black dot at the end. Skin scrapings or material under fingernails can be observed via microscope for detection of the mite or eggs as well (Chosidow, 2000; Estrada, 2003). Scrapings are best obtained from interdigital areas or from flexor surfaces of the wrist. Potassium hydroxide is not used, because it will dissolve the mites, eggs, and feces. Instead a few drops of mineral oil are applied to a lesion before scraping it with the edge of a scalpel. Scabies can imitate other skin disorders such as contact dermatitis, insect bites, or atopic eczema (Orion, Matz, & Wolf, 2004). Misdiagnosis of the scabies rash is common resulting in the use of a topical steroid cream. This can lead to diffuse erythema and crusting of lesions (Flinders & De Schweinitz, 2004).

Treatment

Scabicides are the drug of choice for scabies infestation. Most topical treatments are applied to cool skin from the neck down after bathing and thoroughly drying skin. Care is given not to apply to eyes, mucous membranes, or the mouth. The creams or lotions should be applied evenly but thinly over the body. Lotions or creams are left on for several hours based on manufacturer specific instructions and then should be washed off thoroughly. Many are recommended to be repeated in 1 week. Pruritus may persist after treatment for several weeks until the stratum corneum is replaced and nodules may persist for months (Estrada, 2003; Orion et al., 2004). Antihistamines may be administered to help reduce pruritus.

Scabicide Medications

Lindane (1%)
Lindane 1% lotion (Kwell) is a prescription medication generally effective in treating scabies in children over 2 years but there is increased reporting of resistance (Orion et al., 2004). Also, lindane has the potential for neurotoxic effects and the risks of this are increased if the child has breaks in the skin or if it is applied improperly. Generally, lindane is not the drug of choice because of these risks. As with treatment of pediculosis capitus, patients should only be treated with lindane if other treatments fail and it should not be used on children at risk for seizures or with seizure disorders (Flinders & De Schweinitz, 2004).

Crotamiton (10%)
Crotamiton 10% (Eurax) is a scabicidal and antipruritic agent available as a cream or lotion for topical use by prescription only. Crotamiton (10%) is applied to the scabies lesions and is not removed for 24 hours. Mild burning or stinging may occur upon application. Eurax should be used with caution if the skin is broken or inflamed because of its potential to irritate (Parks & Smith, 1989). The treatment is repeated again in 24 hours (Orion et al., 2006).

Benzyl Benzoate
Benzyl benzoate 10% or 25% lotion is used widely around the world. This OTC compound is a product of benzoic acid and benzyl alcohol. This lotion should be washed thoroughly 12 to 24 hours after application and generally has few adverse reactions if used correctly except for skin irritation (Orion et al., 2006).

Permethrin (5%)
Permethrin 5% cream (Elimite) is considered by many health care providers to be the first-line therapy for children older than 2 months due to its high efficacy and low toxicity. Some studies show that use of OTC permethrin 5% results in less treatment failures than lindane or crotamiton with a lower risk of adverse effects (Strong & Johnstone, 2007).

Ivermectin

Evidence suggests that oral ivermectin may be a safe and effective treatment for scabies in adults; however, ivermectin is not FDA approved for this use (Pilger et al., 2010). Oral ivermectin has been reported effective in the treatment of crusted scabies and in adults with HIV. The mechanism of action of ivermectin is that it interrupts *Sarcoptes scabiei* neurotransmission. The dosage of ivermectin is 200 mcg/kg orally. It should be taken on an empty stomach with water. A total of two or more doses at least 7 days apart may be necessary to eliminate a scabies infestation (Fawcett, 2003). The safety of ivermectin in children weighing less than 15 kg and in pregnant women has not been established. Compared with topical benzyl benzoate in the treatment of scabies, ivermectin was at least as effective and led to more rapid improvement in one study (Sule & Thacher, 2007).

Environmental Measures

Transmission of scabies is mainly by close skin-to-skin contact with family members or through sexual contact (Strong & Johnstone, 2007). Live nits can be found on bed linens so it is imperative that all clothes, towels, and bed linens of the affected child and house members be washed in hot water (130°F or hotter) and dried in a hot dryer. Any items that cannot be washed should be sealed in a plastic bag for 5 days. If the environment is not treated then reinfestation is possible (Orion et al., 2006).

TUBERCULOSIS (TB)

TB is caused by *Mycobacterium tuberculosis*, an aerobic, acid-fast bacillus, and is spread through exposure to aerosolized droplets of an infected person (Cruz & Starke, 2010). After inhaling the droplets, they implant in either a bronchiole or alveolus and then multiply. After exposure to an infected person, the incubation period is 2 to 10 weeks. The bacteria *M. tuberculosis* invade tissues and cause inflammation, stimulating a T-cell-mediated immune response. This response can cause calcium deposits and cavities left by drained fluid called cavitations. Dry porous lung tissue (caseation) and even tissue death may ensue. Tuberculosis typically affects the respiratory system but also may spread to the genitourinary, gastrointestinal, neurological, cardiovascular, or lymphatic systems referred to as extrapulmonary TB. Erosion of blood vessels by the primary lesion can cause widespread dissemination to near and distant sites (military TB). Young children are susceptible to TB meningitis (Cruz & Starke, 2010). TB infection may remain dormant and latent or become active. In many areas of the world, the prevalence of TB is increasing due to the AIDS epidemic, which renders patients more vulnerable to TB infection. Close or prolonged exposure to high-risk adults is the main risk factor for TB acquired by youth (Swaminathan & Rekha, 2010). TB also disproportionately affects individuals from disadvantaged populations, including those who lack health care, are from low-income areas, are malnourished, and/or reside in areas with inadequate ventilation, thus rendering the trafficked child particularly vulnerable (Dharmadhikari, Gupta, Decker, Rag, & Silverman, 2009). TB affects boys and girls equally until adolescence when the disease becomes more common in girls.

Diagnosis

Diagnosis of TB among children and adolescents is complicated by several factors, including the absence of symptoms or the presence of nonspecific symptoms, and the difficulty in obtaining sputum samples in the very young. Diagnosis relies mainly on clinical presentation, tuberculin skin testing (TST), and chest x-rays. Diagnosis of TB is particularly difficult in human immunodeficiency virus (HIV)-infected youth because of the similarity in the symptoms caused by both diseases and the fact that the TST is less sensitive in immune-compromised patients (Marais, Gupta, Starke, & El Sony, 2010). Potential complications include multiorgan involvement, particularly of the lymph nodes and/or the central nervous system, and tuberculosis pneumonia.

The clinical presentation of TB in children and adolescents differs from that of TB in adults. Risk of developing active TB is higher in infants, young children, and older adolescents compared with children 5 to 14 years of age. The interval between infection and the onset of the active form of TB can be several months to years and activation of the latent form of TB to the active form is rare in children younger than 10 years (Swaminathan & Rekha, 2010). Most children with TB have the latent form and even those with abnormal x-rays are often asymptomatic. Further, this population is at increased risk of developing extrapulmonary TB.

Following TST, an induration of 5 mm or greater is generally interpreted as a positive test result and may reflect TB infection as early as 2 to 12 weeks after initial exposure (Menzies, Madhukar, & Comstock, 2007). Sputum culture and smear are used to diagnose active TB. Scant sputum production in children may make samples difficult to obtain, so bronchoscopy or early morning gastric washings may be necessary to obtain fluids (Reznik & Ozwah, 2005). Serum calcium and erythrocyte sedimentation rate (ESR) may be elevated. Pleural fluid analyses and staining may reveal elevated WBC, decreased glucose, and the presence of *M. tuberculosis*. Chest x-ray may reveal enlarged hilar lymph nodes, lung tissue cavitation (particularly in the lung apices), or atelectasis. Lymph node calcification may be seen. CT or MRI scans may show presence of lung damage (Cruz & Starke, 2010).

The bacillus Calmette-Guerin (BCG) vaccine is administered routinely in most countries, with the exceptions of the United States and the Netherlands. Vaccination has been shown to decrease the risk of life-threatening forms of infant TB. The BCG vaccine has not been proven effective outside the infant age group. False-positive results of a TST occur primarily in children exposed to nontuberculous mycobacteria or in those who have recently received a BCG vaccine (Menzies et al., 2007).

Treatment

Children with a positive exposure of TB are generally classified into one of three groups. The first group is children with an unknown diagnosis, possibly waiting on results of TST. The second group includes children with the diagnosis of latent TB (LTBI). They have a positive TST result but have no physical symptoms or radiographic findings consistent with TB. It is recommended that children with LTBI be treated with a course of medication to prevent the progression of future TB. The third group includes children with clinical symptoms of the disease. Patients in this group are treated with a multiple drug combination (Cruz & Starke, 2010).

Children with LTBI are typically treated with isoniazid (INH) for a 9-month course (Cruz & Starke, 2010; Gray, Zar, & Cotton, 2009). If the child is intolerant of INH then rifampin may be given for 6 months. Medication therapy for LTBI can be daily and self-administered or intermittent (2–3 times a week) and supervised through directly observed therapy (DOT). Self-administered intermittent therapy is not recommended because of the increased risk of missed dosages, thus increasing the chance of unsuccessful treatment and also encouragement of resistant isolates. This is particularly a concern in children suspected of being current victims of trafficking who may not return for future visits or be able to be located by public health workers.

Children diagnosed with TB disease have a higher organism burden, and the chance of their having resistant organism is higher than that of an adult. Therefore, any child suspected of having TB disease should be started on combination therapy. All cases of TB disease should have medication administered via DOT by a public health worker providing direct supervision of medication administration. The most common combination is the use of four medications: INH, rifampin, pyrazinamide (PZA), and ethambutol. These medications are known to have high efficacy and are generally well tolerated in children. Medications are administered daily for the first 2 to 4 weeks and then may be changed to biweekly. Younger children may develop medication intolerance and vomiting when switching to bi-weekly dosage and may benefit from staying on daily dosing. Treatment for TB is typically 6 months but may be up to 18 months or longer depending on the severity and location of the disease (Reznik & Ozwah, 2005).

The possibility of drug-resistant (DR) TB should be suspected if certain risk factors are present, including known DR-TB in a probable source case, a history of unsuccessful treatment or relapse with positive sputum smears after 2 months of the usual combination medication. Multidrug-resistant (MDR) TB is defined as resistance to at least two of the first-line TB medications, INH and rifampin (Marais et al., 2010).

Children infected with both HIV and TB present with a number of treatment challenges. These include higher mortality rates; increased likelihood of poor absorption of TB medications; drug–drug interactions between rifampin and many antiretrovirals (protease inhibitors and nonnucleoside reverse transcriptase inhibitors); and worsening of symptoms after initiating symptoms due to an altered immune inflammatory response (Gray et al., 2009). Sex trafficked girls in brothel-type situations confront extraordinary risks of acquiring both TB and HIV through close contact of others housed with them (Dharmadhikari et al., 2009). Treatment of an HIV-infected child who also has TB should be directed by subspecialists experienced in the care of both diseases.

The child on TB medications should be assessed closely for side effects, including liver toxicity (from pyrazinamide, rifampicin, or INH), and optic neuritis including color blindness (from ethambutal). The caregiver should be informed to report any side effects or adverse reactions. Children should be monitored monthly while receiving therapy to document medication tolerance, adherence, and symptoms of disease (Marais et al., 2010). Chest radiography should be repeated 1 to 2 months after treatment is initiated. Nutritional status and weight should be watched closely, plus encouraging a healthy well-balanced diet as well as adequate hydration.

Preventive Measures and Prognosis

TB is a mandatory reporting disease. The local public health department should be contacted to help determine sources and screen other contacts. Younger children with active disease may not need to be isolated due to insufficient cough and low organism burden in the airways. Older children and adolescents, however, may need to be isolated from those not exposed until effective therapy has been initiated, cough has diminished, and sputum AFB (acid-fast bacilli) smears convert to negative. Prevention practices involve proper identification and management of individuals and contacts with LTBI and active disease (Loeffler, 2003). The prognosis of preventing future disease in LTBI children is close to 100% in those who adhere to prescribed therapy. Prompt treatment of active disease in children with drug susceptible TB disease results in cure rates between 95% and 100% (Cruz & Starke, 2010).

CASE STUDY: FELICIA

Felicia is a 12-year-old Hispanic girl rescued from a child trafficking ring 3 days ago. She was born in an urban area of the United States and has never been outside this country. It is suspected that her mother, who cannot be located, sold her to a trafficking ring 2 years ago. Along with symptoms of physical, sexual, and emotional abuse, she also has complications from living in an overcrowded living situation. She reported sleeping on a mat on the floor of a small room with 12 other girls and was rarely given the chance to bathe or wear clean clothes. She is currently living in a temporary foster group home.

(continued)

After her initial assessment and emergency care 3 days ago, she has returned for a follow-up visit and reading of TST with the foster mother from the group home. She is small for age and withdrawn. She is scratching her scalp and arms and appears restless. The foster mother reports that she has been putting hydrocortisone cream on the rash since she arrived 3 days ago but the rash has worsened and the itching has increased at night. Her initial chest radiology was within normal limits and revealed no signs of hilar or mediastinal adenopathy, infiltrates, atelectasis, pleural effusions, cavities, or military disease. Initial HIV testing, hepatitis, and rapid sputum results were negative. Urinalysis and serum results are within normal limits.

Upon assessment she is noted to be at the 25th percentile for height and below the 3rd percentile for weight. Her cardiovascular, neurological, and abdominal assessments are within normal limits. Breath sounds are clear to auscultation bilaterally. A papular rash covers most of her arms and abdomen as well as her wrists, popliteal folds, and interdigital spaces. She also has a few pustules and some grayish-black burrows on her wrists. Scrapings are gently removed from her wrist with the dull edge of a scalpel. Microscopic exam reveals evidence of scabies infestation. Her scalp has scratch marks and several grayish-white nits are noted on hair shafts at the nape of her neck and behind both ears. Her TST site reveals induration of 10 mm at 72 hours.

APPLICATION OF BEST PRACTICES

Felicia and her foster mother are notified that she has head lice, scabies, and a positive TST and the plan of care is reviewed with them. OTC permethrin 1% (Nix) is prescribed for Felicia's pediculosis capitis. She and her foster mother are instructed to apply to damp hair that was first shampooed with a nonconditioning shampoo. The product should be left on for 10 minutes and then rinsed thoroughly. Combing through her hair with a fine toothed comb may be useful in removing old nit casings or some live nits. The treatment should be repeated in 9 days but should not be repeated again after the second application.

OTC permethrin 5% (Elimite) is prescribed for Felicia's scabies infestation. They are instructed to apply the Elimite to cool dry skin after bathing from the neck down, being careful to include all areas, including interdigital areas and folds. After leaving on for 8 to 14 hours, rinsed thoroughly. The hydrocortisone cream should be stopped. An OTC antihistamine can be given to decrease itching such as oral diphenhydramine (Benadryl) 25 mg every 8 hours. Felicia and her foster mother are told that the itching may persist for several weeks after the treatment as the skin continues to heal.

Special environmental instructions are given to Felicia and her foster mother due to the ectoparasitic infections. All towels, linens, and clothing should be washed in hot water (130° or hotter) as well as Felicia's combs, brushes, and hair ornaments. Any items that cannot be washed should be placed in an enclosed plastic bag for 2 weeks. Carpets, car upholstery, and furniture should be vacuumed thoroughly to remove any fallen nits. Felicia's foster mother was assessed and did not exhibit any signs of lice or scabies at this time. She was instructed to check all other family members and they would need to be treated as well if symptoms develop. Felicia does not share a bed with any foster family members.

Because Felicia's TST is positive but she has no other signs of tuberculosis disease at this time she is considered to have LTBI. Felicia and her foster mother are given this information and informed that she will need to begin taking INH (10–15 mg/kg/d) for 9 months to prevent the active disease from developing. Her liver function will be evaluated for hepatic toxicity while on the medication. The significance of taking the medication daily and not skipping any dosages is explained and emphasized. The local health department is notified of the diagnosis of LTBI and they will evaluate for the potential need for DOT intermittent therapy as well as any possible sources.

Felicia is placed on a liquid nutritional supplement and she is referred to a nutritionist for detailed diet planning due to her being significantly underweight. Felicia and her mother are also told that proper hydration is important especially since she will be taking INH. She will be followed on a monthly basis while on the medication. If problems with lice and scabies are not resolved or if any adverse effects are noticed from taking the medication, then she will be followed more frequently. She will continue to be followed by gynecological and pediatric mental health specialists as well as a social worker.

REFERENCES

Barker, S. C., & Altman, P. (2010). A randomized, assessor blind, parallel group comparative efficacy trial of head lice in children—Melaleuca oil and lavender oil, pyrethrins and piperonyl butoxide, and a "suffocation" product. *BMC Dermatology, 10*, 1–7.

Burkhart, C. G. (2004). Relationship of treatment-resistant head lice to the safety and efficacy of pediculicides. *Mayo Clinic Proceedings, 79*, 661–666.

Chosidow, O. (2000). Scabies and pediculosis. *Lancet, 355*, 819–826.

Chunge, R. N., Scott, F. E., Underwood, J. E., & Zaverella, K. J. (1991). A review of the epidemiology, public health importance, treatment and control of head lice. *Canadian Journal of Public Health, 82*, 196–200.

Cruz, A. T., & Starke, J. R. (2010). Pediatric tuberculosis. *Pediatrics in Review, 31*(13), 1–13.

Dharmadhikari, A. S., Gupta, J., Decker, M., Rag, A., & Silverman, J. (2009). Tuberculosis and HIV: A global menace exacerbated via sex trafficking. *International Journal of Infectious Diseases, 13*, 543–546.

Dodd, C. S. (2001). Interventions for treating head lice. *Cochrane Database of Systems Review*, CD001165. Doi: 10.1002/14651858.CD001165.pub2.

Downs, A. M., Harvey, I., & Kennedy, C. T. C. (1999). The epidemiology of head lice and scabies in the UK. *Epidemiology & Infections, 122*, 471–477.

Estrada, B. (2003). Ectoparasitic infestations in homeless children. *Seminars in Pediatric Infectious Disease, 14*(1), 20–24.

Farr, K. (2005). *Sex trafficking: The global market in women.* New York, NY: Worth Publishers.

Fawcett, R. S. (2003). Ivermectin use in scabies. *American Family Physician, 68*(6), 1089–2003.

Flinders, D. C., & De Schweinitz, P. (2004). Pediculosis and scabies. *American Family Physician, 69*(2), 341–348.

Frankowski, B. L., & Bocchini, J. A. (2010). Head lice. *Pediatrics, 126*(2), 392–403.

Frankowski, B. L., & Weiner, L. B. (2002). Committee on School Health, Committee on Infectious diseases, American Academy of Pediatrics. Head lice. *Pediatrics, 110,* 638–643.

Gray, D. M., Zar, H., & Cotton, M. (2009). Impact of tuberculosis preventive therapy on tuberculosis and mortality in HIV-infected children. *Cochrane Database of Systematic Reviews, 1,* CD006418.

Hansen, R. C. (2000). Working groups on the treatment of resistant pediculosis. Guidelines for the treatment of resistant pediculosis. *Contemporary Pediatrics, 17*(Suppl), 1–10.

Jones, K. N., & English, J. C. (2003). Review of common therapeutic options in the US for the treatment of pediculosis capitis. *Clinical of Infectious Disease, 36*(11), 1355–1361.

Ko, C. J., & Elston, D. M. (2004). Pediculosis. *Journal of American Academy of Dermatology, 50*(1), 1–11.

Koch, T., Brown, M., Selim, P., & Isam, C. (2000). Towards the eradication of head lice: Literature review and research agenda. *Journal of Clinical Nursing, 10,* 364–371.

Loeffler, A. M. (2003). Pediatric tuberculosis. *Seminars in Respiratory Infections, 18*(4), 272–291.

Magee, J. (1996). Unsafe practices in the treatment of pediculosis capitis. *Journal of School Health, 12*(1), 17–20.

Marais, B. J., Gupta, A., Starke, J. R., & El Sony, A. (2010). Tuberculosis in women and children. *Lancet, 375,* 2051–2059.

Meinking, T. L., Clineschmidt, C. M., Chen, C., Kolber, M. A., Tipping, R. W., Funek, C. I. et al. (2002a). An observer-blinding study of 1% permethrin crème rinse with and without adjunctive combing in patients with head lice. *Journal of Pediatrics, 141,* 665–670.

Meinking, T. L., Serrano, L., Hard, B. et al. (2002b). Comparative in-vitro pediculicidal efficacy of treatments in a resistant head lice population on the US. *Archives of Dermatology, 138*(2), 220–224.

Meinking, T. L., Taplin, D., Kalter, D. C., & Egerle, M. W. (1986). Comparative efficacy of treatments for pediculosis capitis infestations. *Archives of Dermatology, 122*(3), 267–271.

Meinking, T. L., Villar, M. E., Vicaria, M., Eyerdam, D. H., Paquet, D., Mertz-Rivera, K., Rivera, H. F., Hiriart, J., & Reyna, S. (2010). The clinical trials supporting benzyl alcohol lotion 5% (Ulesfia): A safe and effective topical treatment of head lice (pediculosis humanus capitis). *Pediatric Dermatology, 27*(1), 19–24.

Menzies, D., Madhukar, P., & Comstock, G. (2007). Meta-analysis: New tests for the diagnosis of latent tuberculosis infection: Areas of uncertainty and recommendations for research. *Annals of Internal Medicine, 146*(5), 340–354.

Mumcuoglu, K. Y., Friger, M., Ioffe-Uspensky, I., Ben-Ishai, F., & Miller, J. (2001). Louse comb versus direct visual examination for the diagnosis of head louse infestations. *Pediatric Dermatology, 18*(1), 9–12.

O'Connell Davidson, J. (2005). *Children in the global sex trade*. Cambridge, UK: Polity Publishing.

Orion, E., Marcos, B., Davidovici, B., & Wolf, R. (2006). Itch and scratch: Scabies and pediculosis. *Clinics in Dermatology, 24*, 168–175.

Orion, E., Matz, H., & Wolf, R. (2004). Ectoparasitic sexually transmitted diseases: Scabies and pediculosis. *Clinics in Dermatology, 22*, 513–519.

Parks, B. R., & Smith, D. (1989). Pediatric drug information: Treatment of head lice and scabies infestations in children. *Pediatric Nursing, 15*(5), 522–524.

Pilger, D., Heukelbach, J., Khakban, A., Oliveira, F. A., Fengler, G., & Feldmeier, H. (2010). Household-wide ivermectin treatment for head lice in an impoverished community: Randomized observer-blinded controlled trial. *Bulletin of the World Health Organization, 88*, 90–96.

Plastow, L., Luthra, M., Powell, R., Wright, J., Russell, D., & Marshall, M. (2001). Head lice infestation: Bug busting vs. traditional treatment. *Journal of Clinical Nursing, 10*, 775–783.

Reznik, M., & Ozwah, P. O. (2005). A prudent approach to screening for and treating tuberculosis. *Contemporary Pediatrics, 22*(11), 73–88.

Strong, M., & Johnstone, P. W. (2007). Interventions for treating scabies. *Cochrane Database of Systematic Review, 3*, CD000320.

Sule, H. M., & Thacher, T. D. (2007). Comparison of ivermectin and benzyl benzoate lotion for scabies in Nigerian patients. *American Journal of Tropical Medicine and Hygiene, 76*(2), 392–395.

Swaminathan, S., & Rekha, B. (2010). Pediatric tuberculosis: Global overview and challenges. *Clinical Infectious Diseases, 50*(3), 184–194.

Vander Stichele, R. H., Gyssels, L., Bracke, C., Meersschaut, F., Blokland, I., Wittouchk, E. et al. (2002). Wet combing for head lice: Feasibility in mass screening, treatment preference and outcome. *Journal of the Royal Society of Medicine, 95*, 348–352.

CHAPTER 18

Policy and Procedures Guide for Emergency Departments and Community-Based Clinics

MARY DE CHESNAY AND NANCY CAPPONI

*T*his chapter will focus on how health care providers can recognize and intervene when trafficking victims present in the settings they are likely to use for
health care: emergency departments (ED) and community-based clinics. Some
traffickers have relationships with physicians or others with some health care
training and who practice in private offices or back rooms. They may or may
not be licensed in this country. The latter practices are often supported by the
traffickers who pay for health providers to look the other way when treating
the victims. However, for the most part, trafficking victims will appear in the
ED with major injuries or illnesses. Unless the staff are knowledgeable about trafficking, they will not know how to recognize and treat these patients.

Human trafficking does not appear to be in the minds of ED and free clinic
personnel who often work under chaotic and difficult conditions trying to treat
a variety of patients. Certainly the literature is lacking on how to recognize and
treat this vulnerable population and nursing and medical schools do not teach
how to work with victims of trafficking. Few nurses have written about the
health care issues of the population. Among them are Sabella (2011), Thomas
(2011), and Trout (2010). Yet, in a San Francisco study examining the heaviest
uninsured users of ED services, 40 were found to be prostitutes, costing the
agencies $5 million per year (Hughes, 2004). In another study of 200 women
in San Francisco from 10 years old to over 21 with 70% being under 21, the
level of injuries was severe with 70% of the 200 prostitutes studied stating
that they had been raped an average of 31 times by men who did not want to
pay or "just got off on it" (Silbert & Pines, 1981). Whether victims of forced

labor or sex trafficking, these patients experience injuries similar to victims of intimate partner violence and, like domestic violence patients, may avoid disclosing the nature and origin of their injuries due to fear of further harm by their exploiters.

Prevention

People who control their own bodies, money, nutrition, and living arrangements can be taught strategies for primary prevention of illnesses and injuries. For example, wearing condoms to prevent sexually transmitted infections (STIs) is not an option for sex trafficking women and children whose pimps receive more money for sex without condoms. Delaying pregnancy until later adolescence is not an option for child brides, a common occurrence in Africa, Pakistan, and India. Sanitation and nutritious food is not an option for migrant laborers who live in close quarters with others, sleep on cots with 50 men in a room, and are given only diluted soup or rice twice a day.

Minor Injuries or Illnesses

Many sex-trafficked women and children report that they have no way to obtain medical care for simple injuries or illnesses or chronic conditions. One patient told me that her pimp broke her finger during a beating when she failed to earn her quota that night. She had no first-aid training and her pimp was not about to take her to the ED, but somehow she knew that it hurts less if she immobilized it so she duct-taped it to the next finger. Another patient overdosed on aspirin when she tried to keep working with severe back pain. When asked about her suicide attempt, she denied that she tried to kill herself and said that she was a streetwalker who was forced to wear stiletto heels and her pimp would not allow her to wear low heels until her back felt better.

Victims who present in the ED or free clinics tend to be those with severe injuries, pain, or illness because they have not had the opportunity to seek help when their condition is less severe. When they present in the ED they may also not be able to ask for help escaping. In fact they may actively resist attempts to "rescue" them from a life they view as their only choice. They are usually accompanied by the pimp/trafficker, or a trusted accomplice called a "bottom girl." This person can be trusted to protect the pimp from exposure and make sure the girl returns to work. Unless the staff are aware of the signs of trafficking, have procedures in place to intervene safely, and have resources for the victims, they will perpetuate the tragic lives of the victims. This chapter will present assessment strategies and suggest procedures that can be adapted by nurse managers at such settings. Recommended policy information is found in Appendices A, B, C, and D and a curriculum plan is found in Appendix E. Managers are encouraged to read these critically and adapt the materials for their own agencies in such a way as to be consistent with the American Nurses' Association Code of Ethics (ANA, 2010).

RECOGNITION

Assessment tools and suggested protocols for approaching potential victims of human trafficking are available and will be discussed in this chapter and the chapter by Crane, but they are useless if the staff does not recognize the need to look for trafficking symptoms in specific patients. In this chapter, we present some common aspects of how patients might present and what to do when trafficking is suspected.

How do health care providers know to ask the right questions? Victims of sex trafficking may look like any other young patients. Dress alone is not a reliable indicator. The stereotypical costume of stiletto heels or platform sandals, short shorts, and bra-like tops is worn by many teenagers; yet, when prostituted children present in the ED, they may dress more conservatively so as not to draw attention to themselves.

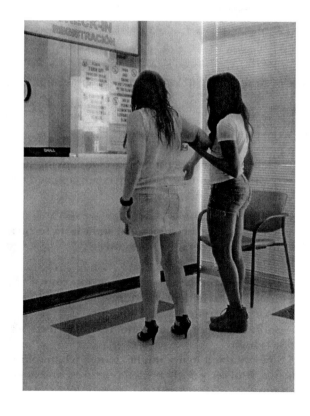

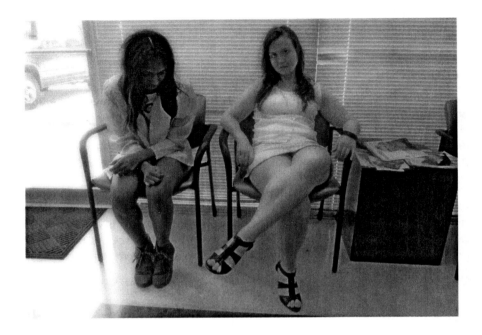

ED nurses are accustomed to do what they call "an across-the-room assessment." This technique incorporates observation of the patient before they even greet or touch the person. For trafficking victims, a nurse might notice the following red flags:

- Older man or woman with a young patient
- Accompanying person dominates
- Patient seems to defer or cower before the accompanying person
- Patient seems withdrawn, frightened, or conversely agitated with signs of high anxiety such as nail biting or fidgeting.

Once the nurse is with the patient, additional indicators to observe serve as a guide for the staff to ask more detailed questions:

- Accompanied by a companion who attempts to control the interview by answering questions for the patient or offering to translate
- Eyes downcast—poor eye contact with providers
- Minimal conversation with providers and fearful affect; alternately might appear hostile or "tough"
- Vague story of how obtained injury might change when told to different staff
- Old injuries such as bruises, poorly healed fractures, and abrasions
- Evidence of self-mutilation (small cuts on arms or legs)

- Presence of tattoos of names—many pimps brand their victims with their own names
- Bad teeth

These characteristics can be observed without direct questions by the staff. If any of the above is present, the staff should ask some key questions to determine if the person is a victim of trafficking or another type of abuse.

The careful attention needed by commercially sexually exploited children (CSEC) places additional stress on already burdened EDs. In communities without easy access to children's advocacy centers, it would be helpful to be able to triage CSEC and other pediatric victims of sexual assault to determine urgency of assessment and treatment. Floyed, Hirsh, Greenbaum, and Simon (2012) conducted a retrospective case record review of 163 cases of pediatric sexual assault of prepubescent children to develop a screening tool that can be used to decide quickly that sexual assault pediatric patients do not require immediate ED screening if timely follow-up can be arranged. While they recommend prospective testing on their tool, the investigators do seem to have a quick screening tool that could be used to determine whether immediate emergency care is needed based upon the following: (a) incident happened within past 72 hours and included oral contact, genital–genital contact, or genital–anal contact, (b) presence of genital or rectal pain, bleeding or discharge, or known genital injury, (c) immediate concern for child's safety, and (d) an unrelated emergency medical condition.

Safety and Rapport

Disrupting the business of human trafficking to provide services to victims is inherently risky and precautions must be taken for both victims and staff (IOM, 2007). Unlike "regular" patients who also come to the ED or clinic in pain and fear, sex trafficking victims have a lower level of trust and do not live in a safe environment where they can count on family and friends to help them. They know we are busy and have many patients to help and do not have reason to trust that we will make their needs a priority. It is critical to be sensitive to their special circumstances.

The first consideration is to create a safe environment to conduct the assessment. Safety involves both the patient and the staff. Protecting the staff is a critical aspect of any agency policy. While traffickers are not likely to be threatening to the staff initially, they walk a fine line between getting help for their victim and protecting their investment.

Safety for the Patient

Find a way to separate the patient from anyone who accompanied her. You can say that hospital policy is to examine patients alone and you need the other person to complete paperwork. If the person resists and argues, simply walk the patient down the hall for a urine sample or to draw blood. While doing this, you can ask the three key questions below. Speak respectfully and nonjudg-mentally. Ask permission to conduct each step of the physical exam as a way of showing respect—they do not control their own bodies and will appreciate this gesture. Slow down the process and take your time with them. Explain pro-cedures before touching the patient. Some patients are quite comfortable with touch; others are not. One patient reported that a nurse hugged her and that was the kindest thing anyone had done in a long time. Another, though, shied away from being touched. Be empathetic without showing pity. Avoid invasive questions about the details of her abuse. This is a time for assessment and refer-ral, not psychotherapy.

Safety for Staff
If a security guard is available, ask the person to be inconspicuous but nearby while the patient is in the agency. Larger agencies may have many staff and a formal policy on dealing with violent patients. Smaller agency staff need to be particularly careful not to frighten the victim into leaving before treatment or to alienate the accompanying person. It may be necessary to involve law enforcement.

Establishing Rapport
A caring, nonjudgmental attitude is the key to establishing rapport with traffick-ing victims (Cooper et al., 2007). If the patient is an immigrant, she may lack understanding of American health care systems and be likely to fear authorities since the traffickers control victims with threats of deportation if they try to escape. Even American patients may fear disclosure. Until law enforcement is educated about trafficking and services for victims are in place, arrest and deten-tion may be the only option to rescue victims.

Observation of nonverbal behavior is critical to establishing rapport because it allows the nurse to pace the interview by backing-off from questions that raise the anxiety level too high. Pay attention to the patient's nonverbal com-munication. Does she maintain a closed posture? Is her tone of voice soft and depressed or loud and hostile? Does she fidget when certain questions are asked? Does her tone or story change when asked about her presenting problem? All of these responses should be noted and charted.

Identification
Several sources have described ways to identify victims of sex trafficking (Clawson, 2008; Polaris Project, 2012; Rescue and Restore, 2006). These are listed in several chapters in the book, particularly the chapter by Crane, who helped to develop the identification protocols. In a busy ED or other clinical prac-tice setting, it is likely that there will not be time for a lengthy interview. The fol-lowing questions might serve as a quick, initial way to determine if further interviewing for CSEC is needed. These questions are not definitive but can be asked quickly and quietly in a way that does not threaten the patient and the

responses would be reason to ask further questions. These questions should never be asked in the presence of the accompanying person, however.

1. Can you come and go whenever you like?
2. Do you control your own money and identification?
3. Do you have to ask permission of anyone for how you spend your time?

If these answers indicate that someone else is in control of her time, freedom of movement, or money, then further exploration is necessary. Whether the patient is an American or immigrant, she probably does not control her money and identification. Expect young victims to claim to be older but they probably will not have a driver's license even if they are old enough to drive. Sometimes the foreign-born are brought in legally for what they believe are legitimate jobs. When they arrive on legal visas, their passports are held by the traffickers until they pay-off their debt, but their debt escalates and will never be paid. Traffickers charge for every item or service. Some victims have said they are charged for a place to sleep, every blanket or pillow, and every glass of water.

Trafficking victims do not control their time and schedules. They are forced to work long hours and prostituted women may be disoriented to time and place from sleep deprivation and malnourishment. As a means of control, pimps tend to have many rules, including such trivial rules as how much toilet paper to use, what kind of dress they must wear (no underwear), when they are allowed to bathe, and what and when they can eat.

If they are not locked up during their nonworking time periods, they are not likely to be free to come and go. They might be assigned other responsibilities by the pimp such as care of children born to the pimp and women in his "stable." Look for evidence of handcuffs or rope burns around the wrists and ankles. For a detailed plan for identification and assessment, review the chapter by Crane.

Policy

The characteristics of a good policy are that it states the rule regarding the phenomenon, that the procedures for implementing the policy are clear, and that the policy reaches the right people. Avoid jargon and "legalese" and use language that anyone who is expected to adhere to the policy can understand.

For a policy designed to service human trafficking patients, there should be a statement of definition so that the staff can recognize human trafficking, a purpose statement that explains why the policy is needed, and a statement of the rule, that is, how patients are to be treated in that agency. The procedures or protocols to be followed can be incorporated into one policy document or written as a separate document. In the example that we provide in Appendix A at the end of this book, we used one document.

Procedures

Procedures will vary according to the organizational culture, but there are several key factors that any agency that treats human trafficking patients should include: (a) training of staff to recognize the signs of human trafficking, (b) providing safety for patient and staff, (c) differentiating victims of trafficking from patients who have experienced other forms of child abuse or intimate partner violence, (d) referring for follow-up, and (e) reporting to authorities.

The minimal training that ED staff should receive is contained in Appendix E. The curriculum plan is designed to be a short lecture discussion that can be given in 30 minutes by anyone in the community who has knowledge of sex trafficking. Social workers, victim service advocates, and employees of child advocacy centers are likely to be experienced at working with this population. Nurses and physicians who have treated patients and survivors who work for shelters are also good resources. However, even nurses who have not specifically worked with these patients could review this book and develop a plan for sharing the basic information with other staff.

Providing safety is critical for both patient and staff. Patients should never be interviewed or asked to disclose in front of the accompanying person. Security personnel should be deployed to the ED if a suspected victim of human

CASE STUDY: STARR

Starr is a 14-year-old Caucasian victim of a trafficker who has moved her around the country for 4 years. Originally from Chicago, she was sold at age 10 by her father to pay gambling debts. She has a history of numerous STIs plus one pregnancy; the baby was taken by her pimp to be sold on the black market. Across-the-room observation reveals that she is submissive to the man who accompanies her, has a frightened look, and hunches over as if she is in great pain. She appears unkempt and malnourished. Presenting problem in ED is numerous abrasions, hematomas, a fractured right clavicle, and head trauma from an alleged car accident. The injuries are not consistent with a car accident, and you suspect she has been beaten. Her laboratory values for red blood cell count, hemoglobin, and hematocrit indicate dehydration. You suspect that she is a trafficking victim and decide you need to talk with her alone to get more information. You manage to convince the man that you need to take her for a CT scan and she discloses that her pimp brought her to the ED after she was severely beaten by a "john." You and the ED physician treat her medically and implement your hospital's policy, which is to notify the ED supervisor who consults briefly with the nursing and medical staffs to formulate a referral. The referral goes to two places: the local police and, because Starr is under the age of majority (18), protective services are also notified.

trafficking appears. Managers of the ED usually have a good relationship with local police and should work closely with law enforcement and the prosecutor's office not just to ensure safety, but also to collect evidence in a way that ensures chain of custody. Adapting the psychiatric liaison model for trafficking patients would help provide a safe environment for the patient to disclose. If the agency has a psychiatric unit, those nurses should work in partnership with ED nurses when trafficking victims appear. Most hospitals would not have a psychiatric unit, but there should be a social worker available to facilitate follow-up.

Differential diagnosis of human trafficking from child abuse and intimate partner violence is easy to establish if the nurse can ask the right questions. The key is commercial exploitation. The trafficker forces or coerces the victim to sell her body for sex. Child sex abusers or intimate partners force sex for their own needs. However, they sometimes do force the victim to have sex with another and if goods or money changes hands, this would fall under the human trafficking definition.

In terms of follow-up, the system of care model is best. A collaborative network of community partners who can jointly develop policies and procedures for the community provides the community focus that is needed to abolish modern slavery in a community. Law enforcement, prosecutors, business community, social services, and medical personnel all have vital roles to play.

Starr's prognosis is good if she can be permanently separated from her pimp and provided with follow-up services to heal her physical and emotional scars. Close coordination among law enforcement, medical personnel, and social services is vital for Starr. If she is placed in a residence with people who do not understand the nature of forced prostitution or in a place that cannot guarantee safety from her pimp, she may sabotage efforts to help her and return to her pimp. The known is less frightening than the unknown.

SUMMARY

In this chapter, we presented information designed to help ED nurses recognize and treat victims of human trafficking. The appendices include a policy and procedures document that can be adapted for the reader's agency and a brief training program outline that can be used to orient ED staff about the problem of human trafficking.

REFERENCES

American Nurses Association (ANA). (2010). *Code of ethics for nurses with interpretive statements*. Silver Spring, MD: Nursesbooks.org.

Cooper, S. W., Estes, R. J., Giardino, A. P., Kellogg, N. D., & Vieth, V. I. (2007). *Quick reference child sexual exploitation for healthcare, social services, and aw enforcement professionals*. St. Louis, MO: G. W. Medical Publishing, Inc.

Clawson, H. J., & Dutch, N. (2008). Identifying victims of human trafficking: Inherent challenges and promising strategies from the field. *Department of Health & Human Services Issue Brief.* Retrieved from http://aspe.hhs.gov/07/humantrafficking/identvict/ib.htm.

Floyed, R. L., Hirsh, D. A., Greenbaum, V. J., & Simon, H. K. (2012). Development of a screening tool for pediatric sexual assault may reduce emergency room visits. *Pediatrics, 128*(2), 221–226.

Hughes, D. (2004). *Best practices to address the demand side of sex trafficking.* Retrieved October 1, 2012 from: http://www.uri.edu/artsci/wms/hughes/demand_sex_trafficking.pdf.

International Organization for Migration (IOM). (2007). *The IOM handbook on direct assistance for victims of trafficking.* Geneva, Switzerland: International Organization for Migration.

Polaris Project. (2012). *Combating human trafficking and modern-day slavery.* Retrieved from the Polaris Project website: http://www.polarisproject.org/human-trafficking.

Sabella, D. (2011). The role of the nurse in combating human trafficking. *American Journal of Nursing, 111*(2), 28–37.

Silbert, M., & Pines, A. (1981). Occupational hazards of street prostitutes. *Criminal Justice and Behavior, 8*(4), 395–399.

Thomas, B. (2011). How to recognize human trafficking in a healthcare setting. *Kentucky Board of Nursing Connection 2011 Spring (27),* 9–10.

Trout, K. K. (2010). Human trafficking the role of nurses in identifying and helping victims. *Penn Nurse, 65*(4), 18–20.

CHAPTER 19

Mental Health Perspectives on the Care of Human Trafficking Victims Within Our Borders

CHERYL ANN LAPP AND NATALIE OVERMANN

*I*n this chapter, the authors provide an overview of the mental health impli-cations of human trafficking, how providers can identify and treat victims, and what programs are available to support victims.

HUMAN TRAFFICKING IN THE UNITED STATES

Involuntary servitude has been illegal in the United States since 1865, yet we need to realize the likelihood that many practicing nurses encounter this very phenomenon at some time within their careers and may not even know it. In a recent classroom discussion about human trafficking, several graduate nursing students could recall practice encounters where self-awareness alerted them to some uncomfortable feeling about a situation and its dynamics, but they could not pinpoint why. One advanced practice student described a case where phys-ical care was given to a young woman on an outpatient basis, yet she intuitively felt that there was something disturbing going on. She had not known how to tackle this and said simply: "It haunts me to this day."

One can read estimates of the thousands of men, women, and children who are trafficked annually into the United States (Clawson, Dutch, Solomon, & Gold-blatt, 2009), but research on the prevalence of human trafficking on both a national and global level is incomplete (Macy & Johns, 2011). This is due to the hidden nature of trafficking as well as inconsistent methodology used to esti-mate numbers of victims (Gajic-Veljanoski & Stewart, 2007). What we do know is that 80% of these victims in the United States are women and minors, and 70%

are trafficked for sexual exploitation (Gajic-Veljanoski & Stewart, 2007; Clawson et al., 2009; Kotrla, 2010). The majority are young adult women in their 20s from southeast Asia, Latin America, Africa, and central and eastern Europe (Family Violence Prevention Fund, 2005; Kara, 2009; Miller, Decker, Silverman, & Raj, 2007). In 2010, the top countries of origin for victims were Thailand, India, Mexico, Philippines, Haiti, Honduras, El Salvador, and the Dominican Republic (U.S. Department of State, 2011). Though the majority of human trafficking victims in the United States are immigrants, domestic victims are also trafficked within the United States. The majority of domestic victims are girls, minors between 12 and 18 years of age, and the average age at which they first become exploited through prostitution is between 12 and 14 years (Barrows & Finger, 2008; Clawson et al., 2009). It is estimated that 199,000 incidences of sexual exploitation of minors occur each year in the United States, and between 244,000 and 325,000 American youth are currently at risk of becoming victims of commercial sexual exploitation (Estes & Weiner, 2001).

Because this is a business that thrives "under the radar" for most Americans, general public awareness is still low, hampered by the fact that accurate, convincing data are extremely difficult to obtain. Americans might know human trafficking as a global issue, and as an international problem it is ranked second to drug trafficking. Although its outcomes are devastating in terms of human misery, analysis of the marketing system of human trafficking reveals it to be highly adaptive environmentally. It has evolved robustly to counteract the usual forms of suppression of illegal activity (Pennington et al., 2009). Whatever is understood about global slavery by average American citizens, including many health providers, most hope or prefer to believe "surely not here."

Essential elements of trafficking include the use of force, fraud, or coercion. Any one of several strategies such as physical confinement, constraint by confiscation of identification papers, physical violence, or threat of bodily harm to family, can effectively silence trafficked victims and immobilize them from seeking help. The media occasionally sheds light on the domestic manifestations of sex trafficking. A recent *New York Times* article (Kristof, 2012) featured the story of a young woman who was formerly trafficked at 16 years of age. She described how she was recruited, held, and sold into the sex trade. She reported that she will always have a scar on her face where a trafficker gouged her with a potato peeler as a warning not to escape or forget. She was branded, she says, "like cattle owners brand their cattle. . . ." Kristof chillingly details this true case that illuminates the recruitment scenario of an underaged girl in New York, and then describes the mechanism of her being offered up to buyers through media websites in the online marketplace. It is an industry with plenty of buyers, difficulties in prosecuting the advertising companies that enable the traffickers, and where millions of dollars are made. For anyone who is paying attention, there is no doubt that human sex trafficking is active and thriving in the land of the free.

THE MENTAL HEALTH PROFILE OF SEXUALLY TRAFFICKED PERSONS

The field of mental health care for trafficked and exploited victims is an emerging specialty, but domestic statistics are notoriously difficult to obtain. Much of the research we have to date involves international subject samples. According to the International Labor Organization estimates, 12.3 million people are in situations of forced or bonded labor, and of these at least half are believed to be women and girls (Hossain, Zimmerman, Abas, Light, & Watts, 2010). Hossain and her research team explored the association between trauma and mental disorders in 207 women and girls trafficked in seven European countries for sexual exploitation and who were now accessing posttrafficking services. There were many forms of physical violence and personal violation likened to torture, the aftermath resulting in both medical and mental health needs. For mental health outcomes, the interview data and two validated instruments for depression and anxiety, and posttraumatic stress disorder (PTSD) were administered. The tools had to be relatively easy to translate, and in many cases, statistical adjustment had to be made for pretrafficking abuse in order to isolate the impact of trafficking-related experiences. Statistical adjustment was also made for differing amounts of time spent in the trafficking situation.

Results indicated that injuries and sexual violence that occurred during trafficking were associated with higher levels of PTSD, depression, and anxiety, either alone or in various combinations of overlap known as comorbidity. Sexual violence was associated with higher levels of PTSD, and more time in trafficking was associated with high levels of depression and anxiety. The significance of looking at comorbidity is that when PTSD is mixed with prior clinical depression, the distress is heightened, and the response to treatment and ultimate recovery is considered less optimistic. Hossain et al. (p. 2447) emphasize that "numerous organizations around the world ... provide care to trafficked persons, yet uncertainty persists regarding the best ways to address their mental health needs." This team recommends that mental health providers and the mental health community must take the lead in moving quickly to develop and test intervention strategies for the mental health aftermath of the trafficking experience.

In another posttrafficking mental health study of 178 returning Moldavian women (Ostrovschi et al., 2011), the authors reiterate that although there are international calls for better psychological support for posttrafficking victims, there is a dearth of clinical evidence on the actual mental health needs of these survivors. They conclude that women found to have comorbid PTSD or other forms of anxiety and depression upon return from trafficking should be offered evidence-based mental health treatment for at least the standard 12-month period of reintegration and rehabilitation. However, these researchers underscore that diagnostic assessment should be tracked over time, beginning with crisis intervention within the first 5 days of posttrafficking, and then comparing diagnoses from 2 to 12 months into the longer-term recovery period. The problem, according to the Ostrovschi team, is that no studies to date have employed clinician-administered diagnostic assessment to describe either primary or comorbid conditions. Their position is that we do not currently have evidence-based research for psychiatric diagnostic assessment to identify the common forms of mental distress among survivors for treatment and recovery posttrafficking. An interesting point that Ostrovschi et al. make is that we should employ caution to avoid adding the burden of stigma by diagnosing them with labels that in other patients might be seen as normal reactions to extremely abnormal events.

Understanding the Process of Victimization

In order to be positioned to identify possible victims of trafficking in the relatively short time they present in urgent care or emergency health care settings, it is important for providers to have some contextual and empathic understanding of the phenomenon. Individuals become victims of human trafficking through deceit, romance, abduction, or even sale by family (Kara, 2009). Often young women and girls in other countries are recruited by traffickers who offer them a better life in the United States through employment opportunities (Kara, 2009; Miller, Decker, Silverman, & Raj, 2007; Patel, Ahn, & Burke, 2010).Traffickers will entice women and girls through false promises of jobs as nannies, maids, dancers, factory or restaurant workers, sale clerks, or models (U.S. Department of State, 2011; Miller et al., 2007; Sabella, 2011).

Women are sometimes seduced with the promise of love by agents who work for traffickers. When targeted women are convinced to move to a wealthier country to start a new life together, the agents typically send them to a location where they are to meet a "friend" who turns out to be the trafficker (Kara, 2009). This chain of travel and the complicated web of transfers effectively obstruct the ability of legal authorities to track the actual perpetrators or locate any single point of origin.

Once in the United States, the traffickers use violence, threats, false promises, debt bondage, or other forms of control and manipulation that keep victims involved in the sex industry (Polaris Project, 2012). Sexual exploitation takes place in street prostitution, massage parlors, brothels, sexual servitude, and servile marriage (Logan, Walker, & Hunt, 2009; U.S. Department of State, 2011). Trafficked women are also frequently moved from one work venue to the next to prevent them from developing any social support or recognition that might allow them to obtain assistance (Miller et al., 2007). But media reports have also suggested that victims are also forced to work in more mainstream businesses such as nail salons and hotels (Logan et al., 2009). Further research is needed to identify other possible sectors where persons are trafficked within the United States.

Several contributing characteristics of trafficking vulnerability, both within the United States and abroad, include circumstances of poverty, lack of employment opportunities, cultural attitudes that allow for mistreatment of women and children, and countries of origin with political instability or natural disasters

(Logan et al., 2009; Miller et al., 2007; Sabella, 2011). Personal factors that can make an individual more vulnerable in addition to youth are lack of education, lack of knowledge of legal rights, or limited access to resources (Gajic-Veljanoski & Stewart, 2007; Logan et al., 2009). Other personal characteristics include a history of physical or sexual abuse, unemployment, lack of family support, placement in foster homes, runaway tendencies, homelessness, and mental health problems (Clawson et al., 2009; Gajic-Veljanoski & Stewart, 2007; Williamson, Dutch, & Clawson, 2009). Substance abuse, isolation, and making poor choices also contribute to overall vulnerability (Logan et al., 2009).

ROLE OF HEALTH CARE PROVIDERS

Nurses are frontline health care workers who could, with astute assessment skills, play an important role in identifying and helping trafficked victims. Although preventive care is not currently realistic for trafficked victims since most of their problems are urgent or life threatening before they present for help, prevention of continued trafficking and caring for victims is the goal. Although health practitioners are in the ideal position to intervene, such efforts still remain challenging. Emergency department (ED) personnel and clinicians are the most likely to encounter trafficked victims, and furthermore, as pointed out by Patel, Ahn, and Burke (2010), these providers can build upon their previously established foundation of identifying and assisting victims of intimate partner violence. Just as intimate partner or domestic violence identification has become a standardized universal assessment protocol in EDs and clinicians' offices, primary care providers are now being urged to refine their skills in preparation for the difficult task of learning how to identify trafficking cases. As Patel et al. explain, the difficulty begins with the reality that there are no classic presenting complaints to provide the diagnostic profile, but rather a variety of physical or mental health conditions. The investigation must include extensive contextual data, sometimes with a reluctant reporter, and often language barriers. The alert clinician must fit many pieces of a puzzle together, all the while providing a secure, private, and reassuring environment for the patient. This is a tall order in a busy emergency department, especially for patients who may not understand their rights or even realize they are victims of a crime.

Within the last 10 years, many initiatives have begun to assist and empower victims of human trafficking. Literature has shown that victims have been identified and helped through law enforcement, community members such as neighbors or customers, and by health or social service contacts (Clawson et al., 2009; Family Violence Prevention Fund, 2005; Logan et al., 2009). Nongovernment and government organizations are working to educate law enforcement, health care providers, social service providers, and even teachers, on how to identify and assist human trafficking victims. Increasingly, media attention and grassroots campaigns against human trafficking are serving to increase public awareness and provide legal protection and services to those affected. Further research in this area is needed to identify effective ways to assist and empower victims to overcome the fear, the lack of knowledge about alternative choices, the isolation, and the physical and psychological confinement that keeps them captive.

Professional organizations and educational institutions are beginning to hold conferences to help educate providers and to promote targeted research. One excellent example is the annual Interdisciplinary Conference on Human Trafficking at the University of Nebraska–Lincoln, now in the planning process for its fourth year. UNL has its own Human Trafficking Team consisting of seven faculty members or alumni who are involved in antitrafficking studies and programs. This interactive conference is formatted for those who have research results or ideas, who wish to inform their peers of relevant nongovernmental or governmental organization, or who wish to fund antitrafficking efforts and research.

Mental Health of Trafficking Victims

Trafficking has detrimental effects on victims' physical and mental health that are often "profound and enduring" (Raymond & Hughes, 2001; Zimmerman et al., 2006). In one study, 95% of trafficking victims interviewed reported that they suffered physical and sexual violence while in captivity (Zimmerman et al., 2003), and these victims suffer many mental health effects directly resulting from the physical abuse and sexual exploitation. Women especially are known to experience health problems due to appalling working and living conditions, psychological abuse, and lack of access to health care (Gajic-Veljanoski & Stewart, 2007). Several categories of health consequences have been identified: physical trauma, sexual and reproductive health problems, noninfectious and infectious disease, and psychological health consequences. It is the latter that is the focus of the following discussion.

Trafficked people face extreme forms of psychological abuse that can lead to mental health problems. As discussed earlier, the cascade of despair reminds one of torture tactics. During early stages of trafficking, traffickers may attempt to control their victims through pacification, brainwashing through rape, physical assaults, or food and water deprivation (Gajic-Veljanoski & Stewart, 2007; Zimmerman et al., 2003). The perpetrators intimidate or mentally defeat victims through blackmail, threats, emotional manipulation, confinement, or isolation (Family Violence Prevention Fund, 2005; Gajic-Veljanoski & Stewart, 2007). Victims experience high levels of fear imposed by their trafficker to keep them from escaping (Logan et al., 2009). Fear tactics can include the threat of intentionally inflicted pain or injury, sexual or physical abuse, violence against loved ones or cessation of money sent to their families, or being jailed or deported (Logan et al., 2009). Victims may often feel that they are to blame for their situation and report feelings of shame, guilt, or worthlessness (Logan et al., 2009; Raymond & Hughes, 2001; Zimmerman et al., 2006). They can also be experiencing culture shock and isolation through language and cultural barriers.

Psychological reactions to the conditions of human trafficking include depression, anxiety, hostility, and PTSD (Hossain, Zimmerman, Abas, Light,

Watts, 2010; Raymond & Hughes, 2001; Zimmerman et al., 2006). Trafficked victims experience depression at much higher rates than the general public (Zimmerman et al., 2006). Suicidal ideation among trafficked victims has been reported to be as high as 38% to 63% (Raymond & Hughes, 2001; Zimmerman et al., 2006). Anxiety symptoms include panic attacks, paranoia, and persistently feeling scared. Hostile or aggressive symptoms may include frequent temper outbursts, becoming easily irritated or angered, having homicidal thoughts, or manifesting acts of aggression such as punching walls or hitting others (Raymond & Hughes, 2001; Zimmerman et al., 2006).

Victims of human trafficking are known to experience PTSD (Bortel, Ellingen, Ellison, Phillips, & Thomas, 2008; Farley, 2003; Farley & Barkan, 1998; Zimmerman et al., 2006). Victims also report comorbid and psychophysiological symptoms related to the anxiety or depression. These can include headaches, body aches, back pain, abdominal pain, dizziness, nausea, and vision disturbances (Stewart & Gajic-Veljanoski, 2005; Zimmerman et al., 2006). Trafficked women also face problems with addictions to drugs and alcohol (Raymond & Hughes, 2001; Zimmerman et al., 2003).

As discussed earlier, the most recently reported studies have analyzed interview data from women attending posttrafficking services for sexual exploitation. There is minimal research and less known about the health care needs of trafficked men.

Health Care Provider Intervention Opportunities

Most early interventions for human trafficking have focused on training law enforcement to identify and help possible trafficking victims. Current literature, however, provides rationale that indicates how health care providers, particularly in EDs, are in a unique and critical position to identify and help victims of human trafficking. A study by Raymond and Hughes (2001), found that 56% of trafficked victims in the United States required ED treatment while in captivity and 25% sought treatment in EDs multiple times. In another study, 28% of victims came into contact with the health care system while in captivity and yet none were identified as victims of human trafficking (Family Violence Prevention Fund, 2005). Each of these visits represents a missed opportunity to rescue a trafficked victim.

Unfortunately, many health care providers currently lack the education to identify and help victims of human trafficking. Results of a survey of ED health care providers indicated that only 13% felt confident that they could identify a trafficking victim and only 3% reported having had training on the topic (Chisolm-Straker & Richardson, 2007). In a recent Canadian study of medical students' awareness and attitudes about human trafficking at the country's largest medical school, fully 93.9% of participants reported that they were not knowledgeable or only somewhat knowledgeable about the subject (Wong, Hong, Leung, & Steward, 2011). Furthermore, the majority of participants (88.9%) at this large and diverse medical school were not familiar with signs and symptoms of trafficked persons, and 93.9% thought that it would be either unlikely or only somewhat likely to encounter or identify a trafficked person in a clinical setting in Canada. Fortunately, over 85% still thought that it was important to learn about the identification and health needs of trafficked persons and felt it should be in their medical education. However, in contrast to this degree of clinical interest, fewer participants felt that it was important to learn about legal and immigration issues, or lobbying and advocacy.

Several organizations including the U.S. Department of Health and Human Services and antitrafficking nongovernment organizations such as the Polaris Project are recognizing the importance of health care providers in the fight against human trafficking. They have developed online toolkits to train health care providers on identifying and assisting victims. Recently, an online international guidance manual, *Caring for Trafficked Persons: Guidance for Health Care Providers* was developed by the International Organization for Migration (IOM) and the London School of Hygiene and Tropical Medicine (LSHTM). The manual presents approaches for safe and appropriate treatment of trafficked persons.

Health care providers need to be educated on how to recognize victims of sex trafficking and how to address not only the immediate health care needs, but also how to collaborate with other disciplines to access resources to plan for the longer term recovery and rehabilitation related to mental trauma. All providers need to recognize victims' limited access to health care follow-up, and make the most of their time together in anticipation of the ongoing exposure to multiple health risks. It is essential that health care providers have awareness of their access to appropriate referral services prior to any attempt at "rescuing" a victim of trafficking. It is critical that providers must not make promises to the victim that cannot be kept.

Barriers to Helping Trafficked Victims

Barriers that health care providers face in responding to the needs of trafficked victims include the lack of awareness of the issue and overall knowledge about human trafficking (Clawson et al., 2009). There is a lack of staff education as well as adequate screening and response protocols in health care facilities (Bortel et al., 2008). Another barrier is that victims have few opportunities to disclose their situation. Most are accompanied to health care facilities by traffickers, who often present themselves as relatives. Usually the traffickers communicate with the health care providers on the victim's behalf, so that victims are less likely to have a chance to speak privately with the provider (Baldwin, Eisenman, Sayles, Ryan, & Chuang, 2011). Language is also a barrier, and as a matter of course and convenience, the traffickers may be unwittingly utilized as the victims' translators. Culturally appropriate care would include the provision of professional or neutral interpreter services.

Another barrier is the possibility that victims of trafficking may not identify themselves to others as victims. In a study by Baldwin (2011), reasons for lack of disclosure to health care providers included lack of trust, feelings of shame, guilt, embarrassment, hopelessness, and fear. Victims may suspect that providers will not believe their stories, are working for the traffickers, or will turn them into authorities. Many are afraid of retaliation by their traffickers that could endanger their own safety or their families' safety. Often victims do not recognize themselves as victims or recognize that their traffickers are breaking the law. Victims in Baldwin's study also reported that providers did not inquire about high-risk behaviors when being treated multiple times for sexually transmitted infections (STIs) or even assess their personal safety.

Identifying Victims

Protocols have been developed to assist with identification of trafficked victims. The U.S. Department of Health and Human Services (2012) developed a campaign called "Rescue and Restore" to assist in the identification and rescue of trafficked victims. The Polaris Project (2012) also developed a toolkit that identifies red flag warning indicators that an individual may be a victim of human trafficking.

Providers at the point of contact should ensure the safety of the patients, themselves, and other staff. This means never asking trafficking-related questions in front of the patient's companions, as this could lead to inaccurate answers and could put victims in danger (Sabella, 2011). One technique is to show assessment questions so that the client can point to the appropriate box of fixed response "yes/no" answers, out of view of a suspected trafficker. Responses can help health care providers discern whether the patient may be a victim of human trafficking. Key questions to ask, adapted from the United States Department of State (2009), include:

1. Are you paid for the work you do?
2. Can you leave your job if you want to?
3. Can you come and go as you please?
4. Have you or your family been threatened?
5. Do you have to ask permission to eat, sleep, or go to the restroom?
6. Are there locks on the doors and windows where you live or work so that you cannot get out?
7. Has your identification or documentation been taken from you?

Guidelines for Interacting With Victims of Human Trafficking

The IOM together with the LSHTM (International Organization of Migration, 2009), have developed guiding principles for health care professionals involved with persons who have been trafficked. The primary concern of the provider should be to prioritize and treat the patient's health problems and ensure their safety. The history and exam should take place alone with the patient, and psychological disorders such as anxiety and depression as well as suicidal ideation should also be assessed. It is important that the provider be aware that if the patient is believed to be a crime victim, the provider cannot force the victim to report it. The health care provider is not mandated by law to report the crime and can do so only with the victim's permission, with the exception that, if the victim is a minor, the health care provider is legally obligated to contact child protection services (Dovydaitis, 2010).

Skillful providers need to engage their patients through respectful and culturally sensitive care in order to establish trust. Their verbal interaction is characterized by remaining calm, patient, and nonjudgmental when talking with the potential victim. They should stress that their conversation will be confidential and that they are asking routine screening questions. If trafficking is suspected, providers should reiterate to patients that if they are victims of a crime, it is not their fault, and that the provider wants to help them. In an ideal world, providers should explore the patient's own understanding of their illness and trafficking experience and, if possible, attempt to view the experience in the context of the patient's religious and cultural beliefs. Alert providers also respect patients' wishes for a provider of the same sex if at all possible.

Just as in intimate partner violence, careful documentation is critical where abuse is evident. A detailed description of the injuries and specifics about the abusive incidents should be included, and, when possible, the patient's own words in quotes should be added. Documentation must include whether mandatory reporting was required, such as in the case of a minor, and how it was conducted.

When a victim is identified and provides consent to accept assistance, the health care provider and the victim need to agree to a plan of action. Health care facilities need to develop policies and protocols that give direction for a consistent course of action. Health care facilities need to decide how they are going to address the needs of victims of human trafficking, with the essential component of staff education on how to identify and help victims. The goal is implementation of screening and response protocols is to safely identify, treat, and provide rescue assistance to victims.

Interventions include notifying local law enforcement if the patient consents, especially if the patient is in immediate danger or if the patient is a minor. Social workers and/or case managers should be involved to immediately help connect the victim with emergency shelter, basic necessities, and crisis legal advocacy. The U.S. Department of Health and Human Services (2012) recommends that the provider and the patient call the National Human Trafficking Resource Center Hotline (NHTRC) if trafficking is suspected (1-888-3737-888). The hotline, operated by the Polaris Project, is available 24 hours a day and 7 days a week. Staff of the hotline can help connect the victims to emergency and long-term local services available to them in their state through the Victims of Trafficking and Violence Protection Act (2000). The hotline center should be contacted in advance of assisting victims to establish knowledge of local services.

If patients are unwilling to accept help at the time, they should be encouraged to return if they change their minds. If the provider can arrange time alone with the patient, it should be used to educate them about the physical and mental health risks of their situation. Providers can stress that the patient is a victim of a crime and is not at fault, while explaining that there are community support services available to help. The patient should discretely be given the number for the NHTRC hotline or other local antitrafficking organizations the patient can contact if the patient chooses to seek help later.

Medical organizations are suggesting that human trafficking training should be integrated into continuing education (Williamson et al., 2009). Medical leaders can also serve as leaders within their own communities to help bring awareness of human trafficking. Providers should stay current on local and national efforts to address human trafficking. They can become politically active in helping to advance local or national policies that promote the rights of trafficked victims. Health care providers can also join or initiate public awareness campaigns on sex trafficking, such as the Respect project designed to assist both U.S. citizens and foreign nationals. These campaigns can educate the public on the presence of sex trafficking in the community, on the rights of victims, and about specific services available in the local area. One example is an initiative to post the NHTRC's toll free number throughout the community in emergency departments, outpatient clinics, public restrooms, and on public transportation.

Developing a Mental Health Plan of Action

The mental and emotional consequences for human sex trafficking are devastating for victims and their needs can no longer be overlooked. One way to view intervention is to use the treatment guidelines of trauma-informed care. Recent trauma studies describe a complex range of posttrauma symptoms and identify the interactions of the multiple factors contributing to their seriousness (Briere & Spinazzola, 2005). Trauma exposure occurs along a continuum of complexity where more serious symptoms are associated with histories of multiple victimizations, often beginning in childhood. Unlike forms of PTSD that may interrupt a normal adult life following a triggering event such as a combat experience or rape, parental or other victimization in childhood complicates the goal of finding a new "normal" when conventional understandings of normal may never have existed for that person. Even a more profound impact results with co-occurring factors such as substance abuse disorders. Briere and Spinazzola conceptualize the complexity continuum from the less complex, single adult-onset incident where all else is relatively stable in a person's life, to repeated and intrusive trauma. This complex trauma becomes highly personal when compounded by stigma and shame, and renders a person extremely vulnerable to its effects. It is on this far end of the continuum where victims of sex trafficking are placed (Briere & Spinazzola, 2005).

Trauma-informed care means several things, but first is to know something about the history of past and current abuse in the life of your clients, in order to find a more integrated, appropriate, and culturally sensitive approach to meeting their needs. Second, to be trauma-informed is to understand the role that violence and victimization plays in the lives of most people, and to design service systems that accommodate the resulting vulnerabilities in such a way as to gain client participation in his or her own treatment (Harris & Fallot, 2001). Harris and Fallot outline the core principles of trauma-informed care as: Trauma is a defining life event, (2) the victim's complaints, behaviors, and symptoms are coping mechanisms, (3) the primary goals of services are empowerment and recovery, and (4) the service relationship is collaborative. As reviewed by Clawson, Salomon, and Goldblatt (2008), the specific core components of practice that build upon these principles include such things as reviewing current agency policies and procedures to remove any that are potentially unsafe or harmful to trafficking victims, to educate and train the staff in both direct and referred systems of care, and the use of culturally sensitive screening for trauma while ensuring safety.

Particularly relevant for mental health is to institute a mechanism for building long-term sustained relationships. This is a strategy to provide opportunities for building trust in regaining or reshaping a victim's sense of self and attainment of a valued social role. It is not enough to attend to basic needs, but ongoing attention needs to be paid to making peer models and social supports available. Just as returning military personnel frequently prefer to seek solace and support from comrades who have been there rather than nonmilitary friends or family, victims of human trafficking may also be most comfortable with peers who understand and have lived their own struggles.

Programs for human trafficking victims are starting to experience success with engaging human trafficking survivors in programming and in peer group counseling or mentoring support. Lastly, a powerful contribution to treatment that is recognized in trauma-informed care is the use of alternative and complementary therapies. This could include such healing therapies as acupuncture, meditation, massage, or a variety of techniques such as art, music, or drama therapy, journaling, poetry, or yoga to encourage self-expression and self-esteem, and reconnection with the self in positive and holistic ways. The St. Paul Healing Center, part of the Minnesota Center for Victims of Torture (CVT), is experienced in the treatment of politically motivated global forms of physical violence and emotional damage. The CVT continues to actively explore alternative therapies while thoughtfully considering how they might be integrated into a more long-term rehabilitative program.

Although the experiences of sex trafficking victims (often referred to as survivors) are varied in duration and complexity, the psychic impact is characteristically enduring and devastating. It is perhaps most appropriate to review trauma-informed services along with integrative and interdisciplinary healing services used for torture victims. The CVT, established in Minnesota in 1985 by then-governor Rudy Perpich, was the first in the nation and only the third worldwide. Among its working principles is the belief that survivors of torture can recover from the traumas that have been inflicted on them, are capable of restoring themselves in contexts of relationships with others, and may even go on to thrive.

This brings to mind the goal of restoration being manifested by the concept of resilience as opposed to recovery or hardiness. Perhaps, as in alcohol treatment, one is never fully "recovered" once and for all, but can be restored within a maintenance state of recovery. Hardiness is a trait that allows individuals to endure significant adversity, but there is not necessarily a positive change in the outcome because survivors may be blocked from growth by anger and blame (Earvolino-Ramirez, 2007). Resilience, on the other hand, enables people to heal from painful wounds, take charge of their lives, and go on to live in a positive manner (Walsh, 1998). Resilient individuals tend to negotiate an abundance of emotionally hazardous experiences proactively rather than reactively (Oconnol-Higgens, 1994), and perhaps the most hopeful feature of all, resilience appears to be a process that can be developed at any time during the life span (Gillespie, 2007).

CONCLUSION

Health care providers might be among the first people to have the opportunity to identify, treat, and possibly rescue victims of sex trafficking. This is no easy task, but even a beginning intervention, with astute assessment and sharing of resources such as the hotline number, can set in motion the process of reclaiming a life. We have the responsibility to educate ourselves about how to identify possible victims and meet their complex health care needs, both short and long term. Primary health care providers can begin to accomplish this at first contact, by actively listening to our patients, and, as Ganley (1998) had suggested for domestic violence intervention, offering validating messages similar to these:

- You do not deserve this; you deserve better than this.
- I care. I am glad you told me. We can work together to keep you safe and healthy.
- You are not alone in figuring this out. I would like to help you.

Indeed, we may be the only chance that victims have for escaping their traffickers and embarking on the long journey toward regaining their lives.

REFERENCES

Baldwin, S., Eisenman, D., Sayles, J., Ryan, G., & Chuang, K. (2011). Identification of human trafficking victims in health care settings. *Health and Human Rights, 13*(1), 1–14. Retrieved from http://www.hhrjournal.org/index.php/hhr/article/viewFile/409/612

Barrows, J., & Finger, R. (2008). Human trafficking and the healthcare professional. *Southern Medical Journal, 101*(5), 521–524.

Bortel, A., Ellingen, M., Ellison, M., Phillips, R., & Thomas, C. (2008). Sex trafficking needs assessment for the state of Minnesota. *The Advocate of Human Rights*. Retrieved from http://www.theadvocatesforhumanrights.org/sites/608a3887-dd53-4796-8904- 997 a0131ca54/uploads/REPORT_FINAL.10.13.08.pdf

Briere, J., & Spinazzola, J. (2005). Phenomenology and psychological assessment of complex posttraumatic states. *Journal of Traumatic Stress, 18*(5), 401–412.

Chisolm-Straker, M., & Richardson, L. (2007). Assessment of emergency provider knowledge about human trafficking victims in the ED. *Academic Emerging Medicine, 14*(5), Supp. 134.

Clawson, H., Dutch, N., Salomon, A., & Goldblatt, G. L. (2009). *Human trafficking into and within the United States: A review of the literature.* Washington, DC: U.S. Department of Health and Human Services. Retrieved from http://aspe.hhs.gov/hsp/07/HumanTrafficking/LitRev/

Clawson, H., Salomon, A., & Goldblatt, G. L. (2008). *Treating the hidden wounds: Trauma treatment and mental health recovery for victims of human trafficking.* Washington, DC: U.S. Department of Health and Human Services, Office of the Assistant Secretary for Planning and Evaluation.

Dovydaitis, T. (2010). Human trafficking: The role of the health care provider. *Journal of Midwifery & Women's Health, 55*(5), 462–467.

Earvolino-Ramirez, M. (2007). Resiliency: A concept analysis. *Nursing Forum, 42*(2), 73–83.

Estes, R., & Weiner, N. (2001). The commercial sexual exploitation of children in the U.S., Canada, and Mexico. Philadelphia: University of Pennsylvania. Retrieved from http://www.sp2.upenn.edu/restes/CSEC_Files/Abstract_010918.PDF

Family Violence Prevention Fund. (2005). *Turning pain into power: Trafficking survivors' perspectives on early intervention strategies.* Family Violence Prevention Fund. Retrieved from http://www.futureswithoutviolence.org/userfiles/file/Immigrant Women/Turning%20Pain%20intoPower.pdf

Farley, M., & Barkan, H. (1998). Prostitution, violence against women, and posttraumatic stress disorder. *Women & Health, 27*(3), 37–49.

Farley, M. (Ed.), (2003). *Prostitution, trafficking, and traumatic stress.* Binghamton, NY: Haworth Press.

Gajic-Veljanoski, O., & Stewart, D. (2007). Women trafficked into prostitution: Determinants, human rights and health needs. *Transcultural Psychiatry, 44*(3), 338–358.

Ganley, A. (1998). *Improving the health care response to domestic violence: A trainer's manual for health care providers.* The Family Violence Prevention Fund. Retrieved from: http://www.futureswithoutviolence.org/userfiles/file/HealthCare/improving_healthcare_healthtrainer.pdf

Gillespie, B. M. (2007). Development of a theoretically derived model of resilience through concept analysis. *Contemporary Nurse: A Journal for the Australian Nursing Profession, 3*(2), 124–135.

Harris, M., & Fallot, R. D. (Eds.), (2001). *Using trauma theory to design service systems: New directions for mental health services.* New York: Jossey-Bass Publishers.

Hossain, M., Zimmerman, C., Abas, M., Light, M., & Watts, C. (2010). The relationship of trauma to mental disorders among trafficked and sexually exploited girls and women. *Journal of Public Health, 100*(12), 2442–2448.

International Organization of Migration, London School of Hygiene and Tropical Medicine, & United Nations global initiative to fight trafficking in persons. (2009). *Caring for trafficked persons: Guidance for health providers.* International Organization for Migration: Geneva, Switzerland. Retrieved from http://genderviolence.lshtm.ac.uk/files/2009/10/Caring-for-Trafficked-Persons Handbook.pdf

Kara, S. (2009). *Sex trafficking: Inside the business of modern slavery.* New York: Columbia University Press.

Kotrla, K. (2010). Domestic minor sex trafficking in the United States. *Social Work, 55*(2), 181–187.

Kristof, N. D. (2012, March 18). Where pimps peddle their goods. *The New York Times,* 11.

Logan, T., Walker, R., & Hunt, G. (2009). Understanding human trafficking in the United States. *Trauma, Violence, & Abuse, 10*(1), 3–30.

Macy, R., & Johns, N. (2011). Aftercare services for international sex trafficking survivors: Informing U.S. services and program development in an emerging practice area. *Trauma, Violence, & Abuse, 12*(2), 87–98.

Miller, E., Decker, M., Silverman, J., & Raj, A. (2007). Migration, sexual exploitation, and women's health: A case report from a community health center. *Violence Against Women, 13*(5), 486–497.

Oconnol-Higgens, G. (1994). *Resilient adults.* San Francisco: Jossey-Bass Publishers.

Ostrovschi, N., Prince, M., Zimmerman, C., Hotineanu, M., Gorceag, L., Flach, C., & Abas, M. (2011). Women in post-trafficking services in Moldova: Diagnostic interviews over two time periods to assess returning women's mental health [Electronic version]. *BMC Public Health, 11*(232), 1–9.

Patel, R., Ahn, R., & Burke, T. (2010). Human trafficking in the emergency department. *Western Journal of Emergency Medicine, 11*(5), 402–404.

Pennington, J. R., Ball, A. D., Hampton, R., & Soulakova, J. (2009). The Cross-national market in human beings. *Journal of Macromarketing, 29*(119), 119–134.

Polaris Project. (2012). *Understanding victims' mindsets.* Retrieved from Polaris Project website: http://www.polarisproject.org/resources/tools-for-service-providers-and-law-enforcement

Polaris Project. (2012). *Polaris Project: Tools for law enforcement and service providers.* Retrieved from http://www.polarisproject.org/resources/tools-for-service-providers-and-law-enforcement

Raymond, J., & Hughes, D. (2001). *Sex trafficking of women in the United States: International and domestic trends. Coalition against trafficking in women.* Retrieved October 2, 2012 from http://www.uri.edu/artsci/wms/hughes/sex_traff_us.pdf

Sabella, D. (2011). The role of the nurse in combating human trafficking. *American Journal of Nursing, 111*(2), 28–37.

Stewart, D., & Gajic-Veljanoski, O. (2005). Trafficking in women: The Canadian perspective. *Canadian Medical Association Journal, 173*(1), 25–26.

U.S. Department of Health and Human Services. (2012). *The campaign to rescue and restore victims of human trafficking.* Retrieved from http://www.acf.hhs.gov/trafficking/

U.S. Department of State. (2011). *Trafficking in persons report 2011.* Retrieved from http://www.state.gov/j/tip/rls/tiprpt/2011/

Victims of Trafficking and Violence Protection Act. (2000). Retrieved http://www.state.gov/documents/organization/10492.pdf

Walsh, F. (1998). *Strengthening family resilience.* New York: The Guilford Press.

Williamson, E., Dutch, N., & Clawson, H. (2009). National symposium of the health needs of human trafficking victims: Post-symposium brief. Office of the Assistant Secretary for Planning and Evaluation, U.S. Department of Health and Human Services. Retrieved from http://aspe.hhs.gov/hsp/07/humantrafficking/Symposium/ib.shtml

Wong, J., Hong, J., Leung, P., & Steward, D. (2011). Human trafficking: An evaluation of Canadian medical students' awareness and attitudes. *Education for Health*, *24*(1). Retrieved from http://www.educationforhealth.net/

Zimmerman, C., Hossain, M., Yun, K., Gajdadziev, V., Guzun, N., Tchomarova, M. et al. (2008). The health of trafficked women: A survey of women entering posttrafficking services in Europe. *American Journal of Public Health*, *98*(1), 55–59.

Zimmerman, C., Hossain, M., Yun, K., Roche, B., Morison, L., & Watts, C. (2006). *Stolen smiles: A summary report on the physical and psychological health consequences of women and adolescents trafficked in Europe.* London: The London School of Hygiene & Tropical Medicine. Retrieved from http://genderviolence.lshtm.ac.uk/files/Stolen-Smiles-Summary.pdf

Zimmerman, C., Yun, K., Shvab, I., Watts, C., Trappolin, L., Treppete, M. et al. (2003). *The health risks and consequences of trafficking in women and adolescents: Findings from a European study.* London: London School of Hygiene & Tropical Medicine (LSHTM). Retrieved from http://genderviolence.lshtm.ac.uk/files/health_risks__consequences_trafficking.pdf

CHAPTER 20

Mental Health Intervention: Clinical Cases

MARY DE CHESNAY

*I*n the previous chapter, the authors presented an overview of the background literature on mental health issues related to sex trafficking. This chapter presents several cases that illustrate various treatment plans that were successful in treating specific clients. All identifying information has been changed to protect the privacy of the clients. A variety of therapeutic methods are presented as options for therapists working with sex trafficking survivors. It must be stressed that clients vary widely and treatment must be individualized for each based upon cultural factors, extent of abuse, available resources, strengths of the client, therapist's style, and experience and training of the therapist in specific methods.

Some methods are more convenient and comfortable for certain therapists and others require specialized training in the techniques. For example, social workers tend to be well-trained in trauma-focused cognitive behavioral therapy (TFCBT). Nurse-psychotherapists also have training in psychopharmacology and medications can take the edge off symptoms while more cognitive work can be done. Eye movement desensitization and reprocessing (EMDR) requires special training and it is wise not to use it without the training.

The following clinical cases are presented. Marta experienced posttraumatic stress disorder (PTSD) long after she had left the life. Cissy presented with anxiety disorder with depression shortly after she had been rescued. Michael was functioning as a male prostitute and worked for a pimp, and he had been sold commercially by his grandfather as a young child. His therapeutic goal was focused on a specific problem. Several examples of other treatments are drawn from the literature to illustrate specific therapeutic techniques. The therapy methods discussed here are only an overview and readers are encouraged to review the original sources.

REVIEW OF THERAPEUTIC METHODS

At this writing, best practices for mental health treatment of sex trafficking victims are not well documented and are largely anecdotal, yet a few methods have some basis for claims of efficacy. While evidence-based treatment is not thoroughly defined for this population, there are some techniques that have received attention in the literature and that have an evidence base for conditions with similar patients, for example, torture survivors and victims of incest. These are TFCBT and dialectical TFCBT.

Family therapy is useful if the client can return to the family of origin or if the early family issues that led to trafficking can be addressed. Family therapy can be practiced with individuals to resolve old issues and explore how current patterns were set by old issues. Peer support in the form of survivor-led groups can provide a sense of connectedness with others who have survived trafficking and reassurance of hope for a different future. EMDR is an interesting technique that can have dramatic effects and has been successful in treating PTSD. For some patients, psychopharmacology can take the edge off high anxiety and ease depression preparatory to psychotherapy.

Finally, expressive therapies can be helpful to provide a safe path to verbalization. Sand tray therapy, art therapy, music therapy, poetry therapy, and animal-assisted therapy are used to assist clients who are not comfortable with verbalization early in the therapeutic relationship.

Trauma-Focused Cognitive Behavioral Therapy (TFCBT)

Developed in the 1980s, TFCBT was first developed to help children with PTSD as a result of childhood sexual abuse (Classon et al., 2001; Cohen & Mannarino, 1996 a, b; Cohen & Mannarino, 1997). The method is to work with nonoffending parents and children in weekly sessions in which the child is guided through the management of trauma with the ongoing support of parents. The sessions progress from educating the client about the nature of trauma to understanding the thoughts and feelings connected with the trauma, reexperiencing the feelings associated with the trauma, and enhancing personal safety skills. Teaching relaxation skills helps the child to manage therapy, which is accomplished in 12 to 16 weeks (Grasso, Joselow, Marquez, & Webb, 2011).

Somewhat controversial in TFCBT is whether the therapist should introduce the topic of the trauma during the first session. This is more about the therapist's preference than about what is best for the child. I am in favor of establishing rapport with a positive story that the client remembers as making him or her feel good. Then follow-up with asking the client to tell the story of the trauma just like the first story—with thoughts, feelings, and actions. This method can be a diagnostic test to determine whether the client is ready to talk, but also conveys that the therapist is not going to be shocked or judgmental about the trauma and the client's reactions.

A particularly good source for learning about trauma-focused cognitive behavior therapy (TFCBY) is Rubin and Springer's (2009) edition of case presentations. They provide an overview of the method but explain the therapeutic challenges through discussion of cases with people who present with a variety of trauma conditions. They have a section on EMDR and PTSD that presents special considerations when using EMDR with children.

There are numerous publications and training seminars for TFCBT. One online source developed with a grant from the Substance Abuse and Mental Health Services Administration (SAMHSA), U.S. Department of Health and Human Services (DHHS) is offered online by the Medical University of South Carolina (http://tfcbt.musc.edu/). Continuing education credits can be earned.

Dialectical TFCBT

Linehan (1993), Linehan et al., (2006) developed a variation of TFCBT to work with people who had borderline personality and self-injurious behavior. DTFCBT has the same characteristics as its parent theory but focuses less on change and more on acceptance of self. She found that clients often sabotaged therapy because they believed they were not able to change (Swales, M., 2009). They would not return or would not verbalize during therapy, so she decided that more work needed to be done on helping the client accept herself as is, before considering whether and how to change.

DTFCBT is an evidence-based treatment that has been documented to be effective in at least seven studies (Lynch et al., 2006). In a randomized clinical trial with 28 women drug abusers, Linehan and her associates (1999) found that DTFCBT was more effective at treating drug abuse than the control group, which received treatment as usual in the community. Effects were documented at intervals for 1 year through interviews and urinalysis.

Sweezy (2011) recommended combining DTFCBT with internal family therapy as a way of helping clients overcome childhood trauma when they are not ready for change. She teaches skills in how to tolerate the distress, how to reorient attention away from shame and guilt to accepting that the base experience cannot be changed but the emotional reaction to the trauma can be managed.

Family Therapy

The goal of family therapy is to promote healthier ways of interacting within one's family. The variety of family therapy theories and methods present a long menu of options for therapists trained to work with family groups, but not all prostituted women or children can be successfully reintegrated into their families of origin. In many developing countries, it is common for parents to sell their children or to give them to traffickers who promise a better life for the child (Trafficking Children: Recruitment and Extraction, 2012). In the United States and other developed countries, there are many examples in the news of parents who sell their children (KCBD INVESTIGATES: Children sold for sex in Lubbock, 2012; Shaniya Davis found dead).

Family therapy can be approached from the standpoint of helping the family cope with the traumatic experiences of one of its members and helping the victim to reintegrate into the family. TFCBT might include family therapy. In family therapy with sex trafficking clients, the priority emphasis should be on the trauma rather than other family therapy goals. The following family therapy models can be adapted for use with sex trafficking victims if therapists are trained in their use and if the other aftercare and trauma services are also provided. This is not to say that other family therapies should not be used, but these have a long track record of success that provides a base for best practice. Family therapists who practice from other models might want to publish case studies of how they were used with sex trafficking clients in order to begin to build the evidence base for this population.

- Intergenerational theory: (Murray Bowen) a family system approach in which the focus is on family patterns through generations (Bowen, 1988)
- Structural theory: (Salvador Minuchin) a system approach in which the therapist "joins" the family to observe and disrupt unhealthy patterns of interaction as a way to guide the family into healthier patterns (Minuchin, 1974)
- Strategic theory: (Jay Haley) a system approach in which the therapist helps the family solve problems identified in therapy (Haley, 1963/2006)
- Communication theory: (Satir, Whitaker) a system approach that focuses on changing patterns of overt and covert communication among family members, particularly between parents and their children (Satir, 1983)
- Solution-focused (Watzlawick, Steve de Shazer) a system approach in which the therapist helps the client family to manage change in order to obtain the future they wish for themselves (Watzlawick, 1974)

Peer Support Groups

Peer support is a highly effective way to establish agency practices that are relevant and respectful to trafficked clients. Access to peer support is important during successful exiting and haling (Cooper et al., 2007). Many organizations were founded by survivors to help other survivors. Here are a few (See also Table 20.1):

- Girls Education and Mentoring Services (GEMS) in New York City—Rachel Lloyd
- Courtney's House serves Washington, DC, northern Virginia, and southern Maryland—Tina Frundt
- Somaly Mam Foundation in Cambodia—Somaly Mam
- Destiny House in Las Vegas—Annie Lobert
- Rahab's Hideaway in Columbus, Ohio—Marlene Carson
- Partners Against Human Trafficking (PATH) in Little Rock, Arkansas—Louise Allison

The survivors who founded the services speak to the need for trust and nonjudgmental attitude on the part of staff. While it is not necessary to have lived through

TABLE 20.1   Websites for Shelters Opened by Survivors

Organization	Website
GEMS	www.gems-girls.org/
Courtney's House	www.courtneyshouse.org/
Somaly Mam	www.somaly.org/whoweare
Destiny House	www.hookersforjesus.net/contentpages/13471/ 56d8edbc-a4e1-4f63-95da-6d3f88d22774/DestinyHouse.aspx
Rahab's Hideaway	http://rahabshideaway.org/news
PATH	http://thepathinitiative.com/

an experience in order to help others, there is certainly credibility from interacting with others who can share *how* they survived.

Eye Movement Desensitization and Reprocessing

EMDR is a technique with some evidence that it can alleviate PTSD. Developed in the 1980s, EMDR was developed to relieve the anxiety associated with traumatic memories (Shapiro, 1989). Maxfield (2003) described EMDR as an eight-phase process that progresses in phases 1 and 2 from assessment (history-taking, setting treatment goals) to preparation (ensuring safety, managing affect, self-calming). Phase 3 begins the processing of the memories by systematically eliciting the power of the memories and meaning to the client. The client learns to link the memories to the feelings and responses that arise during the recounting of the traumatic events. In this phase, the client learns to distinguish feeling from thoughts from actions. Phases 4 to 6 involve learning how to focus on the painful memory and allow the feelings and thoughts to come to the surface to be examined. This is done while the therapist moves his or her fingers from side to side while the client follows the movement with the eyes. Periodically the therapist asks the client to process the experience and to review what is happening and how the client is feeling. This activity of alternatively following the movement with rapid eye movement (focusing attention on the memory) and debriefing is repeated many times until the client's anxiety is reduced. In the final phases, the client records impressions between sessions in a journal, which is then reviewed with the therapist.

There is some evidence that EMDR is effective with adults, but not established as effective with children, though one study has provided some hope for children who are victims of disasters (Chemtob, Nakashima, & Carlson, 2002; D'Anca, 1997; Maxfield, 2003). Seidler and Wagner (2006) conducted a meta-analysis of studies comparing EMDR with TFCBY. They found similar therapeutic outcomes for both treatments but cautioned that treatment should be individualized to the patients.

Tripp (2007) used art therapy in conjunction with a modification of EMDR. As the eye movement session progressed through phases, the client was asked to make a series of drawings that could be used to bring material to consciousness for discussion with the therapist.

Psychopharmacology

Prostituted women and children are particularly vulnerable to a host of psychological conditions such as depression, dissociation, anxiety, attention deficit disorder, and psychosis. They may also be pregnant or of child-bearing age and may abuse alcohol or illegal drugs. These factors complicate prescription psychopharmacologic treatment. Careful assessment and history taking are vital. If it is determined that the client can benefit from medication, it might be useful to review some of the best medications for treating several conditions they are likely to experience. There are so many options available that clinicians should refer to experienced practitioners and prescribing guides such as those from the National Institute of Mental Health (NIMH). The following are a few examples found on the NIMH website (NIMH, n.d.):

- Combination antianxiety and antipsychotic (Prozac, Ziprexa)
- Antipsychotic (Abilify, Clozaril, Haldol, Loxitane, Navane, Risperdol, Stelazine, Thorazine)
- Antidepressants—sometimes also antianxiety agents (Aventyl, Cymbalta, Elavil, Marplan, Nardil, Paxil, Prozac, Sinequan, Tofranil, Zoloft)
- Mood-stabilizing and anticonvulsant (Depakote, Lithium, Tegretol)
- Antianxiety (Ativan, Librium, Tranxene, Valium, Xanax)
- ADHD stimulants (Desoxyn, Dexadrine, Focalin, Ritalin)

These drugs should only be prescribed by clinicians who are knowledgeable in their use, interactions, and side effects.

Expressive Therapies

The following therapy modalities are used to help clients verbalize their thoughts and feelings. Traumatized individuals may have difficulty relating to therapists who they fear might judge them and, at the least, might not understand them. Expressive therapies, or projective techniques, are best used to encourage the client to express feelings without the dangers associated with verbalization. Using these techniques helps to establish rapport and build trust.

Art Therapy

Art therapy has been used effectively with children who have been traumatized, particularly, in sexual abuse, in conjunction with cognitive behavioral therapy (Haygood, 2000; Pifalo, 2007). Chapman et al. (2001) used art therapy to reduce the symptoms of PTSD in children who had been traumatized. In a 10-year prospective study in San Francisco, 85 children admitted to the trauma unit were studied in a randomized cohort study with 31 receiving the art therapy intervention. Although the findings did not suggest that art therapy reduced symptoms of PTSD, the results did show a significant decrease in the number of acute stress symptoms.

It is important to understand that the usefulness of art therapy is not in the therapist's ability to interpret but in the client's expression of feelings through art. There can be variance in how art therapy is done. For example, some therapists might ask the client to draw something specific, as in the case of sexually abused 5-year-old abused by her teenage brother. "Draw your house and everyone who lives there." This child drew a simple three-level home with three bedrooms upstairs—one for her parents, one for herself, and one for her brother. Then she was asked to draw where everyone sleeps and she drew herself and her brother in the basement. When she was able to verbalize the abuse she told me that her brother would enter her room at night and take her to the basement where he abused her.

I asked a trafficked teenage client to draw her home with everyone who lived there and she drew the apartment where she lived with her pimp and four other girls. Then I asked her to draw where everyone sleeps. She thought for a moment and drew a series of 5 separate pictures with the pimp in a bed with each girl. Then she started laughing bitterly and said: "Who gets to sleep? If we ain't working, we doing chores for Daddy."

Another approach might be to ask the client to draw anything she wishes. This is a good technique with clients who are nonverbal and have difficulty even conversing with the therapist. Typically, these pictures look chaotic and are highly symbolic. It is important not to guess at what is being expressed. The therapist should instead ask the client to explain the picture. Maxine was a 17-year-old with a long history of physical abuse by her pimp and many johns. When she came to me she was dissociated and not able to verbalize so I asked her to draw a picture of anything she wished. She drew a primitive oval blob on the ground in black against a red background with gray vertical lines on either side. When she was able to explain it she told me that was her lying in a pool of her own blood in an alley after being beaten and gang-raped by her last customer and his friends.

Music Therapy

Strehlow (2009) described phases of music therapy to relieve distress in an 8-year-old who had been sexually abused by her mother's partner, a convicted pornographer. Though many children present with anger and destructive behavior, Kelly was conforming, sad, and withdrawn. In the first music session after two sessions of establishing rapport, Kelly chose the music and the therapist was not allowed to participate or speak to her. In this way, the child established control. By the eighth session, which included music for the second time, Kelly is a little calmer and allows the therapist to parallel play with her. A more secure environment and relationship is beginning to be established. In session 18, the traumatic memories are coming to the surface and the music becomes louder as Kelly recreates the trauma of lying in bed between the mother and her partner while the man molested her. Kelly pretended to be asleep and her mother slept through this and did not believe Kelly. By session 28, Kelly is experimenting with a different kind of relationship and this is reflected in her music by allowing more participation with the therapist. In session 32, Kelly is actively engaging with the therapist and having fun.

Poetry Therapy

A clinical case study of poetry therapy was reported by Bowman and Halfacre (1994). The client was a young man who had endured a life of sexual abuse since being abandoned by his mother at age 3 and raised in abusive foster homes until age 14 when he was placed with a nurturing family. At age 19, he was finally able to express his victimization. The primary treatment modality was individual psychotherapy designed to move toward self-actualization and poetry was used as a vehicle for expression of feelings. Four poems with the client's description of his learning are presented. The poems show a progression of insight from the pain of keeping secrets to healing and optimism for the future.

Sand Tray Therapy

Sand tray (or sand play) therapy originated in Britain in the 1930s by Lowenfeld who established the London School of Child Psychology (Lowenfeld, 1979). The technique involves using two shallow trays of sand (dry and damp) with dozens of miniature figures (people, animals, objects, food, etc.) with which the child plays (Allen & Berry, 1987; Pickford, 1992; Sachs, 1990; Zhang, 1998). The child selects and places the miniatures in the trays in any way he or she wishes. Typically, the first session or two involves dumping a few to several hundred miniatures into the tray-representing *chaos*. Following chaos is *struggle* as the child works out conflicts among the figures. The child will show fighting among figures or people being devoured by animals. Finally, the child *resolves* the struggles and edits the figures, placing them in a more organized way that makes sense in the real world. For example, animals are in their natural habitats and there is order and balance in the tray.

Animal-Assisted Therapy

Animal-assisted therapy is documented to show positive effects with many who have experienced trauma or who have limited musculoskeletal development such as the use of equine therapy (also called hippotherapy) for children with autism and cerebral palsy (Benda, McGibbon, & Grant, 2003; Keilholz, 2005). In a participatory ethnography, Burgon (2011) demonstrated how equine therapy can improve self-esteem and trust in at-risk children. Similarly, in a study with victims of intimate partner violence, Froeschle (2009) showed how these women could be helped to move past their insecurities and self-doubts to problem solving and career planning. Two of the residential treatment homes (Natalie's House and Wellspring Living), which are discussed in the Resources chapter, use equine therapy for exploited children. Natalie's House also assigns a chicken to each girl in order to teach caring for animals (as well as producing fresh eggs for the group).

Pet therapy has long been used in hospitals and nursing homes to bring comfort to the sick and aged (Horowitz, 2010; Moretti et al., 2011; Rossetti & King, 2011). The author reports a situation that shows how a dog can be an effective "co-therapist." While working with 8-year-old Lisa (pseudonym), who had been sexually abused by her father and then rented to his friends, the author could not establish enough rapport with the child during the first three sessions for her to verbalize the extent of the abuse. Lisa had said she wanted to be a veterinarian and take care of animals when she grew up so I brought my dog to the fourth session at Lisa's home and asked Lisa and her mother to help me walk him around her neighborhood. He was a big Airedale, but gentle, and the mother and I watched carefully to make sure Lisa could handle him. After about 20 minutes, I said to Lisa that I understood that I was a stranger and that she might not be comfortable telling me or even her mother about what her father had done, but would she tell the dog? I explained that he was a good listener and never judged me when I told him my problems. She was silent for a few blocks more, but then her mother and I noticed she was talking to the dog. She told him everything. Once she told the dog her story, she was able to open up to therapy. As a result, I was able to provide enough information to the appropriate officials to ensure that the father would be held accountable. I remain convinced that the breakthrough could not have happened had she not told the dog her story.

AFTERCARE SERVICES

All of the previous modalities of treatment can be used by trained individual clinicians, but successful aftercare for sex trafficking victims needs to be continuous and coordinated. In order to identify practice recommendations for international survivors of sex trafficking, Macy and Johns (2012) conducted a systematic review of journal databases and citations in articles on sex trafficking. Their search yielded 49 articles for possible review. However, at first only three articles were relevant to their topic of aftercare services for international victims identified in the United States, so they expanded the search to include grant reports and documents used by agencies serving victims. The final sample was 20 documents. Although the study involved international survivors, most of the following are relevant to domestic survivors. They found that sex trafficking survivors:

- Have many needs that are best addressed through comprehensive services
- Have needs that change over time
- Have an immediate need for safe shelter but once safe, they need long-term housing as they work to build new lives

- Immediate needs are basic necessities, language interpretation, medical care and legal help
- Needs evolve into support for immigration, transitional housing, job training life skills, and language training
- May need substance abuse treatment, repatriation, reunification with families permanent housing if staying in the United States

There was consensus in the literature that service providers should provide safety conduct a comprehensive needs assessment, ensure confidentiality, provide trauma-focused care, coordinate services with other professionals, and provide culturally appropriate services. Most authors stress that every effort should be made to provide care in the native languages of survivors or that competent interpreters trained to be sensitive to the needs of sex trafficking survivors be present during interviews.

On the surface this sounds like a good idea, but there are several issues that should be considered. First, accompanying persons should not be allowed to interpret unless they have been ruled out as traffickers or other trafficking survivors who might be in league with the traffickers. Even family members or "friends" might have been involved in the victimization. Second, language does not always ensure cultural competence. For example, caste systems in different cultures might produce unfair judgments if the victims and interpreters are of different socioeconomic groups. Third, training of interpreters is essential, not just about how to ensure confidentiality but also about the nature of human trafficking. The shame and guilt experienced by many victims could easily be exacerbated when the person is interacting with someone of the same culture.

The U.S. Department of State's Office to Monitor and Combat Human Trafficking (2008) sponsored a symposium of experts in victim services to determine priorities for aftercare. Consensus was reached on the following services and what they mean. Table 20.2 was designed to categorize the recommendations.

TABLE 20.2 Consensus on Aftercare Services

Shelter safety measures	Physical safety measures such as bulletproof glass, female trained security guards, no-visitor policy, controlled entry, 24-hour staff
Safety protocols	The Coalition to Abolish Slavery and Trafficking (CAST publishes: *The CAST Social Services Manual: A Guidebook to Serving Survivors of Human Trafficking in Los Angeles* with much helpful information on screening and personal safety protocols
Program policies and procedures	Agencies must have clear policies and train staff carefully

(continued

TABLE 20.2 Consensus on Aftercare Services (*continued*)

Legal and victims services case planning	Critical to restore legal documents to victims and to develop legal services plan as well as victims services plan
Psychological first aid	Emphasizes the trauma endured by victims and need for crisis intervention
Trauma-informed treatment for young victims	Recognizes possible pattern of victimization and need to develop trust with clients
Comprehensive medical care	Need for thorough physical assessment; multiple traumas, illnesses, STIs, untreated injuries are common
Mentoring	Peer support can be a vital and effective part of treatment to show victims that others have rebuilt their lives
"Soft skills" training	Many victims need help understanding the basics of living—how to shop for food, how to cook for themselves, how to present themselves for a job interview prior to "hard skills" training that focuses on choosing and preparing for a vocation
Microcredit loans	To address the root problem of poverty, loans are made from individuals or nongoverment organization (not financial institutions) for obtaining an education or starting a small business to rebuild lives
Cooperative agreement	Coordinated efforts are needed among many agencies—business, law, medical, social service
Comprehensive repatriation services	Coordinated effort to return trafficked victims to country of origin
Guidelines for safe return	Critical to put in place measures to accompany victims who are returning home since traffickers may intercept them
Comprehensive guidelines for reintegration	Help to communities in which victims are returned to monitor safe reintegration and prevent future trafficking
Survivor advisory caucus	Activism by survivors not only to mentor newly rescued victims but also to participate in policy and legislative efforts

Adapted from U.S. Department of State Office to Monitor and Combat Human Trafficking (2008). *Developing a consensus on aftercare services for victims of human trafficking*. Retrieved July 10, 2012 from http://2001-2009.state.gov/g/tip/rls/fs/08/111378.htm.

CLINICAL EXAMPLES

The following case studies were drawn from former clients of the author, but their names and identifying information have been disguised. Although the cases focus on one psychiatric condition, their history revealed long-standing suffering from multiple health issues. The complexity of their issues illustrates the nature of trauma and the necessity of a caring, nonjudgmental approach from trained therapists.

CASE STUDY: MARTA

Marta is a 23-year-old woman who escaped the sex trade after being trafficked from Mexico to the United States. At the age of 12, she was kidnapped from her village while on her way to school. For 7 years, she lived in captivity in various western cities in the United States, was forced to service a quota of 25 men per night, and endured torture in the form of beatings, cigarette burns, food and sleep deprivation, gang rapes, and being dragged by her hair around the room. The trafficker maintained control by showing her a photograph of himself with her little niece in Mexico. The child was smiling up at him and holding a new doll that he had given her. The implication was clear that he would take the child if Marta resisted or tried to escape. At 19, Marta was deemed trustworthy enough to be sent on errands to recruit younger girls. She did so under threat of death to her family in Mexico but was arrested and jailed. Fortunately, the police in that community had access to victim services and were more interested in arresting the trafficker than in treating her as a criminal. She received services that enabled her to make a good start on pulling her life together.

While in community college studying social work, she experienced flashbacks for which she sought help from a nurse-psychotherapist. Although Spanish was her first language, she was fluent in English and sessions were conducted in English. When she did not know how to express a concept in English, she wrote down the Spanish and the therapist had it translated confidentially. She presented with "bad dreams" and flashbacks but expressed the wish to talk about her painful experiences in order to "get past the past." The therapist was impressed with her strength of character that she did not seem to recognize in herself. When first rescued she had been placed on antidepressants, which she discontinued when she felt her symptoms were improved. She did not like taking medication and expressed the fear of becoming "addicted like so many of the other girls." The flashbacks took the form of feeling as if she was locked in her room with a particularly brutal regular customer who beat her and burned her with cigarettes. She was not a smoker and reported that the smell of cigarettes made her nauseated.

Therapy progressed for 14 weeks with the first two sessions serving as basic rapport-building, background information, genogram data, and information about TFCBT. She asked a few questions and seemed eager to proceed. In sessions 3 and 4 we explored in order of priority the traumatic memories that she most feared and wanted to control. We also discussed her coping mechanisms—how she handled the memories when they arose in daily living. One thing that particularly troubled her was being

(continued)

around other people who smoke and her best friend was a smoker. Since Marta could not bring herself to confide her past to this friend, she feared that the friend thought she would reject her if she avoided the smoking. She did not want to tell the friend she was allergic to smoke because "this would be lying to a friend and that is worse than the smoke."

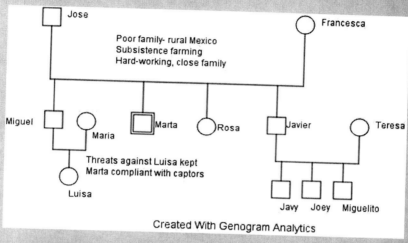

Created With Genogram Analytics

CASE STUDY: CISSY

Cissy was a 25-year-old Caucasian woman of European descent with blond hair and blue eyes that made her attractive to the traffickers. She came from an affluent family in a large East coast city and had completed high school but she wanted to see the world before going to college and she took a back-packing trip to Europe with her boyfriend. They had an argument in Rome over her stated need to return home to take care of her mother. Her father had died many years earlier and her mother's cancer had progressed to the point that she needed more personal care. Her boyfriend called her mother "manipulative" and accused Cissy of wanting to leave him. She then became angry and they separated but she had planned to meet him later in the day to tell him she was cutting her trip short and returning to New York because her mother was truly ill and that he could stay in Europe if he did not want to go home.

She went to a café alone where she met a charming young man who was a kindly and attentive listener as she confided in him about the argument. She was pleased that he clearly took her side in the argument and they talked for several hours. He then told her he would like to ask her to dinner, but couldn't because he had to catch a plane for New York. It did

(continued)

not occur to her that he had listened carefully to her story and checked out the flights, discovering there was only one flight she would logically take. They parted and she said goodbye but then saw him at the airport where he expressed delighted astonishment that they were on the same flight. Eagerly, she agreed to sit with him. She became very drowsy during the flight and he helped her leave the airport where he had a car meeting him. He took her to an apartment where several men raped her and one of them announced he had bought her from her new "friend." Following several weeks of enduring continuous beatings and rape, she "broke" when he told her he knew about her mother and would kill her if Cissy tried to escape. He claimed though, that he was sending money to her mother for medical treatment until the mother died. She lived a life of prostitution until she was too battered to work when after a final beating, her pimp tossed her out of his car on the highway, thinking she was dead. She managed to move to another city where she made a new life for herself and sought help for depression with anxiety and low-self-esteem.

Cissy's stated treatment goals were to "learn not to hate myself for what I've done" and to "go to college to become a nurse and help people." She expressed shame and guilt over not being available to her mother who died without Cissy's support but who "thankfully never knew" about her exploitation. Despite her series of violent pimps and Johns, Cissy demonstrated strength that she attributed to a wonderful childhood and the love and support of her family. She was articulate and sad, but well-differentiated in terms of being able to distinguish thoughts and feelings from behavior. At some level, she knew none of what happened to her was her fault, but she felt depressed that she should have been able to escape and be with her mother when she died.

Cissy had an aunt (her mother's sister) who lived in a distant city from where Cissy was trafficked. Strategic family therapy was the method of choice to help Cissy overcome the trauma, with a good bit of helping her recall the most painful memories and to be reconnected with her aunt. Problems were identified by Cissy, solutions worked out in conjunction with the therapist, who served as a coach, and decisions were made by Cissy that firmly placed her in control of her life.

After 11 sessions, Cissy felt strong enough to connect with her aunt and to tell her about her exploitation. The aunt flew to the therapist's city and sessions were scheduled with the two of them to allow Cissy to tell her story and to deal with the aunt's response. To Cissy's wonderment, the aunt reacted in complete support of Cissy with empathy toward her and anger directed at the traffickers and johns. Two sessions were needed to allow Cissy to tell her story and to give her aunt and Cissy time to reconnect. The outcome was that Cissy decided to accept her aunt's invitation to live

(continued)

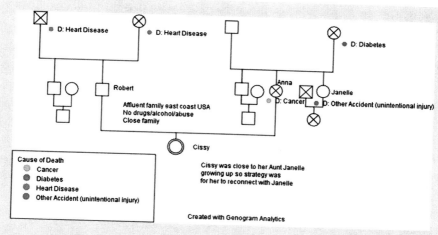

Cause of Death
- Cancer
- Diabetes
- Heart Disease
- Other Accident (unintentional injury)

Cissy was close to her Aunt Janelle
growing up so strategy was
for her to reconnect with Janelle

Created with Genogram Analytics

with her while attending school in the new city. I provided a list of potential therapists in the new city, but Cissy preferred to stay connected with me through phone calls. Several phone interviews were conducted over the next two years when Cissy needed to talk about a situation that recalled her days in the life, but she came to a sense of peace and hope for the future.

CASE STUDY: MICHAEL

Michael was a young man of 24 who had been sexually abused by his grandfather beginning at the age of 6 and then photographed for the entertainment of the grandfather's pedophile friends. He managed to escape his home life by running away and maintained a life of survival sex on the streets, first connecting with a pimp, and later on his own. He described himself as heterosexual and maintained a double life with days spent with a girlfriend and nights spent at his "job" engaging in sex with customers his pimp found at a local park. Although he had experienced violence from rough customers, he and his pimp had worked out a compromise arrangement about money that he thought was fair, and he reported that they both "stuck to the deal" and he had no need of "discipline." He denied any mental health issues and reported frequent checks for STIs. He presented a picture of a young man, ashamed of his lifestyle and not wanting to continue but taking responsibility for his current choices, and he seemed to have a clear understanding that his past exploitation was not his fault, though he said he had wrestled with that for years.

He came to see me because he wanted to marry his girlfriend and needed to figure out how to ask her—he wanted to be honest about his lifestyle but planned "to quit and go to college and settle down and raise a

(continued)

family with her." He had heard that I worked with people on the street and decided I could help him. At first I was reluctant since I had not worked with adult men who had been trafficked—only women and children—but he persisted and I agreed to meet with him in a marathon session of 3 hours (not a traditional format for therapy) I listened to him tell his story and then asked pertinent questions about what he wanted to do—he came up with a plan that we refined until he was satisfied that this approach was best. The approach was to bring the girlfriend in and tell her his story in my presence. He told the story factually and chronologically as he had told it to me. The girl listened carefully without interrupting, started crying at one point, but then she said: "All I can think to say is that I love you." Michael called some time later to tell me he had married her and moved to another city where he was not known "to start over." He was attending college and had a job at the school, which gave him a tuition break. I never heard from him again but did have the chance to give him a referral in his new city.

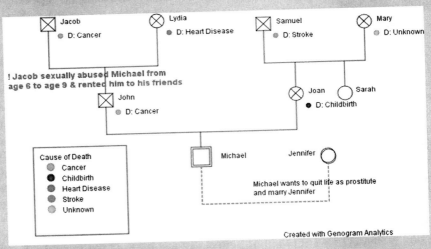

This situation was resolved to Michael's satisfaction without intensive therapy. Since the only living relative that he could name was his mother's sister, Aunt Sarah, she could have been a resource for him in family therapy. However, he accomplished his own therapeutic goal, which was relief at having Jennifer know what he did and accept him despite his past.

SUMMARY

This chapter has presented a menu of treatment options for sex trafficki clients. Although there is evidence that trauma-focused care represents b practice to date, clinicians are encouraged to test and improve upon the modalities presented here and to design new treatments that can be tested empirically. In particular, outcome studies are needed, but even case reports that are published and discussed by clinicians can help to establish the base of evidence for efficacy of treatment.

REFERENCES

Allen, J., & Berry, P. (1987). Sand play. *Elementary School Guidance and Counseling, 21*(4), 301–306.

Benda, W., McGibbon, N., & Grant, K. (2003). Improvements in muscle symmetry in children with cerebral palsy after equine-assisted therapy (hippotherapy). *The Journal of Alternative and Complementary Medicine, 9*(6), 817–825.

Bowen, M. (1988). *Family evaluation: An approach based on Bowen theory,* co-written with Kerr, M.E. at The Family Center at Georgetown University Hospital, New York: Norton & Co.

Bowman, D., & Halfacre, D. (1994). Poetry therapy with the sexually abused adolescent: A case study. *The Arts in Psychotherapy, 21*(1), 11–16.

Burgon, H. (2011). "Queen of the world:" Experiences of at-risk young people participating in equine assisted learning/therapy. *Journal of Social Work Practice, 25*(2), 165–183.

Chapman, L., Morabito, D., Ladakakos, C., Schreier, H., & Knudson, M. (2001). The effectiveness of art therapy interventions in reducing post-traumatic stress disorder (PTSD) symptoms in pediatric trauma patients. *Art Therapy: Journal of the American Art Therapy Association, 18*(2), 100–104.

Chemtob, C. M., Nakashima, J., & Carlson, J. G. (2002). Brief-treatment for elementary school children with disaster-related PTSD: A field study. *Journal of Clinical Psychology, 58,* 99–112.

Classon, C., Koopman, C., Nevill-Manning, K., & Spiegel, D. (2001). A preliminary report Comparing trauma-focused and present-focused group therapy against a wait-listed condition among childhood sexual abuse survivors with PTSD. *Journal of Aggression, Maltreatment & Trauma, 4*(2), 265–288.

Cohen, J. A., & Mannarino, A. P. (1996a). A treatment outcome study for sexually abused Preschool children: Initial findings. *Journal of the American Academy of Child and Adolescent Psychiatry, 35*(1), 42–50.

Cohen, J. A., & Mannarino, A. P. (1996b). Factors that mediate treatment outcome in sexually abused preschool children. *Journal of the American Academy of Child and Adolescent Psychiatry, 35*(10), 1402–1410.

Cohen, J. A., & Mannarino, A. P. (1997). A treatment study of sexually abused preschool children: Outcome during one year follow-up. *Journal of the American Academy of Child and Adolescent Psychiatry, 36*(9), 1228–1235.

Cooper, S., Estes, R., Giardino, A., Kellogg, N., & Vieth, V. (2007). *Quick reference: Child sexual exploitation.* St. Louis: G. W. Medical Publishing, Inc.

D'Anca, J. A. (1997). Employing eye movement desensitization/reorientation. *Dissertation Abstracts International: Section B: The Sciences and Engineering, 57*(8B), 5321. Retrieved June 20, 2012 from http://www.ebscohost.com.proxy.kennesaw.edu/ehost/delivery?sid=a78acaf1-7a34-460e-9e.

Froeschle, J. (2009). Empowering abused women through equine-assisted career therapy. *Journal of Creativity in Mental Health, 4*, 181–190.

Haley, J. (1963/2006). *Strategies of psychotherapy*. Norwalk, CT: Crown House Publishing Ltd.

Haygood, M. (2000). *The use of art in counseling child and adult survivors of sexual abuse*. London: Jessica Kingsley Publishers.

Horowitz, S. (2010). Animal-assisted therapy for inpatients. *Alternative and Complementary Therapies, 16*(6), 339–343.

Grasso, D., Joselow, B., Marquez, Y., & Webb, C. (2011). Trauma-focused cognitive behavioral therapy of a child with posttraumatic stress disorder. *Psychotherapy, 48*(2), 188–197.

KCBD Investigates: Children sold for sex in Lubbock (2012). Retrieved July 13, 2012 from http://www.kcbd.com/story/18169510/kcbd-investigates-children-sold-for-sex-in-lubbock.

Keilholz, N. (2005). Children with disabilities and hippotherapy. In M. de Chesnay (Ed.), *Caring for the vulnerable* (pp. 399–400). Sudbury, MA: Jones and Bartlett, Inc.

Linehan, M. (1993). *Cognitive-behavioural treatment of borderline personality disorder*. New York: Guildford.

Linehan, M., Comtois, K., Murray, A., Brown, M., Gallop, R., Heard, H. et al. (2006). Two-year randomized controlled trial and follow-up of dialectical behavior therapy vs therapy by experts for suicidal behaviors and borderline personality disorder. *Archives of General Psychiatry, 63*, 757–766.

Linehan, M. M., Schmidt, H., Dimeff, L. A., Craft, J. C., Kanter, J., & Comtois, K. A. (1999). Dialectical behavior therapy for patients with borderline personality disorder and drug dependence. *The American Journal on Addictions, 8*(4), 279–292.

Lowenfeld, M. (1979). *The world technique*. London: George Allen & Unwin.

Lynch, T. R., Chapman, A. L., Rosenthal, M. Z., Kuo, J. R., & Linehan, M. M. (2006). Mechanisms of change in dialectical behavioral therapy: Theoretical and empirical observations. *Journal of Clinical Psychology, 62*, 459–480.

Macy, R., & Johns, N. (2011). Aftercare services for international sex trafficking survivors: Informing U.S. service and program development in an emerging practice area. *Trauma, Violence and Abuse, 12*(2), 87–98.

Maxfield, L. (2003). Clinical implications and recommendations arising from EMDR research findings. *Journal of Trauma Practice, 2*(1), 61–81.

Medical University of South Carolina. Retrieved July 12, 2012 from http://tfcbt.musc.edu/.

Minuchin, S. (1974). *Families and family therapy*. Boston, MA: Harvard University Press.

Moretti, F., De Ronchi, D., Bernabel, V., Marchetti, L., Ferrari, B., Forlani, C. et al. (2011). Pet therapy in elderly patients with mental illness. *Psychogeriatrics, 11*, 125–129.

National Institute of Mental Health. (n.d.). *Mental health medications*. Retrieved May 22, 2012 from http://www.nimh.nih.gov/health/publications/mental-health-medications/nimh-mental-health-medications.pdf.

Pickford, R. (1992). The sand tray: Update 1970–1990. *British Journal of Projective Psychiatry, 37*(2), 26–32.

Pifalo, T. (2007). Jogging the clogs: Trauma-focused art therapy and cognitive behavioral therapy with sexually abused children. *Art Therapy: Journal of the American Art Therapy Association, 24*(4), 170–175.

Rossetti, J., & King, C. (2010). Use of animal-assisted therapy with psychiatric patients: A literature review. *Journal of Psychosocial Nursing, 48*(11), 4448.

Rubin, A., & Springer, D. (2009). *Treatment of traumatized adults and children.* Hoboken, NJ: John Wiley & Sons.

Sachs, R. (1990). The sand tray technique in the treatment of patients with dissociative disorders: Recommendations for occupational therapists. *American Journal of Occupational Therapy, 44*(11), 1045–1047.

Satir, V. (1983). *Conjoint family therapy.* Palo Alto, CA: Science and Behavior Books.

Seidler, G., & Wagner, F. (2006). Comparing the efficacy of EMDR and trauma-focused cognitive-behavioral therapy in the treatment of PTSD: A meta-analytic study. *Psychological Medicine, 36*, 1515–1522.

Shaniya Davis found dead: Mother turned little girl into sex slave. The Huffington Post. First Posted: 03/18/10 06:12 AM ET Updated: 05/25/11 03:40 PM ET. Retrieved October 2 from http://www.huffingtonpost.com/2009/11/17/shaniya-davis-story-5-yea_n_360942. html

Shapiro, F. (1989). Efficacy of the eye movement desensitization procedure in the treatment of traumatic memories. *Journal of Traumatic Stress Studies, 2*, 199–223.

Strehlow, G. (2009). The use of music therapy in treating sexually abused children. *Nordic Journal of Music Therapy, 18*(2), 167–183.

Swales, M. (2009). Dialectical behaviour therapy: Description, research and future directions. *International Journal of Behavioral Consultation and Therapy, 5*(2), 164–177.

Sweezy, M. (2011). Treating trauma after dialectical behavioral therapy. *Journal of Psychotherapy Integration, 21*(1), 90–102.

Trafficking children: Recruitment and extraction. (2012). Not for Sale website. Retrieved July 10, 2012 from http://www.notforsalecampaign.org/about/slavery/#rs_4.

Tripp, T. (2007). A short-term therapy approach to processing trauma: Art therapy with bilateral stimulation. *Art Therapy: Journal of the American Art Therapy Association, 24*(4), 176–183.

U.S. Department of State Office to Monitor and Combat Human Trafficking. (2008). *Developing a consensus on aftercare services for victims of human trafficking* Retrieved July 10, 2012 from http://2001-2009.state.gov/g/tip/rls/fs/08/111378.htm.

Watzlawick, P., Weakland, J., & Fisch, R. (1974). *Change.* New York, NY: W.W. Norton.

Zhang, R. (1998). Sand play therapy. *Psychological Science, 21*(6), 544–547.

Appendix A: Policy and Procedures for the ED on Human Trafficking

MEDICAL CENTER

SUBJECT: HUMAN TRAFFICKING

POLICY #:
SUPERSEDES: REVISED: *Date*
FORMULATED BY:
STAKEHOLDERS:
ATTACHMENTS:

POLICY

The ethical standards inherent to the nursing practice are the responsibility of nurses to uphold.

The wellbeing and safety of patients, the public and healthcare providers are promoted through standards of care.

PURPOSE

It is the policy of this facility to care for victims of alleged child or adult abuse, human trafficking, sexual exploitation, domestic abuse or sexual assault in a supportive manner. Provision for the medical, physical, emotional and spiritual needs of the patients and staff will be completed and managed in a appropriate, ethical manner. All Emergency Department personal will provide care to patients presenting with the complaint of alleged abuse, neglect, or sexual assault or those with injuries or conditions due to these circumstances in accordance with legal requirements, while protecting the privacy and dignity of the patient. All patients will be assessed for physical injuries, mental and emotional status, and a forensic examination may be completed. The processes for staff to identify and report possible victims of alleged/suspected human trafficking.

PRINCIPLES:

See Appendix B

342

PROTOCOL

A. Identification and Recognition of Trafficking Victim (The term trafficking is a broad topic that includes forced labor but for the purposes of this protocol, the focus is on sex trafficking as women and children who present to the Emergency Department or other clinics are usually victims of sex trafficking.)

  1. Red Flags

    a. No one sign can indicate with certainty that a person is being trafficked but the presence of any of the following indicators or red flags listed in Table 18.1 should prompt further investigation.

    b. General red flags.

    c. Signs of physical abuse.

    d. Signs of psychological abuse

    e. Signs of child abuse (also refer to facility abuse/neglect policy and procedures).

    f. Signs of isolation.

  2. <u>Common</u> Complaints, Signs and Symptoms (refer to Table 18.2)

    a. Physical

    b. Psychological

  3. Common Health Issues Associated with Victims of Human Trafficking

    a. HIV/AIDS

    b. Sexually transmitted diseases

    c. Posttraumatic stress disorder

    d. Infertility

    e. Undetected or untreated chronic diseases such as diabetes mellitus, hypertension, cancer, and cardiovascular or respiratory conditions.

    f. Chronic malnutrition and overall poor health

    g. Substance abuse

    h. Physical consequences of early pregnancy

    i. Skin diseases from being locked up in dark rooms with insufficient oxygen and lack of proper sanitation

    j. Chronic psychological problems

  4. Screening

    a. Things to remember when talking with a potential human trafficking victim (refer to Appendix D for more detailed guidance)

      • Only staff trained in the special needs and rights of children should question child victims (after initial screening).

      • Child victims should be questioned by staff of the same sex but if a male child is examined by a male provider, a female should be present in the room as male children are most likely to have been abused by men.

      • Work to earn the trust of the patient – communicate that one's intention is to help and attempt to gain the victim's trust. Build trust using the nurse-patient bond.

      • Ensure privacy

      • Create an environment of safety

        ○ Safety questions to ask

          –*Is it safe for you to talk with me right now?*

TABLE 18.1   Red Flags that may Indicate a Human Trafficking Victim

General	Signs Physical Abuse	Signs Psychological Abuse	Signs of Child Abuse	Signs of Isolation or Social Signs
Injury that does not match explanation of injury	Sexual assault	Fearful	Involved in the sex industry in any form or fashion and is under 18 years of age	Not allowed to leave home or work without knowledge and permission of employer or sponsor
Numerous inconsistencies in story or lied or provides canned story	Burns	Anxious, depressed, tense, nervous, paranoid	Sexually transmitted diseases, pregnancy, history of abortion	Freedom restricted or not allowed to move about the community freely
Reluctant to give information about self, injury, home or work environment	Signs of torture or restraint and/or confinement	Expresses fear of leaving living or employment situation	Children cannot give consent for any acts	High security measures at work and/or in living conditions
Inappropriately fearful of authority figures, employer, sponsor	Malnourished	Avoids eye contact	Lack of personal care or hygiene	Has few or no personal possessions or has clothing, jewelry or a cell phone that cannot afford
Likely will not self-identify as victim or that what is being done to him/her is a crime	Lacks health care	Unusually fearful or anxious when topic of law enforcement is discussed	Inappropriate sexual behaviors such as demonstrating overly sexualized behavior or use of explicit sexual language	Not in control of his/her money, no financial records, no bank account
Person with patient does not allow patient to be alone with provider	May have multiple abusers	Uncooperative with healthcare provider		Is not in control of his/her own identification documents or is using false identification papers
Accompanying person answers questions for patient	Poor hygiene	May be defensive, aloof, or dissociated		Unsure of where he/she lives (claims "just visiting" and unable to clarify where he/she is staying)

Presence of older boyfriend or there is age disparity in relationship (not a guardian)

If see patient more than once, clothing may be the same, clothing mended, poor hygiene persists

Fear and mistrust of adult or people in positions of authority (including health care providers)

Lack of knowledge about he/she is and doesn't know what city he/she is in

Loss of sense of self and/or time/space and has disjointed memories

Homelessness

Criminal trespassing

Shoplifting

Giving a false name

Runaway or throwaway child/adolescent

Open DFCS case

Violation of probation

Problems at school such as truancy, suspension, academic failures

Substance abuse or other risk-taking behaviors (alcohol use, carrying a weapon)

Inappropriate clothing for age or for weather conditions

Tattoo/branding

TABLE 18.2   Common Complaints, Signs and Symptoms (not all Inclusive)

Physical	Psychological
Sexually transmitted diseases	Depression
Vaginal & rectal trauma (could be in various stages of healing)	Anxiety
Unintended pregnancy(ies)	Hostility
Infertility	Posttraumatic stress disorder (PTSD)
Urinary tract infections	Suicidal ideation
Bald patches on scalp	Addiction
Lacerations, bruises, scars, burns, bite marks, muscle strains and sprains, joint pain, poorly healed fractures	Severe mood swings
Chronic back pain	Dissociative identity disorder
Malnutrition, dehydration, weight loss, exhaustion	Terror
Dental issues including poor hygiene and tooth loss	Intense shame
Vision problems	Appears disoriented
Headaches and dizzy spells	
Abdominal pain, diarrhea, vomiting	
Jaw and neck pain	
Rashes, itching, skin sores	

–Are there times when you don't feel safe?
–Do you feel like you are in any kind of danger while speaking to me here?
–Is there anything that would help you to feel safer while we talk?
- Non-judgmental attitude
- Have patience
- Remember that it is not important to get the entire story in the ED at this time
- It is not up to the health care provider to prove that trafficking is occurring

b. Initial
   i. ICE technique
      I – isolate the victim without increasing suspicions from the person with them.
      C – confidentiality must be ensured
      E – enlist the help of a trusted translator if needed
   ii. Ask 3 questions as a screening and, based on the responses, are reason to ask further questions at some point. These questions can be asked quickly and in a way that does not threaten the suspected victim.
      Do you control your own money and identification?

Do you have to ask permission of anyone for how you spend your time?

Can you come and go whenever you like?

   iii. Secondary Assessment

General health questions should be asked.

Past medical history, treatment for any medical conditions or trauma, medications, allergies.

Obtain brief history of any injuries – enough to treat the injury/ condition and any potential sequelae.

Determine immunization status for all childhood inoculations, especially tetanus.

B. Provision of Care

  1. Goals/Objectives of Care

    a. Victim-centered approach that addresses rescue, rehabilitation, and reintegration of victims into society.

    b. Victims require advocacy similar to victims of domestic violence including possibility of multiple supports and assistance to get used a new, more structured environment that doesn't involve violence and confinement.

    c. These victims may have fear that they are leaving one coercive situation into another with people unknown to them or that the victim will owe something to their rescuers.

    d. Safety is primary concern for the suspected victim and healthcare providers.

  2. Safety

    a. Never confront a suspected trafficker directly – contact law enforcement.

    b. Determine when a trafficker may return or if the person's communications are being monitored.

    c. Notify local law enforcement or protective services if a minor.

    d. Notify hospital security per facility protocol.

  3. Medical Management

    a. Recognition of potential or suspected human trafficking victim.

    b. Care of medical needs and treatment completed.

      i. Life-threatening emergency care first. Treatment of medical or other health conditions requiring urgent care.

      ii. Forensic examination – may be performed by the Emergency Department physician as indicated or as medical condition warrants. Recommendation that this examination especially on children is performed by a trained physician or nurse practitioner who specializes in examinations and interviews with traumatized children.

      iii. Medical management of chronic medical and health issues as appropriate in the Emergency Department setting per facility and department protocols.

Admission to hospital versus outpatient care.

    c. Assessment of potential danger to the suspected victim and/or healthcare providers.

    d. Assessment questions regarding human trafficking.

    e. Assistance from protective services per facility protocol in determining appropriate law enforcement contacts (see Appendix C).

4. Nursing Implications

    a. Nurses can intervene during the initial encounter with a suspected human trafficking victim by being trained and educated on the recognition of potential victims in the Emergency Department, physicians' offices, and dentists' offices.

    b. Prioritize and treat the person's health problems first and foremost.

    c. Provide suspected victims of human trafficking with small palm-sized cards with instructions in several languages for calling the NHTRC hotline number.

    d. Posters in the Emergency Department waiting rooms and bathrooms with information about trafficking and the NHTRC hotline number.

    e. Expand facility policies on Intimate Partner Violence, Abuse/Neglect, and/or Sexual Assault to include guidelines for human trafficking.

    f. Emergency Department staff education on the issue of human trafficking, recognition of victims, and what to do if suspect a trafficking situation. NOTE: Researchers in a study by the Family Violence Prevention Fund found that 28% of the survivors of human trafficking surveyed had contact with healthcare providers during their enslavement (Sabella, 2011).

5. Cultural competence

    a. Need to remember ethnic and cultural considerations in assisting the victim of human trafficking.

    b. Be sensitive to the victim's age, race, gender, sexual orientation, national origin, and mental status.

    c. The healthcare provider as well as the victim will have their own cultural lens or viewpoint.

    d. Healthcare provider's own cultural lens may affect their ability to recognize and connect with the trafficking victim:

        i. Stereotyping

        ii. Language and literacy barriers can lead to ineffective communication

        iii. May have different expectations of the roles of the healthcare provider and the victim from what the victim does.

Appendix B: Principles and Definitions

Human trafficking is a form of modern-day slavery in which people profit from the control and exploitation of others. The common themes present in any human trafficking situation are force, fraud, or coercion that are used to control the victim.

Domestic trafficking human trafficking that occurs within a country with its own citizens or permanent residents.

Child sex tourism travel to another country (usually) for the intent of engaging in a commercial sex act with a child.

Child pornography the use of pictures of children in seductive poses or engaged in some type of sexual act for the purpose of eliciting a sexual response from the viewer of the pictures.

Commercial sexual exploitation of children (CSEC) the use of sexual exploitation of a child for the purpose of financial or other economic gain and supporting practices that allow a person (usually an adult) to achieve sexual gratification, financial gain, or advancement in society.

Prostitution performing sexual acts for the purpose of profit.

Victim someone who is forced to work or provide commercial sex against their will. Victims can be men or women, adults or children, educated or illiterate, and foreign nationals or U.S. citizens.

Traffickers anyone who is willing to exploit someone else for profit. Includes people who recruit, transport, harbor, obtain, and exploit victims. Traffickers can be male or female, family members or friends, intimate partners, acquaintances or strangers, and U.S. citizens or foreign nationals. Traffickers use force, threats, lies, and other physical or psychological type of control over victims.

Facilitators industries or business that enable, support, or facilitate human trafficking including individuals, organizations, businesses and corporations, and internet sites. These facilitators may also assist in concealing victims and make it more difficult for a victim to get help.

Appendix C: Patient Referrals

A. *Inpatient or observation hospital admission*
  1. Medical management
     a. May need admission to a medical facility (adult or pediatric) for management of medical issues or trauma care.
     b. May require inpatient medical care.
  2. Psychiatric management
     a. May need admission to a psychiatric facility (adult or pediatric) for management of psychological issues.
     b. May require emergency psychiatric evaluation for psychiatric trauma or substance abuse (10:13 or 20:13 in Georgia)
B. *Referral Agencies*
  1. Outpatient care with appropriate medical, psychiatric, and social service referrals.
     The referral agencies vary by city. Some agencies may accept both domestic and international victims. Others specialize in one or the other. The national hotline at 888-3737-888 will be able to advise.
     a. Obstetrics/Gynecology follow-up
     b. Mental Health follow up – per facility protocol
     c. Other specialty physician follow up
     d. Immunization follow ups
  2. Law enforcement
     a. If patient is less than 18 years of age, mandatory reporting.
     b. For state of Georgia only: Georgia Care Connection Office 404-602-0068
     c. National Human Trafficking Hotline 1-888-373-7888 (1-888-3737-888). Access 24/7 and 170 languages are available.
     d. Witness protection – through law enforcement or prosecutor's office
     e. Protective services
C. *Continuity of Care*
   Unique to the state of Georgia, the Georgia Care Connection Office (GCCO) provides referrals to all appropriate care modalities for the victim of human trafficking including medical, psychiatric, legal, and social agencies. The GCCO provides guidance for healthcare providers for rescuing, recovery, and rehabilitation of human trafficking victims (survivors). In other states city-wide responses are coordinated through one or two service agencies and law enforcement.

Appendix D: Tertiary Screening and Interviewing

This interview should be performed by a trained interviewer, not necessarily in the Emergency Department or clinic setting.

1. What type of work do you do?
2. What country are you from?
3. Who assaulted you? (Intimate partner, stranger, or employer.)
4. Is anyone forcing you to do anything that you do not want to do?
5. Are you allowed to talk to people outside of your home/job?
6. Are you being paid?
7. How did you get your job?
8. Can you leave your job?
9. Have you or your family ever been threatened?
10. What is your working and living conditions like?
11. Have you/Are you being forced to have sex or perform sex acts?
12. Are there locks on your doors/windows that you cannot unlock?
13. Has your identification or documentation been taken from you?
14. Questions about fraud, coercion, debt/monetary issues, force, sex trafficking, intimate partner and inter-familial trafficking, pimp-controlled trafficking, commercial front or residential brothels should be asked by a trained interviewer.

Appendix E: Curriculum Plan for Staff Development on Human Trafficking

INTRODUCTION

We recognize that busy ED and clinic nurses do not have time for full courses on human trafficking. The following outline is a short course for staff development that managers of emergency departments or community-based clinics might adapt for their settings. The session can be offered in 30 minutes or expanded to include content specific to the type of agency or locale. For example, if children under age 18 are seen exclusively, then more information about interacting with protective services in that state should be included. If the practice includes psychiatric services, then more detailed psychotherapeutic strategies can be included. All material in this book can be used for teaching the content.

OUTLINE

(I) Overview of Human Trafficking: Introduction to importance of topic
   a. *Why should nurses know about human trafficking?* Nurses in the ED or community-based clinics may be the first-line responders for victims who present with serious injuries or illnesses. Traffickers do not make primary prevention or treatment of "minor" illnesses or injuries a priority because seeking treatment detracts from income produced. Their concern is to make the most money from their victims.
   b. *What do nurses need to know about human trafficking?* Human trafficking is a global pandemic affecting at least 27 million people who currently live in slavery. Human trafficking is the fastest-growing criminal enterprise and accounts for $32 billion per year in revenue to the traffickers.
   c. *What is human trafficking?* The two types of human trafficking are forced labor (e.g. agricultural, domestic servitude, child soldiers) and sex trafficking. Debt bondage is a way of controlling all slaves (escalating debt from traffickers charging the victims for every resource consumed (such as food, clothing, toilet paper.) About 80% of human trafficking includes women and children, most of whom are engaged in the sex trade. *Human trafficking* by forced labor is the recruitment, harboring, transportation, provision or obtaining of a person for labor or services through

the use of force, fraud or coercion for the purpose of involuntary servitude, peonage, debt bondage or slavery. *Sex trafficking* is the recruitment, harboring, transportation, provision or obtaining of a person for the purpose of a commercial sex act in which the act is induced by force, fraud or coercion or in which the person is under the age of 18.

d. *CSEC.* Commercial sex exploitation of children is a growth business with an average entry point between 12 and 14 years of age, though children much younger are forced into the sex trade. It is estimated that between 100,000-300,000 children in the U.S. and 2 million globally are CSEC victims.

(II) Human Trafficking and Health Care Professionals

a. *Recognition.* Nurses should observe for any of the following red flags, some of which are similar to intimate partner violence and child abuse:
   - Patient accompanied by a person who dominates
   - Old injuries, poorly healed fractures, malnutrition, poor dentition
   - Patient may lie about age
   - Disoriented to time or place
   - Inconsistencies in accounts of injury/illness
   - Presence of tattoos with men's names (branding)
   - Fearful or highly anxious/submissive
   - Not in control of own documents
   - STIs or frequent bacterial/ yeast infections

b. *Safety.* It is critical to provide for safety of both patient and staff, especially in the presence of any accompanying person, who is likely to be the pimp or a trusted accomplice. Establishing rapport and trust in a non-judgmental way is critical. Do not question about safety or status in front of the accompanying person but try to find a ruse to separate the patient from the other: e.g. say it is "hospital policy" to examine her alone, or take her into a bathroom for a urine sample, to the lab for blood work, or for a CT scan if head injury. Agencies that have security back-up for psychotic patients should have the security guard in the ED or exam area if trafficking is suspected.

c. *Action Plan.* Treat the medical condition. Stay calm and document observations of any recognition signs in notes. Follow agency protocol for child abuse reporting if patient is under the age of 18. If adult, offer to help but respect her wishes as to whether she is ready to leave. Call the national hotline at 888-3737-888 for advice even if she refuses help. They can sometimes follow up with local authorities. The trafficking policy and procedures guide in this chapter can be adapted for use in any agency.

(III) Case Study

a. Present case study from Chapter 18
b. Open discussion of cases seen in ED

Appendix F: Common Emergency Room Lab Values

Lab	Normal Value	High Value Causes	Low Value Causes
Glucose	70–110	Diabetic ketoacidosis; hyperglycemic non-ketotic coma	Insulin overdose
Creatinine	0.6–1.3	Renal disease	
Blood urea nitrogen (BUN)	7–18	Renal disease	
Sodium (Na)	135–145	Sweating, diarrhea, diabetes	Congenital heart failure, cirrhosis; renal failure; nausea, vomiting, and diarrhea; excess water intake
Potassium (K)	3.5–5.1	Metabolic acidosis	Poor potassium intake; diuretics; nausea, vomiting and diarrhea
CO_2	21–32	Respiratory acidosis	
Aspartate aminotransferase/serum glutamic oxaloacetic transaminase (AST/SGOT)	15–37	Liver damage	
Alanine aminotransferase/serum glutamic pyruvic transaminase (ALT/SGPT)	30–65	Liver damage	
Lipase	114–286	Pancreatitis; cholecystitis	
Amylase	25–115	Pancreatitis; cholecystitis	
White blood cell count (WBC)	4–11	Infection; inflammation; leukemia-very high levels	Neutropenia
Red blood cell count (RBC)	4.2–5.5	Dehydration	Anemia

(Continued)

Lab	Normal Value	High Value Causes	Low Value Causes
Hemoglobin (HGB)	12–16	Dehydration	Anemia
Hematocrit (HTC)	37–47	Dehydration	Anemia; gastrointestinal bleeding
Platelets (PLT)	140–440	Chronic inflammation	Thrombocytopenia
Troponin	0–0.10	Myocardial infarction	
Creatinine-kinase MB (CKMB)	0–3.6	Myocardial infarction	
D-dimer	0–682	Congestive heart failure; pulmonary embolism	
Partial thromboplastin time (PTT)	18–41 varies	Hemophilia; heparin overdose; disseminated intravascular coagulation (DIC)	
Prothrombin time (PT)	11–14 varies	Coumadin overdose; decreased potassium; liver disease	
Calcium (Ca)	8.5–10.6	Hyperthyroidism; tuberculosis; too much vitamin D	Pancreatitis; parathyroid trauma; alcohol abuse; renal failure

Buettner. J. (2010). *Fast facts for the ER nurse* New York: Springer Publishing Co., pp 243–6. Reprinted with permission from Springer Publishing Company.

Index

AA. *See* Alcoholics Anonymous
ABC. *See* airway, breathing, and circulation
abortion. *See also* adolescent pregnancy
  methods, 197
  unsafe, 197, 198
acid-fast bacilli (AFB), 290
acquired immunodeficiency syndrome
    (AIDS), 243
  ART medications, 245
  confirmatory test, 244
  medical visit, 244
  primary HIV infection, 244
  unprotected sexual intercourse, 244
ADHD stimulants, 326
adolescent pregnancy, 192
  baby farming, 193
  medical plan, 195
  nutrition, 192
  primary prevention, 192
  Rh status, 192–193
  uncomplicated pregnancy, 194
AFB. *See* acid-fast bacilli
AIDS. *See* acquired immunodeficiency
    syndrome
airway, breathing, and circulation
    (ABC), 272
alcohol, 229. *See also* cocaine
  alcoholism, 232
  benzyl, 284

case study, 234, 235–236
coerced or forced use, 184
dangers of alcohol abuse, 232–233
diagnosis, 231
drinking patterns, 230
effects, 230, 231, 233
nurse screening, 233
physical withdrawal, 231–232
production, 229
respondent, 210, 211
signs of intoxication, 230
street names, 229
support groups, 234, 235
treatments, 233–234
withdrawal criterion, 210
Alcoholics Anonymous (AA), 223, 234
alcoholism, 232
Alien Prostitution Importation
    Act, 75–76
American Nurses Association (ANA),
    8, 146
ANA. *See* American Nurses Association
animal-assisted therapy, 328–329
ANTI-Slavery International, 25
antianxiety, 326
antibiotics, 241, 248
  for BV treatment, 245
  in pregnancy, 17–18
antidepressants, 326

antihuman trafficking law, 82
   state sex trafficking
      legislation, 82
   TVPA, 27
antipsychotic, 326
antiretroviral medications (ART
   medications), 245
antitrafficking legislation, 53, 82
ART medications. *See* antiretroviral
   medications
art therapy, 325, 326–327

baby farming, 193
bacillus Calmette-Guerin vaccine (BCG
   vaccine), 288
bacterial vaginosis (BV), 245
BCG vaccine. *See* bacillus Calmette-Guerin
   vaccine
behavioral health referral, 122, 123
benzyl alcohol, 284
benzyl benzoate, 286
beta-HCG hormone. *See* beta-human
   chorionic gonadotropic hormone
beta-human chorionic gonadotropic
   hormone (beta-HCG
   hormone), 196
bio-psychosocial spiritual assessment,
   122, 123
BJS report. *See* Bureau of Justice Statistics
   report
Black Women's Agenda, 114
BMI. *See* body mass index
body mass index (BMI), 185
bonded labor, 4, 40, 117, 154
brain development review, 214
brothel operation, 31
brutality, 138–139
Bureau of Justice Statistics report (BJS
   report), 116
   child sex transportation, 89
   human trafficking cases, 91
burns, 223, 272
   acid, 134
   cigarette, 145
   lip, 133
BV. *See* bacterial vaginosis

Cable News Network (CNN), 28
cab operation, 31

CAI Instrumentation. *See*
   Computer-Assisted Interviewing
   Instrumentation
call operation, 31
CBT. *See* cognitive behavioral therapy
CCISC approach. *See* Comprehensive
   Continuous Integrated System of
   Care approach
CDC. *See* Centers for Disease Control and
   Prevention
Center for Victims of Torture (CVT), 316
Centers for Disease Control and Prevention
   (CDC), 239
central nervous system (CNS), 217
CEOS. *See* Child Exploitation and
   Obscenity Section
Cervarix, 246, 251
cervical cancers, 246
Child Exploitation and Obscenity Section
   (CEOS), 64, 89
child
   labor, 43, 154
   pornography, 349
   prostitution, 33
   sex abusers, 303
   sex tourism, 7, 349
   sexual exploitation, 33–34
child soldiers, 4, 43–44
   female, 154
   global conversation on issue of, 45
Child Soldiers Protection Act (CSPA), 44
child trafficking, 110, 281
   application of best practices, 291–292
   case study, 290–291
Chinese Laogai, 38–39
chlamydia, 246–247
Civil Rights Division (CRD), 89
CIW. *See* Coalition of Immokalee Workers
clap. *See* gonorrhea
clinical assessment strategies, 209. *See also*
   drug-abused women and children
   conversation, 210
   NSDUH CAI instrument, 210
   screening tools, 211
   structured interviews, 210
   withdrawal criterion and respondent,
     210, 211
clinicians
   challenges in human trafficking, 167

genogram tool, 122
    intervention models for, 133
    primary prevention toolkit for, 170
CNN. *See* Cable News Network
CNS. *See* central nervous system
co-occurring disorders (COD), 236–237
Coalition of Immokalee Workers (CIW), 39
cocaine. *See also* heroin
    abuse, 220
    appearance, 219–220
    complications of using, 222–223
    diagnosis, 221
    effects on body, 222
    feeling, 221
    history, 218–219
    long-term effects, 223
    medical treatment, 222
    nursing implications, 224
    opioid dependence, 221
    physical withdrawal, 223
    respondent, 210, 211
    street name, 219
    treatment options, 223–224
    withdrawal criterion, 210
COD. *See* co-occurring disorders
cognitive behavioral therapy (CBT), 223
combat sex trafficking
    international efforts to, 74
    sex trafficking treaties and legislation,
        73–74
    state antitrafficking legislation, 82
    UN protocol, 74
commercial sex act, 77, 91–92
    practice of transporting individuals
        for, 81
    sex trafficking, 155
commercial sexual exploitation of children
        (CSEC), 4, 33, 191, 263, 349
    attention, 299
    issues for CSEC victims, 9
    patient's presenting problems, 264
    special considerations, 264, 265
    victims rights, 191
communication theory, 324
community-based clinics, 295
    care based on, 299
    minor injuries, 296–297
    observation of patient, 298–299
    policy, 301

prevention, 296
    procedures, 302–303
    safety, 299–300
Comprehensive Continuous Integrated
        System of Care approach (CCISC
        approach), 54
computer-assisted family prostitution, 31
Computer-Assisted Interviewing
        Instrumentation (CAI
        Instrumentation), 210
crab lice. *See Pethirus pubis*
crabs. *See Pethirus pubis*
crack, 219–220
    abuse, 220
    prostitution, 31
    smoking, 220–221
CRD. *See* Civil Rights Division
crime, 23–24
    economic, 45
    sex trafficking, 77, 82
    victimless, 53
    victims, 309, 314, 315
crotamiton, 286
CSEC. *See* commercial sexual exploitation
        of children
CSPA. *See* Child Soldiers Protection Act
cultural competency, 120
cutting, 219
CVT. *See* Center for Victims of Torture

debt bondage. *See* bonded labor
delirium tremens (DT), 235
Democratic Republic of Congo (DRC), 44
Department of Health and Human Services
        (DHHS), 69, 323
    literature review of trafficking
        victims, 132
    literature review projects, 132–133
    printed material for HCPs, 71
Department of Homeland Security
        (DHS), 65
Department of Justice (DOJ), 64
deportation, 77, 177
destination sex trafficking stage, 173
    health problems of victims, 175
    interventions, 174
    screening questions for HCPs,
        174, 175
    trust-building messages, 175, 176

detention, deportation, criminal evidence
stage, 176. *See also* integration and
reintegration stage
  interventions, 177–178
  protections for human trafficking
    victims, 177
detox. *See* detoxification
detoxification, 217–218
DHHS. *See* Department of Health and
  Human Services
DHS. *See* Department of Homeland
  Security
*Diagnostic and Statistical Manual of
  Mental Disorders-IV (DSM-IV)*, 203
  criteria for substance abuse, 216, 231
  substance abuse questions, 210
  substance dependence symptoms, 215
  symptoms of substance abuse, 216
*Diagnostic and Statistical Manual of
  Mental Disorders (DSM)*, 203
dialectical cognitive behavior therapy, 16
dialectical TFCBT (DTFCBT), 323
diamorphine, 224
directly observed therapy (DOT), 289
DMST. *See* domestic minor sex trafficking
DOJ. *See* Department of Justice
domestic minor sex trafficking (DMST), 4,
  155, 171
  GCCO mission, 54
  Innocence Lost, 64
domestic trafficking, 349
DOT. *See* directly observed therapy
DR. *See* drug-resistant
DRC. *See* Democratic Republic of Congo
drip. *See* gonorrhea
drug-abused women and children, 204
  alcohol, 207–208
  cocaine, 206
  COD, 236–237
  hallucinogens, 206–207
  illicit drug use, 205–206
  implications for nursing, 209
drug-resistant (DR), 289
drug addiction in sex trafficking, 204
  barriers to overcoming, 204–205
  barriers to treatment, 218
  prevalence, 205
  recruitment methods and coping,
    208–209
  risk factors, 204
  understanding, 217–218
drugs
  categories, 218
  detoxification, 217–218
  illicit, 205
  injecting, 220
  maladaptive behaviors, 217
  mixing, 222
  physical and psychological
    dependency, 217
  tolerance, 215, 217
  traffickers using, 16
  using in trafficking, 203
  withdrawal, 215, 217, 218
*DSM-IV. See Diagnostic and Statistical
  Manual of Mental Disorders-IV*
*DSM. See Diagnostic and Statistical
  Manual of Mental Disorders*
DT. *See* delirium tremens
DTFCBT. *See* dialectical TFCBT

eco-map, 122–123
ECPAT. *See* End Child Prostitution and
  Trafficking
ectopic pregnancy, 195, 241, 248
  diagnosis, 196
  occurrence, 195
  treatment, 196–197
ED. *See* emergency department
educational design. *See also* health
  professional students
  face-to-face encounter, 108–110
  faculty participation, 105–106
  interdisciplinary education,
    103–104
  preparation for learning, 106–108
  transformational learning, 111
EMDR. *See* eye movement desensitization
  and reprocessing
emergency department (ED), 234, 255,
  263, 295, 309
  care, 299
  complaints, signs and symptoms, 346
  curriculum plan, 352–353
  emergency room lab values, 354–355
  human trafficking victim, 344–345
  minor injuries, 296–297
  observation of patient, 298–299

patient referrals, 350
policy, 301, 342
prevention, 296
principles and definitions, 349
procedures, 302–303
protocol, 343, 346–348
purpose, 342
safety, 299–300
tertiary screening and interviewing, 351
End Child Prostitution and Trafficking
(ECPAT), 8
entrance wound, 278
entrapment, 6
ethnic prostitution, 31
exit wound, 278
exploitation, 5
exposure, discovery, and liberation, 5–6
eye movement desensitization and
reprocessing (EMDR), 16, 321, 322,
325–326

facilitators, 349
family therapy, 16, 322, 323
case study, 332–336
goals, 323, 324
models, 324
FBI. *See* Federal Bureau of Investigation
FCAHT. *See* Florida Coalition Against
Human Trafficking
FDA. *See* Federal Drug Administration;
Food and Drug Administration
federal agencies
FBI, 64, 65
ICE, 64
immigration and customs
enforcement, 65
local law enforcement, 65–66
primary prosecutorial, 64
state police agency, 65
Federal Bureau of Investigation (FBI), 64
Federal Drug Administration (FDA), 222
female condom, 253
Florida Coalition Against Human
Trafficking (FCAHT), 66
Food and Drug Administration (FDA), 283
forced labor, 4, 37–38, 134, 154
in United States, 39–40
victims as economic commodity, 71
forced prostitution, 31

nature of, 303
victims of, 76
freebasing, 219
Free the Captives, 57
Fulton County police officer, 23

gang-related prostitution, 31
Gardasil, 251
GCCO. *See* Georgia Care Connection Office
GEMS. *See* Girls Education and
Mentoring Services
generational prostitution, 31
genital herpes, 247
acyclovir, 248
HSV, 247, 248
lifelong chronic infection, 247–248
in pregnant women, 248
transmission, 247
genital injuries, 267
abrasions, 268
by beatings and torture, 272–276
gunshots, 277–279
hematomas, 268
incised/stab wounds, 276–277
lacerations, 268
perforations, 268
rectal fistula, 271, 272
vesicovaginal fistula, 269–270
Genogram, 122
Georgia Care Connection Office
(GCCO), 54
Girls Education and Mentoring Services
(GEMS), 11, 28, 55, 324
Global law enforcement, 27
gonorrhea, 240. *See also* chlamydia
diagnosis, 241
NAAT, 241
symptoms, 240–241
in urine, 195
Great Imitator, 243
gunshots, 277–279

hangover, 231
HBV. *See* hepatitis B viruses
HCP. *See* health care providers
health care, 121
access to, 119
assistance, 8
biopsychosocial, 169

health care, (*Contd.*)
  in Eastern Europe, 10
  primary prevention, 9
  system for compliance, 17
  torture signs, 9
  trauma-focused CBT, 9
health care providers (HCP), 167, 295, 314
  alcohol treatment, 317
  barriers to helping trafficked victims,
      312–313
  building long-term sustained
      relationships, 316
  challenges for clinicians, 167
  ED personnel and clinicians, 309
  facilities, 314
  health risks, 315
  human trafficking toolkit for, 179–180
  human trafficking victim programs, 316
  interventions, 311–312, 314
  intimate partner violence, 314
  medical organizations, 315
  mental and emotional
      consequences, 315
  mental health of trafficking victims,
      310–311
  mental health plan development, 315
  nongovernment and government
      organizations, 309–310
  nurses role, 309
  psychological disorders, 313–314
  roles in sex trafficking stages,
      167, 168
  screening questions for, 174, 175
  sex trafficking victims, 316
  trauma-informed care, 315–316
  triggering event, 315
  victims identification, 313
health care workers, personal safety
    concerns, 71–72
health issues, 157. *See also* sex trafficking
    victims
  conditions, 159
  drugs and alcohol addiction, 158
  homicide rate, 157
  infectious diseases, 158
  mental health issues, 158
  mortality rate, 157
  nutritional problems, 158
  physical and emotional problems, 157
STIs, 158
UTIs, 158
health professional students, 101, 102
  educational approaches, 102–103
  educational tools, 108
hepatitis B vaccine, 242, 251–252
hepatitis B viruses (HBV), 242
heroin, 224. *See also* alcohol
  abuse, 225
  appearances, 224–225
  complications of using, 227
  diagnosis, 226
  effects on body, 226–227
  feeling, 226
  history, 224
  injection, 225
  nursing implications, 225
  oral ingestion, 225
  physical withdrawal, 227
  respondent, 210, 211
  snorting/insufflation, 225
  street names, 224
  support groups, 228
  treatments for addiction, 227–228
  withdrawal criterion, 210
herpes simplex viruses type 1 (HSV-1), 247
HIV. *See* human immunodeficiency virus
Homeland Security Investigations
    (HSI), 65
HPV. *See* human papillomavirus
HSI. *See* Homeland Security Investigations
HSV-1. *See* herpes simplex viruses type 1
human immunodeficiency virus (HIV),
    242, 243, 288
  ART medications, 245
  infection, 244
  medications, 244
  and STI testing, 244
  unprotected sexual intercourse, 244
human papillomavirus (HPV), 246
human trafficking, 3, 4, 24, 45, 113, 133,
    167, 349
  abject poverty, 46
  Anti-Slavery International, 25
  characteristics, 308–309
  cocoa farms, 46–47
  destination countries, 26
  fair trade, 47
  Fair Trade movement, 46

forced labor, 4
gender-or age specific, 25
Ghanian cocoa seller and chocolate
    developer, 47
individuals become victims, 308
interacting with victims, 313–315
interventions for, 311
labor trafficking, 154–155
law enforcement agency, 25, 26
Maiti personnel and soldiers, 28–29
metro law enforcement agency, 45
modern-day slavery, 25, 48
Palermo Protocol, 27
personal factors, 309
pimp, 24
pop culture lexicon, 24
process stages, 4–5
recognizing signs, 68–70
regional factors, 46
report estimation, 153–154
sex trafficking, 4, 306
shop to stop slavery, 47
slave-like conditions, 24–25
source, transit, and destination, 25–26
traffickers, 66–68, 153
Trafficking in Persons, 152
Trans-Atlantic slave operations, 47
transit countries, 26
TVPA, 27
in United States, 305–306
universal factors, 46
human trafficking victims, 30, 46, 116,
    176, 311
destination stage, 173
health problems of, 175
programs for, 316
protections for, 177
in United States, 306

ICAP. *See* International Center for Alcohol
    Policies
ICE. *See* Immigration and Customs
    Enforcement
ICU. *See* intensive care unit
ILO. *See* International Labour Organization
Immigration and Customs Enforcement
    (ICE), 64, 94
incised wounds, 276–277
injuries. *See also* genital injuries

by beatings and torture, 272
entrance versus exit wound, 278
herbal treatment, 272, 273–275
minor, 296–297
retaliation risk, 276
Innocence Lost program, 64
Institutional Review Board (IRB), 135
institutional sex slavery, 35–37
integration and reintegration stage,
    178–179. *See also* predeparture sex
    trafficking stage
intensive care unit (ICU), 235
interdisciplinary education approach,
    103, 104
Intergenerational theory, 324
international agencies. *See also* sex
    trafficking
CCISC model, 54
Free the Captives, 57
GCCO, 54
GEMS, 55
Johns schools, 53
Maiti Nepal, 56
Natalie's House, 55
New Hope Moldova, 56
Shared Hope International's initiative,
    52, 57
Somaly Mam Foundation, 55–56
Streetlight, 54–55
trafficking victims resources, 58–61
International Center for Alcohol Policies
    (ICAP), 234
International Labour Organization
    (ILO), 33
International Organization for Migration
    (IOM), 312
International Programme on the
    Elimination of Child Labour
    (IPEC), 33
international traffickers, 66
intervention
for destination stage, 174
detention, deportation, criminal
    evidence stage, 177–178
HCP, 311–312, 314
integration and reintegration stage,
    178–179
for predeparture stage, 170–171
for travel and transit stage, 172

intimate partner violence (IPV), 119
   diagnosis of human trafficking, 303
   documentation, 314
   victims identification, 309
involuntary domestic servitude, 41–43
IOM. *See* International Organization for
   Migration
IPEC. *See* International Programme on the
   Elimination of Child Labour
IPV. *See* intimate partner violence
IRB. *See* Institutional Review Board
ivermectin, 287

JCAHO. *See* Joint Commission on
   Accreditation of Health Care
   Organizations
Johns schools, 53
Joint Commission on Accreditation of
   Health Care Organizations
   (JCAHO), 218

labor trafficking, 27, 154–155
lambskin. *See* natural membrane condoms
latent TB (LTBI), 289
law enforcement
   agencies, 63, 64–66
   contact identification, 70
   health care facilities, 71
   task forces, 70–71
   working groups, 70–71
learning preparation, 106. *See also* health
   professional students
   crossing contextual borders,
      107–109
   focusing on resilience, 108
   meaning, 106
   metaphor, 106–107
   veil of ignorance, 106
lice, 281
   diagnosis, 282
   head, 281–282
   pubic, 249
   treatment, 282–283
lindane
   for pediculosis, 283
   for scabies, 286
living in fear, 137
London School of Hygiene and Tropical
   Medicine (LSHTM), 312

Lord's resistance army (LRA), 44–45
LRA. *See* Lord's resistance army
LSD. *See* lysergic acid diethylamide
LSHTM. *See* London School of Hygiene and
   Tropical Medicine
LTBI. *See* latent TB
lysergic acid diethylamide (LSD), 206

mail-order brides, 32–33
Maiti Nepal, 56
Maiti strategy, 28
malathion, 283
male condoms, 252–253
male prostitution, 31
malnutrition, 183
   American Academy of Pediatrics,
      183–184
   assessment, 186–187
   case study, 186
   children and adolescents, 184
   drugs and alcohol, 184
   evaluation, 187
   healthiest diet, 183, 184
   human traffickers, 184
   nursing diagnoses, 187
   nutrition for, 183–185
   outcomes, 187
   plan and implementation, 187
   plant-based foods, 183
   poor nutrition/starvation reversing
      effects, 185–186
   victims of human trafficking, 183, 185
massage parlors, 31–32
Master's of Public Health (MPH), 104
Memorandum of understanding (MOU), 37
mental health, 307
   clinician-administered diagnostic
      assessment, 307–308
   injuries and sexual violence, 307
   posttrafficking mental health study, 307
   PTSD, 307
   trafficked and exploited victims, 307
   trafficking victims, 310–311
   victimization process, 308–309
mental health intervention, 321. *See also*
   sex trafficking victims
   aftercare services, 329–331
   therapy methods, 322–328
military prostitution, 35

Minority Women's Plank, 114
modern-day slavery, 25
  bonded labor, 40
  child labor, 43
  child sexual exploitation, 33–34
  child soldiers, 43–44
  forced labor, 37–40
  forced prostitution, 31
  involuntary domestic servitude, 41, 43
  lord's resistance army, 44–45
  mail-order brides, 32–33
  massage parlors, 31–32
  military prostitution, 35
  sexual servitude, 30
mood-stabilizing and anticonvulsant, 326
morphine, 224
MOU. *See* Memorandum of understanding
MPH. *See* Master's of Public Health
multidisciplinary approach, 121
  behavioral health referral, 123
  bio-psychosocial assessment, 123
  eco-map, 122–123
  genogram, 122
music therapy, 327–328
Mycobacterium tuberculosis, 287
myplate icon, 189

NAAT. *See* nucleic acid amplification test
Natalie's House, 55
National Center for Missing and Exploited
  Children (NCMEC), 64
National Human Trafficking Resource
  Center hotline (NHTRC hotline),
  161, 314–315
National Institute of Allergy and Infectious
  Diseases (NIAID), 242
National Institute of Mental Health
  (NIMH), 326
National Institute on Alcohol Abuse and
  Alcoholism (NIAAA), 233
National Institute on Drug Abuse
  (NIDA), 212
National Institutes of Health (NIH), 213
National Student Nurses Association
  (NSNA), 8
National Survey on Drug Use and Health
  (NSDUH), 205
  CAI instrument, 210
natural membrane condoms, 252

NCMEC. *See* National Center for Missing
  and Exploited Children
New Hope Moldova, 56
NGO. *See* nongovernmental organization
NHTRC hotline. *See* National Human
  Trafficking Resource Center hotline
NIAAA. *See* National Institute on Alcohol
  Abuse and Alcoholism
NIAID. *See* National Institute of Allergy and
  Infectious Diseases
NIDA. *See* National Institute on
  Drug Abuse
NIH. *See* National Institutes of Health
NIMH. *See* National Institute of
  Mental Health
nongovernmental organization (NGO),
  110, 176
NSDUH. *See* National Survey on Drug
  Use and Health
NSNA. *See* National Student Nurses
  Association
nucleic acid amplification test (NAAT),
  241, 247
nurses, 309
  alcohol addict, diagnosis for, 221
  cocaine addict, diagnosis for, 221
  heroin addict, diagnosis for, 221
  implications for nursing, 209
  nursing resources for information, 213
  role in substance abuse screening, 203
nutrition plan
  foods to keep on hand, 188
  for healthy living, 187–188
  myplate icon, 189
  well-stocked pantry, 188, 189

opioid dependence, 221, 226
opium poppy, 224
over-the-counter (OTC), 272
  antihistamine, 291
  benzyl benzoate, 286
  medications, 282
  permethrin, 286, 291

pain relievers
  respondent, 210, 211
  withdrawal criterion, 210
Palermo Protocol, 27
Papaver somniferum, 224

Partners Against Human Trafficking (PATH), 324
PATH. *See* Partners Against Human Trafficking
pay off matrix, 215
PCP. *See* phencyclidine
pediculosis, 281–282
  benzyl alcohol, 284
  diagnosis, 282
  environmental measures, 284–285
  lindane, 283
  malathion, 283
  permethrins, 284
  pyrethrins plus piperonyl butoxide, 284
  treatment, 282–283
pediculus humanus capitis, 281
pelvic inflammatory disease (PID), 195, 241, 248
penicillin G, 243
permethrins, 284
Pethirus pubis, 249
pet therapy, 329
phencyclidine (PCP), 207
physical trauma, 263
  approaching patients, 263–264
  case study, 265–267
  CSEC patients experience, 264, 265
  genital injuries, 267–268
  gunshots, 277–279
  herbal treatment chart, 273–275
  incised/stab wounds, 276–277
  injuries from beatings and torture, 272, 276
  mental health abuse, questions regarding, 265
  rectal fistula/perforation, 271, 272
  reproductive history, questions regarding, 264
  substance abuse, questions regarding, 265
  prior trauma, questions regarding, 265
  treatment best practices for Ife, 270–271
  vaginal fistula, 268–269
PI. *See* principal investigator
PID. *See* pelvic inflammatory disease
pimp, 12, 24, 119
  guerrilla, 95

hierarchy, 95
  renting, 11
pimping, 33, 116, 118
Players' Ball, 12
poetry therapy, 328
Polaris project, 34
  operating NHTRC hotline, 314
  recognizing HCP's importance, 312
  toolkit, 313
polyurethane condoms, 252
posttraumatic stress disorder (PTSD), 9, 307
  case study, 321
  prevalence among sex trafficking population, 158
  psychological and behavorial conditions, 158–159
  symptom clusters, 9
practical street drug information
  alcohol abuse and addiction, 229–236
  cocaine abuse and addiction, 218–224
  drug categories, 218
  heroin abuse and addiction, 224–228
predeparture sex trafficking stage, 169. *See also* travel and transit sex trafficking stage
  intervention, 170–171
  limitations in education, 169, 170
pregnancy, 191
  adolescent, 192–195
  care requirement, 17–18
  ectopic, 195–197
  unsafe abortion, 197–199
primary prevention toolkit
  for destination stage, 174
  detention, deportation, criminal evidence stage, 177–178
  integration and reintegration stage, 178–179
  for predeparture stage, 170–171
  for travel and transit stage, 172
principal investigator (PI), 135
problem-based learning approach, 102–103
Prosecutorial Remedies and Other Tools to end the Exploitation of Children Today Act (PROTECT Act), 81
prostituted children, 192
  costume, 297

health issues, 132
medical insurance problem, 197
suffering by physical trauma, 263
sweeps, 64–65
vulnerability, 326
prostituted women
diagnosis for PTSD, 158
health issues, 132
medical insurance problem, 197
in military, 35
nutritional problem, 192
pregnancy, 193
suffering by physical trauma, 263
vulnerability, 326
prostitution, 349. *See also* pimping
child, 33
exploitation, 4
forced, 31, 76
juvenile, 95–96
sexual servitude, 30
stages of entrapment, 6
voluntary, 77
PROTECT Act. *See* Prosecutorial Remedies
and Other Tools to end the
Exploitation of Children Today Act
psychopharmacology, 322, 326
PTSD. *See* posttraumatic stress disorder
pubic lice, 249
pyrazinamide (PZA), 289
pyrethrins, 284
pyrethrins plus piperonyl butoxide, 284
PZA. *See* pyrazinamide

RAA. *See* Recreation and Amusement
Association
Racketeer Influence and Corrupt
Organizations (RICO), 81
rape
camps, 35
obstetric or traumatic fistula, 269
report, 192
Recreation and Amusement Association
(RAA), 37
recruitment, 5
rectal infection symptoms, 241
rectal–vaginal fistula, 269
red flag identifiers, 211. *See also*
drug-abused women and children
nursing resources for information, 213

personality assessment, 211–212
physical assessment, 212
physical screening methods, 212
reform-through-labor camps. *See* Chinese
Laogai
Reiter's syndrome, 247
resiliency-based learning approach, 103
restavek children, 133
reversing effects of poor nutrition/
starvation, 185–186
RhoGAM, 193, 198
RICO. *See* Racketeer Influence and Corrupt
Organizations
rocks, 220

safety, 299
concerns for HCPs, 71–72
for patient, 299–300
rapport establishment, 300
for staff, 300
salpingitis, 247
SAMHSA. *See* Substance Abuse and Mental
Health Services Administration
sand play therapy. *See* sand tray therapy
sand tray therapy, 328
SANE. *See* sexual assault nurse examiner
sarcoptes scabiei, 285
scabicides, 286
scabies, 285
benzyl benzoate, 286
crotamiton, 286
diagnosis, 285
environmental measures, 287
ivermectin, 287
lindane, 286
symptoms, 285
treatment, 286
serfs, 29
sex tourism, 6
to Caribbean, 7
Code of Conduct, 8
complexity of relationships, 7
to Thailand, 7
sex traffickers, 87. *See also* sex trafficking
prosecutions
cases, 89, 90
convictions, 90, 91
defendants charged, 89, 90
TVPA statutes, 88

sex trafficking, 4, 27, 77, 114, 168, 244, 306
  access to health care, 119–120
  BJS report, 116
  case study, 123–124
  common tactic of, 117
  cultural competence, 12–13
  culture, 10
  destination stage, 173–175, 176
  detention, deportation, criminal
     evidence stage, 176–178
  early trauma/sexualization, 117–118
  ED actions, 15
  federal legislation, 81, 82
  HCP's role, 168, 169
  health care assistance, 8–10, 115
  Homeland Security Act, 81–82
  implications, 125
  indicators of, 173
  integration and reintegration stage,
     178–179
  language, 10–11
  law enforcement, 115
  life-ways and rituals, 12
  media glamorization, 118–119
  mental and emotional
     consequences, 315
  multidisciplinary approach, 121–123
  native women and youth
     experience, 116
  pimps, 12
  Players' Ball, 12
  population growth, 120–121
  poverty, 116–117
  predeparture stage, 169–171
  prevention levels, 169
  PROTECT Act, 81
  RICO, 81
  risk factors, 116
  stages, 168, 169
  statistics on, 114
  travel and transit stage, 171–172
  in United States and Mexican
     border, 116
  victims of, 144
  vulnerabilities, 115, 116
  woman-centered approach, 121
  women and children, 115
sex trafficking legislation, 73
  additional legislation, 81–82

  Alien Prostitution Importation Act, 76
  international and interstate criminal
     activity, 76
  Mann Act, 77
  regulation of immorality, 76
  state sex trafficking legislation, 82–83
  TVPA, 77–79
  TVPA reauthorizations, 79–81
  in United States, 75–76
  victim protection, 76–77
sex trafficking prosecutions, 87
  challenges and barriers, 91–92
  federal prosecution, 88–89
  importance, 87, 88
  number of, 89, 90
  success strategies, 93–98
sex trafficking victims, 155, 156, 316
  of American citizens, 155–156
  barriers to identification, 203
  brutality, 138–139
  control, 139–144
  entry into the life, 137–138
  family experiences, 137
  identification, 300–301
  illnesses and injuries, 131, 135, 136, 13
  interactions, 159–162
  international, 80
  literature review, 132–133
  living in fear, 137
  personal accounts, 135, 136
  psychological issues, 135, 136
  research question, 131–132
  research study methodology, 134–13
  significance of study, 132
  witchcraft, 144–145
sexual assault nurse examiner (SANE), 2(
sexual contact partners, 251
sexual health history, 250–251
sexually transmitted infection (STI), 9, 15
  195, 239
  bacterial vaginosis, 245
  birth control methods, 253
  case studies, 254–257
  chlamydia, 246–247
  condoms, 252, 253
  genital herpes, 247–278
  genital ulcer disease 252
  gonorrhea, 240–241
  hepatitis B, 241–242

hepatitis B vaccine, 251–252
HIV/AIDS, 243–245
HPV vaccines, 251
human papillomavirus, 246
partner notification, 251
pelvic inflammatory disease, 248
prevention and control, 249, 253
prevention counseling, 252
prevention education, 251–253
pubic lice, 249
recommendations, 252
safer sex practices, 239
sexual contact partners, 251
sexual health history, 249–251
strategies, 249
syphilis, 242–243
trichomoniasis, 240
sexual servitude, 30
sexual trafficking, 101, 108
  community efforts on, 110
  crossing contextual borders, 107–109
  face-to-face encounter, 108–110
  faculty participation, 105–106
  focusing on resilience, 108
  health-related projects, 110
  interdisciplinary education, 103–104
  learning experiences, 101, 102
  meaning, 106
  metaphor, 106–107
  preparation for learning, 106–108
  privately funded organization, 108–109
  problem-based learning approach, 102–103
  resiliency-based learning approach, 103
  transformational learning, 111
  veil of ignorance, 106
Shared Hope International's initiative, 52, 57
silent disease. *See* chlamydia
slavery, 29
  contemporary, 29
  institutional sex, 35–37
  modern-day, 25, 48
  shop to stop, 47
smuggling, 92
solution-focused system approach, 324
Somaly Mam Foundation, 55–56
speedball, 219, 222

stab wound, 277
Stages of Change Model, 16, 198. *See also* sex trafficking
  action, 199
  chronic pain, 17
  contemplation, 198
  expectations, 16–17
  health conditions and treatments, 17–18
  maintenance, 199
  precontemplation, 198
  psychotherapeutic process, 16
  relapse, 199
  self-determination, 17
state investigative agency. *See also* state police agency
state police agency, 65
STI. *See* sexually transmitted infection
stimulants
  respondent, 210, 211
  withdrawal criterion, 210
strategic theory, 324
street-level prostitution, 31
Streetlight mission, 54–55
structural theory, 324
substance abuse
  DSM-IV criteria, 216
  NSDUH CAI instrument for, 210
  nurses role in screening, 203
  physical signs of, 216–217
  questions regarding, 265
  for Stages of Change Model, 16
  symptoms of, 216
  treatment for trafficking victims, 16
Substance Abuse and Mental Health Services Administration (SAMHSA), 205, 323
substance use disorder (SUD), 203, 236
SUD. *See* substance use disorder
syphilis, 242–243

TB. *See* tuberculosis
TFCBY. *See* trauma-focused cognitive behavior therapy
therapy methods, 322
  animal-assisted therapy, 328–329
  art therapy, 326–327
  DTFCBT, 323
  EMDR, 322, 325–326

therapy methods, (*Contd.*)
 family therapy, 322–324
 music therapy, 327–328
 peer support groups, 324, 325
 poetry therapy, 328
 psychopharmacology, 326
 sand tray therapy, 328
 TFCBT, 321, 322
TIP. *See* Trafficking in Persons; treatment improvement protocol
trafficked children. *See* child trafficking
traffickers, 153, 349
 challenge, 66–67
 mischaracterizations, 68
 in Peru, 67
 in United States, 67
trafficking, 24, 115
Trafficking in Persons (TIP), 4, 57, 152
Trafficking Victims Protection Act (TVPA), 15, 27, 73, 87, 153
 granting continued presence, 78
 humanitarian interests, 79
 Immigration and Nationality Act, 78
 Interagency Task Force, 79
 international sex trafficking, 77
 interstate and foreign sex trafficking, 77
 labor trafficking, 27
 prosecute sex traffickers, 78
 reauthorizations, 79–81
 sex trafficking, 27, 78
 statutes, 88
 unlawful conduct, 77–78
 U.S. v. O'Connor case, 96–97
 VTVPA and, 77
Trafficking Victims Protection Reauthorization Act (TVPRA), 80
transformational learning approach, 111
transportation, 5, 88
 child sex, 88
 lack of, 119
trauma-focused cognitive behavior therapy (TFCBY), 16, 321, 322
trauma-informed care, 315
trauma, 316, 322
travel and transit sex trafficking stage, 171. *See also* detention, deportation, criminal evidence stage
 acts of violence, 171–172

interventions, 172
 myriad health problems, 172
treatment improvement protocol (TIP), 213, 234
trichomonas vaginalis, 240
trichomoniasis, 240
trust-building interviews, 212, 213. *See also* drug-abused women and children
 brain development review, 214
 familiar with privacy rules, 214
 risk assessment, 215
 symptoms of substance abuse, 215–217
trust-building messages, 175, 176
TST. *See* tuberculin skin testing
tuberculin skin testing (TST), 288
tuberculosis (TB), 227, 281, 287–288
 diagnosis, 288
 medications, 289
 preventive measures, 290
 prognosis, 290
 symptoms, 290
 treatment, 289–290
TVPA. *See* Trafficking Victims Protection Act
TVPRA. *See* Trafficking Victims Protection Reauthorization Act

United Nations Office on Drugs and Crime (UNODC), 26
United States Agency for International Development (USAID), 110
UNODC. *See* United Nations Office on Drugs and Crime
UN protocol, 74
 international agreements, 75
 international treaty, 75
 labor trafficking and organ trafficking, 75
 sex trafficking, 74–75
unsafe abortion, 197
 case, 198
 do-it-yourself method, 197
 Stages of Change Model, 198–199
UNTAC. *See* UN Transitional Authority in Cambodia
UN Transitional Authority in Cambodia (UNTAC), 35
urinary tract infection (UTI), 158

USAID. *See* United States Agency for
International Development
U.S. interaction with global governments
law enforcement agencies, 28
Maiti strategy, 28
progress tiers, 28
restrictions, 28
TVPA minimum standards, 27–28
U.S. Trafficking In Persons Report, 27
UTI. *See* urinary tract infection

vesicovaginal fistula, 269
special considerations, 271
treatment, 270
Victims of Trafficking and Violence
Protection Act of 2000 (VTVPA), 77
VTVPA. *See* Victims of Trafficking and
Violence Protection Act of 2000
vulnerable stage, 5

WHO. *See* World Health Organization
Wilberforce Trafficking Victims Protection
Reauthorization Act, 80–81
witchcraft, 144–145
WOC. *See* Women of color
woman-centered approach, 121
Women of color (WOC), 113–114
analysis, 124–125
BJS report, 116
Black Women's Agenda, 114
case study, 123–124
cultural competency, 120
culture and language, 120
early trauma/sexualization, 117–118

health care, 119, 121
implications, 125
individual self-identification, 121
IPV, 119
lack of education, 119–120
lack of insurance, 120
lack of transportation, 119
law enforcement and health care
systems, 115
media glamorization, 118–119
Medicaid thresholds, 120
Minority Women's Plank, 114
multidisciplinary approach, 121–123
National Women's Conference, 114
population growth, 120–121
poverty, 116–117
practice techniques, 120
prostitution and trafficking of, 115
published materials, 115–116
risk factors, 116
statistics on, 114
vulnerabilities, 115, 116
Western- and European-based cultures,
114
woman-centered approach, 121
women and children, 115
World Health Organization (WHO),
168, 239
wounds, 68
entrance, 278
exit, 278
gunshot, 277–278
incised, 276–277
stab, 277

12 - Cultural Competency
16 - Evidence-based Therapies for CSEC
17 - Guidance re: approaching a victim
to provide services
54 - Best Practice: Integrated model
of Care
88 - Federal Prosecution Statutes
93 - Strategies for Effective Investigations
+ Prosecutions
111 - Transformational Learning
132 - Presenting Health Conditions of
Sex Trafficking Victims
133 - Need for long-term mental heath care
+ for assistance transitioning out
of commercial sexual exploitation
135 - Good quote re: psychological strain
157 - Important stats re: violence during
trafficking
157 - medical symptoms resulting from
sex trafficking
158 -   "   "   "
158 - Finding that delay in medical care
159   can result in death

CPSIA information can be obtained
at www.ICGtesting.com
Printed in the USA
FFOW04n0543080115
10146FF

9 780826 171153